I0131045

Optimal Wellness: Necessary Biological, Psychological, and Social Integrations.
Conceived by: **Dr. Vladimir Friedman** and **Dr. Bob Davis**

Published by: International Publications Media Group (IPMG)

Dr. Vladimir Friedman conceived the necessity and guiding purpose of this book. A Doctor of Chiropractic Medicine with full-year post-graduate studies as a Certified Chiropractic Sports Physician, Certified Clinical Nutritionist, and certified practitioner of Electrodiagnostic Studies, Vlad has been a personal trainer and now is owner-therapist of Accelerated Care Chiropractic and Accelicare Sports Chiropractic in Midtown Manhattan. Driven by a professional need to offer holistic therapy, Vlad has earned over 30 two-day post-grad certifications and over 50 lifetime certifications including EMT, first aid and safety, and lifeguarding.

Dr. Bob Davis, content supervisor, writing coach, and editor of this book, is a Ph. D. in Nineteenth-Century British Literature who taught university English for almost 40 years, principally at Clark University in MA and at NYU, where for 12 years he created, directed, and instructed a four-course program of expository prose for graduate students in the 22 majors of the Professional Studies Program. His published work includes *Your Writing Well: Common-Sense Strategies and Logic-Based Skills, in 15 Essays for the 21st Century*, instructor manuals for five college-level reading and writing anthologies, along with two volumes of literary criticism, style-diverse nonacademic prose, and poetry. As a freelance editor and language consultant for corporate and individual clients, Bob has been copy-chief for AOL Digital City New York, has development- and copy-edited over twenty volumes of literature for Houghton Mifflin's New Riverside Editions, edited online for The College Board and Pearson, and also edited for magazines, advertising agencies, architectural builders, and philanthropic foundations.

Luke Bongiorno, graduate of the University of Melbourne, Australia, is Director of the North American Neuro-Orthopaedic Institute (Noigroup) in New York City and, previously, was co-founder of New York Sports Medicine. Recognized as one of the most prominent physical therapists in NYC, Luke not only is affiliated with the clinical education programs of Columbia University and Touro College and serves as a consultant with the NBA League, but also is internationally recognized for his treatment of professional and Olympic athletes and performing arts and dance company members, and for his consulting with professional European soccer teams

Alex Cooksey, a Princeton graduate of East Asian Studies having recently changed his professional focus to computer software, was founder and trainer of Coaching with Cooksey in New Jersey, where he coached clients to achieve health and fitness goals through fully individualized exercise programming and a collaborative approach to value-based progressive behavior change.

Dr. Rob Curran, D.C. and EMT, is the Injury Prevention Coordinator/ Department of Trauma Surgery at New York Presbyterian/ Weill Cornell Medical Center. In addition to his being the New York City Chapter Coordinator of the Sudden Cardiac Arrest Association and his providing extensive community service organization and instruction, he is or has been an adjunct faculty member and lecturer at seven colleges and universities throughout greater New York City.

Sharon Dominguez, an acupuncturist and founder of Ki Element Theory, is a Godan-ranked Aikido instructor, practitioner of Kototama Life Medicine, integrated strategist for structural, internal, and behavioral wellness, herbalist, non-denominational minister performing weddings and other important rituals, past stone specialist for fashion jewelry, and flute player.

Dr. Marisa Galisteo, former Professor of Chemistry at U de Granada in Spain, biomedical research scientist at MIT and NYU Medical Center, and founder of Scientists as Leaders Training Co., is an international yoga instructor who naturally integrates Eastern thought into her yoga practice's emphasis on the art and science of tapping one's potential, specifically with Body Awake Yoga and Energy Codes. To her yoga instruction she adds eclectic experience as an Executive Coach, Department Manager at Landmark Worldwide, Neurolinguistic Master Practitioner, and authority on the latest applications of Chinese medicine and sound therapy.

Greg Grube's background includes swimming and diving, yoga instruction, and an individualized Pilates apprenticeship with Collette Stewart following the completion of his degree in dance from the University of Wisconsin, Madison; he also has a double-major B.A. in English and art history from UDelaware. While pursuing dance professionally, Greg gathered additional certifications from Eric Franklin (Level I and Level II) and a year-long professional dance program under the direction of Steve Paxton, a leading figure in the contemporary dance world. Already with over 1000 hours of training relevant to Pilates, Greg continues to explore and to study his interests in anatomy, biomechanics, functional movement, and somatic restoration.

Hicham Haouzi, 1988 Moroccan Olympic Taekwando team member and also gold medal Muay Thai winner in The Netherlands and twice in the U.S., is a Life and Personal Coach with over 20 years' experience at Equinox, where he's received a Lifetime Achievement Award and was co-founder of the first Equinox Games. Now, Hicham is General Manager of Hudson Yards' Equinox E Training Studios in Manhattan, the most elite coaching platform offered by Equinox; having designed that studio, Hicham also owns and runs HASTO Home Gyms.

David Jean-Bart is Manager of Equinox's "E Madison Avenue" on the Upper East Side of Manhattan, following his E-Club managerial positions at Columbus Circle in Manhattan and in Greenwich, CT. His Bachelor's degree in computer science, telecommunication, and network technology, his 20+ years with Equinox, and his ongoing accumulation of certifications have furthered his interest in the importance of habit change as a prerequisite to wellness.

Dr. Lanae Mullane, a Doctor of Naturopathic Medicine, is Medical Director at Vejo+ and the Director of Nutrition at Vejo in Santa Monica, CA. Having completed a residency focused in rheumatology, Lanae utilizes biochemistry, genetics, behavioral change, medical history, and specific individualized goals to create a truly personalized program for each of her patients or clients. Vejo+, a team of doctors and nutritionists who formulate a personalized blend of nutrients made just for each client, works with NASA to promote each astronaut's nutritional well-being while in outer space.

Dr. Maria Santoro is a licensed massage therapist and movement therapist with expertise in Swedish, Shiatsu, Thai, reflexology, medical, soft tissue, and deep tissue massage. Her graduate studies include physical anthropology, movement science, and motor learning. Also a Tier-X Equinox fitness trainer, the highest rating for Equinox trainers, Maria taught for the Equinox Training Institute (EFTI). In Korea, she worked at The Point, an exclusive fitness club on the United States Military Base in Seoul, where she was promoted to Lead Athletic Trainer/Athletic Coordinator; also in Seoul, she was an intern in the Physical Therapy Department at 121 Hospital on the same base. While in Korea, Maria earned a 1st Dan Black Belt in Taekwando and completed her training for the American Red Cross, becoming a CPR/First Aid Instructor. In Thailand, she began her studies in Thai massage at the Wat Pho School of Thai Massage in Bangkok and continued in Koh Phangan with a course in Medical Thai massage taught by Nipha Sangkhwai. In India, she studied Iyengar Yoga in Pune. She holds certificates from ISHTA (Integrated Science of Hatha Tantra, and Ayurveda), from a yoga teacher's training program, and from Pilates Mat training at Kinected.

Nicole Visnic is Director of Nutrition at LifeSpan Medicine in Santa Monica, CA and a board-certified clinical nutritionist through the CNCB. With an M.S. in Nutrition from the University of Bridgeport, CT, six years in the Air Force National Guard, managerial duties at the corporate wellness center for Honeywell Aerospace, and work as an adjunct psychology instructor at Brown Mackie College, Nicole also has spent a significant portion of her career working with professional athletes in the NFL, NBA, MLB, and USATE, as well as helping athletes prepare for the Olympics.

Sam Visnic, CMT, is one of the nation's leading practitioners working to solve the complexities of chronic pain. Owner and Director of Release Muscle Therapy in Temecula, CA, and author of the e-book *Why Didn't My Doctor Tell Me That?*, Sam has studied dozens of methodologies for uncovering the root cause of aches and pains, including pain science, hands-on soft tissue massage techniques, myofascial release, and coaching movement.

Conceived as a self-help personal guide for understanding and attaining holistic or integrated comprehensive wellness, *Optimal Wellness: Necessary Biological, Psychological, and Social Integrations* offers a new, convergent approach to understanding and achieving what optimal human health should and can be. Written by 14 doctors, physical and massage therapists, and fitness trainers, this book gives clear explanations of the latest scientific research, medical knowledge, therapeutic innovations, and smart fitness goals, combined with enduring lessons in wellness from around the globe. Containing applicable information and practical tools which young and older adults can work with self-helpfully to repair, develop, and maintain their multifaceted well-being, and to prevent future illness, *Optimal Wellness* also will enable readers to apply its intertwining truths to deal with degenerative behaviors resulting from the pandemic.

Conceptual and practical integrations and syntheses inform all content in the 300-page text. In its parts and as a whole, *Optimal Wellness* provides original educational solutions to the frequent misconceptions and mistakes from people's harmful personal habits and from institutional misguidance and monocular specialism. Because optimal wellness cannot exist without achieved synergies at work in the human body, the scope—the breadth and depth—of each writer's chapter establishes how the biopsychosocial principles of its topical section should be understood. These chapters include an introductory definition of each component's (bio's or psycho's or social's) fundamental principles and of when and how it's braided with aspects of the other two; reasons and ways to implement behavior modification and habit change; pain's reinterpretation and management, with inevitable attention to neuroplasticity in one chapter, and the latest understanding of chronic pain in another; human resilience through better sleep, nutrition, and management of stress, a concern examined by a Doctor of Naturopathy and persisting throughout the book; varying kinds and purposes of massage and touch therapies from around the world; acupuncture and other Eastern approaches to biopsychosocial wellness; yoga, Pilates, and fundamental movement capacities of mobility, balance, coordination, stability, strength, power, speed if applicable, and endurance. Working together, the book's chapters spotlight the larger biopsychosocial perspectives from which complete health is drawn while featuring the proper building blocks to structure readers' future wellness and health programs, whatever a reader's current state of wellness may be.

Because *Optimal Wellness: Necessary Biological, Psychological, and Social Integrations*, represents a paradigm shift for understanding and exercising personal wellness, it will draw an audience **01** ready for—or interested in being ready for—a useful departure not only from our nation's fixed vision of and institutionalized approaches to wellness, but also from the more than two years of biopsychosocial harms from the pandemic. Many prospective readers, already sensing the connections among their social limits, enclosed psychological borders, and physical torpor because of Covid, will want to counteract their behaviors and to improve the total wellness they've partially lost. Reminding readers of and helping them to embody the lasting values of biopsychosocial wellness in their lives, this book offers expansive empowerment to confront and counteract the biopsychosocial setbacks we've all experienced.

Our book aims its enduring truths and facts, lessons and self-help strategies at every demographic except children, although adults can use many of its sage understandings while raising them. *Optimal Wellness* also provides an integral model of biopsychosocially holistic practice that other wellness professionals will want to experience and emulate in whatever ways are practical to them and beneficial to their clients and patients. Our book's global emphases further broaden our reading audience, as they offer insights applicable to the increasingly borderless village of wellness-seekers. Whatever the kind and degree of this book's influence, its authors have been dedicated to establishing for public and peer awareness a consolidated multifaceted understanding of the next step or new wave in well-founded, properly practiced approaches to wellness. It will resound with readers whose wholeness has been neglected or altogether overlooked because reduced to parts-care.

TABLE OF CONTENTS

INTRODUCTION

All of this book's fourteen authors—doctors, physical and massage therapists, fitness trainers—steadfastly believe and practice that wellness of the human body is the multifaceted result of physical, physiological, psychological, emotional, spiritual, and sociocultural factors, and that the human body and the brain with mind must be thought of as a holistic system of convergent functions and interconnections. Each participating writer acknowledges having been a specialist whose specialized education and applied practice to some extent determined—and on occasion limited—her or his professional destiny. Yet as these wellness experts' expertise developed within the restrictions of their specializations, they discovered their need to search beyond established boundaries of their standardized normal knowledge and to lift the lid off their boxed understandings. It wasn't enough for these masters to learn from only their specialized degree or degrees; therefore, reaching out, they borrowed from other ways and means of learning about wellness, from alternative practices, from theoretical and applied possibilities beyond but nonetheless compatible within the range of their specialty. In effect, all writers of this book integrated into their specializations other harmonious modes for wellness in an attempt to promote a more holistic health for their clients.

In "Towards a Definition of Holism," Joshua Freeman explains holistic health or wellness as "the ability to use a biopsychosocial model [George L. Engel's term] taking into account cultural and existential dimensions"; healers and health-promoters, Freeman continues, must acknowledge "that everything affects health [and] we must understand and honour the whole, in each of its parts and with the synergies that are created as they act together" (155). Holistic wellness therefore also must consider a patient's and client's day-to-day lifestyle choices, routines and habits, emotional support systems and how they influence health, and the effects of all environmental and institutional contexts; thus, the well-being and total health of the body becomes inseparable from the brain's mind or psyche itself, while body and mind are influenced by external stimuli. This book uses the term "biopsychosocial" to indicate holistic wellness.

Our emphasis on holism—on integrating parts (at first, sometimes seemingly dissimilar parts) that add up to larger conceptual wholes—signifies a growing trend in human intellectual history's evolution of consciousness, how consciousness operates, and how it collectively imposes mental energy on material existence. For about the past 450 years, since the Renaissance and the birth of the scientific method, the "Newtonian paradigm" has been Westerners' rigorous intellectual model for thinking, perceiving the world, and validating facts and truths. Standard inquiry and analysis have been presupposed and informed by strict material empiricism interested in analyzing matter into single (atomistic) visible parts—sightings microscopic, observable to human eyes, and telescopic. Unchanging, Newton's "clockwork universe" was a non-evolutionary machine constructed by the Great Clockmaker, God, Who gave humans reason (so said the eighteenth-century Age of Reason or Enlightenment) to aid in deconstructing the material world into its fully knowable parts and, with physics, to discern their mechanistic interactions. Only slowly has the Newtonian paradigm yielded to concepts of evolution and everlasting change within the material world. In stages, Western thought has abandoned belief in the mechanical fixity of all living existence and appreciated, correctly, the interrelated, ever-weaving processes of energy contained by the material parts of our organic universe and solar system, planet Earth, and Her plants and animals.

With the aid of computers and the Internet, and with an increased understanding of benefits derived from an escalating focus on theoretical and factual interrelatability, humans have been shifting intellectually to convergent thinking, to a mode of integrative, academically interdisciplinary thought that joins parts into newly formed and understandable wholes. Recurring descriptors throughout this book on holistic or biopsychosocial wellness, "integrated" and "comprehensive" are explained in Josep Galliea's article "Integral Thinking," which "argues about the need to use a new modality of thinking, defined as integral thinking. . . . a kind of thinking that is holistic but also has span and profundity. . . . the kind of thinking appropriated to the contemporary need to think integrally in science, culture, professions, and arts or about the evolution of personal consciousness. It's useful also to be applied in the diverse professional fields, especially when comprehensive approaches are needed" (http://www.integralworld.net/gallifa4. html).

The seeds for this new mode of thought were planted slightly more than two centuries ago in the fertile soil of Western philosophy and art, and botanical and geological science, and today have begun to flower in all fields of human intellectual consideration, physics included. When applied to our lives and our world, convergent thinking merges interplaying ideas whose overlaps and synergies yield broader vision, deeper insight, and more meaningful foresight which, when applied to human existence, are intellectually greater than the sum of their parts and therefore are moving human consciousness upward, frequently raising it and us above the material limitations of our preceding paradigm. Convergence emergence is an unstoppable force of collective mental energy promoting greater sapience in homo sapiens, a truth evidenced in this book and in all that this book adds up to. One can say that whereas the Newtonian paradigm's accumulation of specialized knowledge has made us smarter about the world's material parts in isolation, the increased convergence of that smart knowledge—through integration and synthesis, through comprehensive and holistic thinking—is making us potentially wiser with the wholes which those parts add up to. An obvious example of convergent thinking backed by proof is humans' recent attention to the ecology and ecosystems of planet Earth, also a living body whose large-scale wellness depends on the collective small-scale biopsychosocial health of humans. Presently, neither our planet nor its population of people is commendably well. We're only beginning to apply and enact our new, holistic understandings wisely, sapiently.

Aiming its convergent ideas and comprehensive approaches to the field of integrated human health or holistic wellness, this book is purposed towards readers' biopsychosocial self-supervision, with practical truths providing knowledge and applicable tools with which all people can coach, repair, restore, develop, and maintain their biopsychosocial well-being. Idealism governs this book's intentions, not only because human biopsychosocial wellness is attainable to so many of our readers through careful self-assistance, but also because human wellness as a means for eliminating stress, promoting wisdom, and attaining peace can lead to larger holistic wellness for our societies and our planet.

Helping to explain the practical value of *Optimal Wellness* is the unifying premise of David Epstein's 2019 Range: Why Generalists Triumph in a Specialized World. Epstein argues that in most fields—especially those that are complex and unpredictable—generalists, not specialists, are better prepared to excel. People who think broadly and embrace diverse experiences and perspectives have the kind of sophisticated smarts—the wiser knowledge or sapience—that increasingly will help them to adapt and thrive in our dynamically changing twenty-first century worlds of business, technology, science, and medicine, among other professional pursuits. Creating an antibiotic vaccine against Covid-19 required a new range of convergent thinking, required "applying original thinking across domains" (Kapoor), "collaborative efforts across sectors of society" (Felter), and, for research, "identifying points of integration within a sequential convergent design using text mining to manage large data volumes and studying complex phenomena" (Poth). Already becoming increasingly collaborative and convergent, those worlds and their systems are de-emphasizing what Epstein characterizes as specialization's short-sighted thinking and instead are emphasizing broader, more integrated comprehensive perspectives that result in innovations created from multifaceted synergies. Such is the focused range in the reports by all authors of this book, themselves eclectic generalists even when labeled as specialists.

To more fully inform our understanding of integrative holism, let's set aside a few pages here to explore the limitations of specialization. Of course first we gratefully must appreciate that Western medicine and knowledge of the human body have made notable educational and practical progress in specialist disciplines, and that specialist research and practice have led to diagnoses, preventions, treatments, and cures for specific diseases, illnesses, bodily ailments, injuries, and impairments. But specialism by its nature, and by Western institutional habit, works in isolation and still too often is unaware of or neglects the broader causes and fuller implications—the holistic range—of those aforementioned problem diseases, illnesses, and ailments. "Medical mistakes are far too common because each specialist is treating (or more likely over treating) her own pet organ," says Dr. Allen Frances, Professor Emeritus of Psychiatry and former Chair at Duke University. "No one is considering the whole patient to organize a global, integrated, safe, and effective treatment plan." The patient as a whole is neglected, Frances continues, because "Unfortunately, doctors no longer know their patients. GPs [General Practitioners] are overworked, underpaid, and must shuttle patients in and out of the office . . . . Specialists tend to treat the test, not the patient, and earn their living doing procedures that often are unnecessary." Since 1961, the number of GPs in America has declined by one third, while specialization obviously has increased proportionally. Further problems with this trend are that "Specialty dominated practice also leads to inadequate preventive health services, late detection of diseases, and difficulty managing common chronic conditions such as obesity, diabetes, hypertension, and heart disease." In this context, writers of *Optimal Wellness* intend to serve also as a preventive health service.

As does this book, Frances argues for an educational holism in which, among other institutionalized requirements, "Medical school testing should be comprehensive and integrated [my emphasis], instead of the current common practice of administering exams based on discipline." Lacking a comprehensive overview of the patient, current medical specialism shows how "The doctor/patient relationship has lost its healing power. Doctors are too busy doing the wrong things. Patients have been reduced to a collection of lab test results." The purpose of good doctoring, therapy, and physical training for wellness and health care is a cultural necessity and ethical imperative, not primarily the bolstering of institutions' financial well-being, a trend whose origin in America, Frances explains, is rooted in the Flexner medical reforms of 1910 which despite their high medical standards advanced "a flaw that now haunts and distorts medical education and practice throughout the world." This flaw, based originally on Johns Hopkins University's "great emphasis on departmental specialization and research productivity," has become the model for achieving the financial goals of attracting the most research dollars and of producing the most clinical revenue by doing costly medical and surgical procedures. Conversely, "Primary care teaching and practice has always been deeply devalued by medical centers," Frances concludes, "because it does neither [kind of financial gain advocacy]." Money still talks, and talks loud, even if greater human wellness is being cumulatively silenced. Frances' article's subtitle sums this up: We should be "Putting the patient, not the procedure, in the center of medical care."

Nearly 20 years ago, the authors of "Integrative Medicine: Bringing Medicine Back to Its Roots" noted the irony that, "just when decades of biomedical research are beginning to pay miraculous dividends, public confidence in the medical establishment is eroding" because of "the gap between what many conventional health care providers deliver and what the public wants and needs" (395). Essentially, according to that article, "a public need for holism in medicine is clashing with the industry's most fundamental, reductionist ways," reductionism being the medical industry's emphases on specialization. Dr. Snyderman et al. highlight the need for conventionalized integrative medicine, agreeing with its "calls for restoration of the focus of medicine on health and healings and emphasi[s on] the centrality of the patient-physician relationship" (Snyderman, 396).

Granted, increased numbers of Americans recently have gained access to networks of specialists from top-tier hospitals, comprehensive health care systems, and medical concierge referral services or alliances, specialists working under the same healthcare umbrella and consequently doing better both to improve patients' wellness through teamwork and to upgrade technology for transferring test results and prescriptions. But complementary healthcare systems are principally urban and academic, remain time-consuming and often prohibitively expensive, and still don't eliminate the inherent flaw associated with specialization: its financially skewed perspectives on healthcare.

The disadvantages of specialization's reductionist approaches are best understood when we examine "multimorbidity," the ugly-named condition of patients with multiple chronic diseases, a population of patients "quickly becoming the norm" (The Atlantic). A 2014 study of 60,000 Americans found that 59.6% or three-fifths were typed multimorbid (https://www.jabfm.org/ content/31/4/503). Given the population density of multimorbidity, we should be concerned about how specialization fusnctions when we further learn that

> Not only do multimorbid patients receive suboptimal care, but the unnecessary hospitalizations, redundant tests, and disjointed care they receive put disproportionate pressure on our health system. . . . specialists rarely know how the treatment they administer interacts with other concurrent treatments (*The Atlantic*).

What we learn from our country's medical and therapeutic emphasis on specialization is that a fragmented, piecemeal approach to wellness has not made and never will contribute to making us a healthy nation. "Best Healthcare in the World Population 2020" offers global statistics that use evaluative criteria set by the World Health Organization. Countries having universal healthcare rank notably high in this study; the United States ranks 37th, between Costa Rica and Slovinia, and by global standards looks dismally deprived of effective national medical services and health care, a fact whose roots obviously extend beyond but nonetheless include specialization.

The many contributing causes leading to Americans' unfortunate lack of wellness are being studied and addressed but aren't yet changing in ways leading to improving America's collective wellness. Added to the problems within American health care and its widespread financial inaccessibility are four other contributing deterrents to our national wellness: medication errors and American overuse of prescriptive drugs;[1] unhealthful family habits and behaviors, notably harmful cultural patterns of food consumption and their consequent high levels of obesity and illness;2+3 inherent social conditions promoting unhealthful norms; and inadequate public knowledge of and education programs for teaching wellness. Statistically, it's an obvious conclusion that the U. S. isn't a nation of healthy people, at least not relatively speaking: "Americans live shorter lives and experience more injuries and illnesses than people in other high-income countries. . . . This health disadvantage is particularly striking given the wealth and assets of the United States and the country's enormous level of per capita spending on health care, which far exceeds that of any other country" (National Research Council).

And from a cultural viewpoint it's easy to see that America's wellness is further sidetracked because too many people's brains are overstuffed with visual and verbal marketing that portrays and bespeaks the media's misleadingly idealized, usually unattainable standards for looks, bodies, and lifestyle, marketing that implies our insufficiencies for not appearing like, measuring up to, and living those standards. Subliminal and conscious doubts about our looks, physical bodies, and lifestyle can—and for many people do—affect self-perception, which then becomes their reality; such reality can foster false beliefs about and goals for wellness. Further, this kind of value-laden vision promotes the misconception that attractively formed bodies necessarily indicate fitness or are equal to wellness and health; that, of course, is an empirical fallacy, as countless factors are involved in complete physical wellness, not just pumping iron in a fashionable gym, not just aerobic exercise on a sandy beach in the Hamptons or Malibu, not just stretchability and agility down a snowy slope in Aspen. Pretty frames very possibly obstruct our view of unseen problems that need to be attended to and cared for when wellness is our goal. Wellness is a multi-faceted construct best understood by holists, whose integrationist and broad-range or comprehensive thinking looks into the larger medical, anatomical, and practical pictures within which complete health exists. Moreover, optimal wellness isn't the result only of a healthy body, but also of the well mind and intellect, emotions, psyche or spirit, and stressless interaction with society. Not judging a book by its cover, we must learn to inspect and respect its content and contexts, and to be confident that we author our own book wisely.

Given these national limitations and psychological misconceptions concerning wellness, *Optimal Wellness* is devoted to educating anybody anywhere who wants to improve her or his wellness and health. We offer preventive measures with which to avoid multimorbid complications—and strategies and practices for wellness that can modify or repair such complications. Here you'll find accessible explanations, enduring lessons, and reliable instructions from degreed and certified practitioners whose evolving professional research, scientifically validated learning, and personal ethics regarding the sensible preventions and prudent revitalizing strategies for wellness have enlightened them as holistic thinkers beyond the pale of reductive specialization. In their respective professional fields, all writers of this book have been ahead of the times, moving their practice towards a more integrated comprehensive approach to wellness; together, as a unit, their holism takes on new dimensionality, a deeper and broader overview and understanding of what makes us tick best. While some people may see holism and reductionism as opposites, this book will prove that there is overlap between the two, with room for each in the world of medicine, physical therapy, and fitness training. Holism does not seek to drive out reductionism; instead, it seeks to complement it by recognizing—and then converging—added pieces to the puzzle of wellness or added colors to the full spectrum of health.

The Covid-19 pandemic certainly has forced humans to puzzle out the implications of maintaining their own wellness and the complications from failing to do so, especially when unhealthful habits develop without our noticing. Commonly affected, many of us have experienced directly for ourselves or indirectly among family and friends the decline of physical health, breakdown of dependable psychological security, compromises to financial livelihood at home, collapses of business and industry around us, fragmenting of professional structures and systems, minimizing of interpersonal education, removal of cultural events, and in some instances even the fracturing of family. Undoubtedly a time of increased physical inactivity, psychological pressures, economic hardship, and social distancing, the Covid-19 pandemic has impacted—and has demanded restoration of—our individual and collective biopsychosocial wellness.

Kinds and degrees of social hardship have varied and still vary from country to country and, in the U. S., from state to state, but there's been global frustration about the cancellations or postponements of relied-on sources of entertainment and social diversion. Discontinued large-scale sports and tournaments, closed gyms and swimming pools, dimmed lights for all performing arts, shut movie theaters, prohibited in-house dining, and disrupted celebration of religious and festive events have imposed a social blackout on too much of our world as we once regularly lived in it. People have become estranged from one another. Much of society's service sector hasn't been able to provide their proper services, either. And social existence has been further darkened, distanced, and disconnected by the lockdown of travel, which has imposed limitations both inter- and intra-nationally, with mandatory quarantining and, in some instances, entry bans.

America and all other countries continue to proceed as they must, and when and where they may, with "new normal" operations lessening restrictions and relaxing regulations. Nonetheless, in each of our minds resides the immediate impact and residual consequences of psychological worry and fret—and the stress that comes with it all. For some people, bereavement has been a reality; for many others, isolation and its separations have loomed large because of social distancing. For everyone, fears of future uncertainties and deprivations, changes and adjustments have hit home. Indeterminacies of all kinds have imposed undue stress among many sectors of our society. And what has this added up to? In one way,

> Call it a . . . crisis of productivity, of will, of enthusiasm, of purpose. Call it a bout of existential work-related ennui [boredom] provoked partly by the realization that sitting in the same chair in the same room staring at the same computer for 12 straight months (and counting!) has left many of us feeling like burned-out husks, dimwitted approximations of our once-productive selves.

Clinically known as "behavioral anhedonia," this burned out, dimwitted feeling comes with people's inability to take pleasure in their activities, which in turn causes lethargy and lack of interest, which ultimately slackens their productivity. The less clinical but popular psychological term for this condition is "languishing," the opposite of flourishing, the blahs, with a lack of interest in what typically brings you joy.

Resilience against these kinds of psychological slumps is difficult to summon or to actualize, especially if one's body has been and still is sequestered in relative isolation. Intensifying these psychological slumps, physical inactivity with its accompanying neuromuscular deconditioning has eroded many people's biological fitness during the pandemic. Sedentary habits aren't surprising when people have worked and lived exclusively from home in repetitive stationary positions, with movement bounded. And in many instances the national decline in activity and good health grew worse during the pandemic's first two or three months, when patients were unable to see their doctors, dentists, and other healthcare providers. Post-vaccine, patients with diseases and health problems other than Covid frequently report having experienced neglect, as human care redistributed to fight Covid has created not only an overload on doctors and other healthcare professionals, but also a disruption in the medical supply chain.

Optimal Wellness is timed to coincide with our nation's need to reactivate physically, reassert psychologically, reconnect socially (without neglecting sensible protocols), and self-educate to accomplish this needed new-normalcy with our biopsychosocial habits and behaviors. Wellness education and the self-practices learned from thorough, reliable instruction must become our routine self-expectation. Unfortunately, further downgrading America's standards for wellness is our nation's inadequate physical education institutionally, which in schools ought to be the foundation for people's understandings of wellness and maintaining personal health. Despite this, "An Analysis of Research on Student Health-Related Fitness Knowledge in K–16 Physical Education Programs" observes that

> Two major results [in its study] . . . are misconceptions about fitness and the lack of an adequate amount of human-related fitness (HRF) knowledge among students at all educational levels (i.e., elementary, secondary, and college). These results were essentially the same as those found more than 20 years ago, indicating a persistent deficiency in fitness education (Keating 333).

This contemporary article highlights the inadequacies not only of students' understanding of fitness, but of curricular content and physical educators' instruction—if school systems haven't already eliminated such instruction. Those inadequacies, for many of us, have been our inheritance.

So it's time for each of us to help ourself. But deciding on what's reliable information and practice isn't always easy and can be daunting amid trending fads, opposing views, and far too much unreliable online foolishness. How, then, do we separate the wheat from the chaff, the enduring facts from the trendy fads, the permanently proven from the provisionally experimental? This book already has done that for you, each of its authors offering reliable holistic help for everyone to learn what wellness is and how to accomplish it. Hope exists actively here in this book, where what you learn comes from reliably validated and scientifically replicated research, with instructive explanations and integrated holistic methods and tools to help yourself become a healthier, thus happier person.

Optimal Wellness's foundational principles add up to safe, advisable procedures for laying out your self-help paths to wellness and guiding yourself towards self-maintenance. As with all ethically concerned doctors, therapists, and trainers, this book's authors recommend that you seek specialist help whenever a situation warrants special attention beyond what you can do on your own. That said, this book offers verified guidelines and strategies that will save you time, money, and needless physical and psychological aggravations and that will provide the proper building blocks to structure your future wellness and health programs: frequently our well-being is in our own hands, ours to do with as we see fit—long before professional medicine or therapy or training must intercede. Therefore, Total Wellness's intention is to offer instruction on the bodily, mental, and behavioral additions and modifications that will foster wellness for you, whatever your state of wellness presently may be. In effect, as self-helping instruction containing foundational biopsychosocial wellness principles, this book will assist readers with preventive, curative, and maintenance practices needed for being well and for well-being. Many of us know how Internet research about diagnoses and management of any physical condition can be dead-ended, or confusingly open-ended, and sometimes needlessly alarming to readers, whereas this book's discussions of assured behaviors and dependable practices provide controlled supervision throughout all wellness processes, with wellness developed naturally according to each individual's individual needs.

Optimal Wellness begins with a chapter by Dr. Vladimir Friedman, who conceived its depth of purpose and breadth of investigation. Vlad maps and explains his eclectic personal and professional pursuit of biopsychosocial wellness, a journey whose visited destinations allow for a thorough theoretical and practical understanding of what biopsychosocial wellness means in general and therefore will mean specifically to each of you. The book then explores the enduringly valuable fundamentals or bottom-line necessities to consider when making biopsychosocial wellness one's own; no reader will be able to appreciate the meanings of wellness, to work self-helpfully towards it, and to live well without this fundamental knowledge. To undo your harmful personal traits and to create helpful ones, readers next will become acquainted with strategic skills and practices structured by behavioral conditioning to break bad habits and breed good ones before or during any wellness program. Just as behavior change can occur anytime in one's life, so too can anxiety and pain, and especially chronic pain lasting more than six months; these important topics are explored biopsychosocially by two of this book's experts, who scientifically explain the causes and effects of pain, and how and where to deal therapeutically with it. Following that are multiple discussions devoted to human resilience as maintained by proper nutrition, effective sleep, and stress management, subjects that will benefit all readers, as will our professional observations for people with orthopedic musculoskeletal injuries and in need of massage therapies in clinics or at home, through healing touch and self-massage.

Throughout the book but principally in its final third are Eastern understandings and practices of wellness which meet and converge with those of the West, thus forming a global partnership for smart health that legitimizes *Optimal Wellness's* truly integrated comprehensive presentation. *Optimal Wellness* infuses Asian philosophical lessons and practices, including acupuncture, protocols and guides to live by for wellness, purification ceremonies, ways to mitigate sickness and to attain self-healing balances through body work, meditation, and sounds. Biopsycho self-healing and wellness, and detailed guides for exercise are viewed through the lenses of our experts with yoga, Pilates, and motion and exercise training for fitness, all of whose techniques and tips promote athletic performance not only by identifying weakness in optimal stability and mobility, but also by improving fundamental movement capacities (FMC) of mobility, balance, coordination, stability, strength, power, speed if applicable, and endurance.

To attain genuine total wellness, people need guides whose wisdom-based knowledge is focused purposefully, reasoned comprehensively, and integrated patiently, not haphazard bits and pieces of scattered information fragmented throughout the public domain and in specialist tomes, or popularized by trendy, short-lived fads. This book's accessible outlook, with best-practice lessons from the West and the East, and informed by wellness holists writing about their holistic practices, is heightened and further unified by the "Index of Recurring Subjects" at its end. There, yet another source of holism exists, as readers will be able to create their own thorough overview of important subjects of interest or concern as treated by whichever writers of Total Wellness address them. If for example you're interested in "breathing," "enteric nervous system," maybe "subconscious"or "voices, self-doubting," then under each of those headings you'll find a complete list of pagination leading you through a comprehensive understanding of those subjects from our writers' multiple and diverse but never contradictory points of view. Packed with opportunity, the Index will allow you to create in unity your own tracts for all subjects you'd like to discover more about. This book is devoted to facilitating and guaranteeing your self-education.

Further, we hope *Optimal Wellness* will be useful to other wellness practitioners as a mindful spur to their already existing awareness of the theoretical and practical importance of integrated comprehensive wellness. Some of those practitioners already think convergently but need a catalyst to conjoin with similar thinkers, while other such practitioners may be just beginning to appreciate the functional imperatives of integrated comprehensive wellness and its biopsychosocial components. Whatever the kind and degree of this book's influence, its authors have been dedicated to establishing for public and peer awareness a consolidated multifaceted understanding of the next step or new wave in well-founded, properly practiced biopsychosocial wellness. Just as science historian Peter Watts' 2019 *Convergence* painstakingly details the theoretical and applied developmental overlaps and integrations among the biological and physical sciences from 1859 to the present, so *Optimal Wellness: Necessary Biological, Psychological, and Social Integrations* recognizes and explains the convergent modalities that already exist—even if not yet frequently observed and applied by professionals —in the scientific studies and practices of human wellness.

ENDNOTES

[1]Americans "live in a culture, say the experts [whom Consumer Reports] consulted, encouraged by intense marketing by drug companies and an increasingly harried healthcare system that makes dashing off a prescription the easiest way to address a patient's concerns" (Carr). Wanting and receiving feel-better quick fixes and long-term remedies, we rely on healthcare practitioners to responsibly know about and to ethically administer our drugs; consequently, we're inclined to feel safe about consuming them. Due to this over-reliance on drugs coupled with our assumption of their safety and proper prescription, "The percentage of Americans taking more than five prescription medications has nearly tripled in the past 20 years, according to the Centers for Disease Control and Prevention"; Dr. Michael Hochman adds that unfortunately "The risk of adverse events increases exponentially after someone is on four or more medications" (Carr). This exponential increase happens more commonly when multimorbid patients have multiple specialists. It's fair to conclude that prescription drug misuse is prevalent in America. "The reasons for the high prevalence of prescription drug misuse vary by age, gender, and other factors," says the National Institute on Drug Abuse, "but likely include ease of access" (https://www.drugabuse.gov/publications/research-reports/misuse-prescription-drugs/what-scope-prescription-drug-misuse).

While it's true that "Prescription opioids, also known as prescription painkillers, have become a popular staple in medicine cabinets across the United States, resulting in devastating misuse, addiction and overdose" (Carr), we'd be naïve to assume that full responsibility for inflated use of these drugs is attributable alone to bad decisions by patients. Ease of access to prescription drugs is attributable also to America's bedeviling pharma-drug production. A 2019 Drugwatch reported that "Prescription drug use is a global problem, and the U.S. is the world's biggest addict"; we consume 99% of the world's Vicodin, 80% of Percoset and OxyContin, and 60% of Dilaudid (Elkins). Since 1999, American deaths by overdose of prescribed painkillers have quadrupled; recent data show "The amount of harm stemming from inappropriate prescription medication is staggering. Almost 1.3 million people went to U.S. emergency rooms due to adverse drug effects in 2014, and about 124,000 died from those events. That's according to estimates based on data from the Centers for Disease Control and Prevention and the Food and Drug Administration" (Carr). More than 6.5 million people use prescription medication for non-medical reasons, which is more than cocaine, heroin, and hallucinogens combined. Further, overuse of antibiotics and antidepressants continues to skyrocket. And what has this added up to? "[T]he paths to high-quantity prescriptions and dependencies collided in the 21st century" (Elkins). And it's a proven fact that high-quantity prescriptions are further generated by a knowing collusion between pharma's drug manufacturing and many doctors' casually immoderate drug prescribing, yet another unfortunate fact contributing to increased abuse, addiction, and death.

Further, frequent medication errors both in hospitals and at pharmacies cause unnecessary illness and death in the United States. "Medical errors," occurring at multiple points in the prescription process at hospitals—for reasons as avoidable as indecipherable handwriting—"are considered the third leading cause of death in the United States" according to a 2016 Johns Hopkins study; "The American Association for Justice estimates that 440,000 errors resulting in death occur each year" (https://scartelli.com/pharmaceutical-errors/).Pharmaceutically, letters to state regulatory boards and interviews with The New York Times reveal that pharmacists at CVS, Rite Aid, and Walgreens, among other major drugstore chains, "described understaffed, chaotic workplaces and said it had become difficult to perform their jobs safely, putting the public at risk of medication errors." Nearly fifteen years ago was the last comprehensive study of pharmaceutical medication errors, when "The Institute of Medicine estimated in 2006 that such mistakes harmed at least 1.5 million Americans each year" (The New York Times Morning Brief). Annually in the United States 7,000 to 9,000 people die as a result of a pharmacy medication error, and "The total cost of looking after patients with medication-associated errors exceeds $40 billion each year (Tariq). Additionally, hundreds of thousands of other patients experience but often do not report an adverse reaction or other complication related to a medication. And it's likely that the mishandling of meds has become worse, because "One of the major causes for medication errors is distraction. Nearly 75% of medication errors have been attributed to this cause" (Tariq); it follows that if a pharmaceutical workplace is "chaotic," just as most hospitals necessarily are, then errors of distraction are more likely to ensue. No statistics yet exist for Covid-occasioned prescriptive mishandlings, but the pandemic likely has increased the chaos.

[2+3]Not altogether surprising, the relationship between easy access to and overconsumption of drugs is paralleled in Americans' easy access to and overconsumption of food, particularly unhealthful food at take-out restaurants. According to a December 2018 report, "Every day, more than 1 in 3 U.S. adults [84.8 million, or 37%] eat some type of restaurant fast food, according to a recent report from the National Center for Health Statistics" (Safety Health); this report reveals also that about the same percentage of children daily consume fast food. A major health concern, "Fast-food consumption has been associated with increased intake of calories, fat and sodium, which can lead to obesity, diabetes and other health issues, according to the researchers" (Safety Health); not unexpectedly, fast food is "low in several key nutrients that adult bodies need to flourish and that children's bodies need to grow" (ABC Action News). Exacerbating this trend of too many children eating too much unhealthful food, "American public schools have problems with putting out healthy meals" (Cheung). Supersizing ourselves, many Americans become obese.

Obesity is defined as a person having a body mass index (BMI) of 30 and up. Measuring body fat as based on a weight to height ratio, the BMI includes three ascending Classes for obesity, with Class 3 having a BMI of 40 and over. The normal range for one's BMI is 18.5 to <24.9. People between a 25 and 30 BMI are classified as "overweight." In most high-income countries, around two-thirds of adults are overweight or obese. In the US, 70% are; worse, a 2018 article in Our World in Data notes that American obesity "nearly tripled between 1975 and 2016" (Ritchie). The October 2019 World Population Review's global rating of population obesity ranks the United States in 16th position, a ranking that included all age groups ("U.S. Obesity Rates"). Closer examination of this statistic shows that of the 15 countries with greater obesity, nine have a total population under 65,000 people, most of them living on tropical islands; another five countries are populated between 100,000 and 200,000, about the size of Dayton OH; and one, Kuwait, has slightly over four million people. Because all 15 more obese countries' populations total slightly over five million people, the 16th-place ranking of the U.S., which has over 330 million people, is deceptive; it misleadingly neglects to emphasize the widespread mass of obesity throughout our country.

The pandemic's impact on consumers has increased global reliance on fast food, not curbed it. Nathaniel Ashby's study hypothesizes that the pandemic increased feelings of stress and anxiety that led and still leads to the emotional eating of unhealthy foods (Ashby). Skyrocketing grocery store prices sent consumers back to fast-food restaurants, now more convenient because of restarted drive-through and mobile pickup operations (Myers). And "It isn't just the price that makes fast food attractive. Parents are juggling working and looking after their kids who are spending more time at home. . . . These time-strapped Americans are turning to the convenience of takeout food, and many delivery services are soaring.

Domino's reported that its US same-store sales . . . generated $240 million in net income - 30% higher than in 2019 (Dean). And throughout the pandemic, fast-food convenience continues to increase technologically with app proliferation and the food-marketers' ability to connect with customers through automated ordering and payments.

WORKS CITED

ABC Action News, Lifestyle Section, "CDC report: 84.8 million U.S. adults consume fast food every day and other startling findings," Oct 03, 2018

American Cancer Society, Cancer Action Network, "Increasing and Improving Physical Education and Physical Activity in Schools: Benefits for Children's Health and Educational Outcomes"
https://www.fightcancer.org/policy-resources/keeping-children-healthy-recommendations-promoting-physical-education-and-physical

Ashby Nathaniel J. S. "The impact of the COVID-19 pandemic on unhealthy eating in populations with obesity." Obesity, 2020. doi:10.1002/oby.22940

Best Healthcare in the World Population 2020 (2019-10-24) from
http://worldpopulationreview.com/countries/best-healthcare-in-the-world/

British Journal of General Practice. 2005; 55 (511): 154-155

Carr, Teresa, "Too Many Meds? America's Love Affair With Prescription Medication." Consumer Reports, August 3, 2017
https://www.consumerreports.org/prescription-drugs/too-many-meds-americas-love-affair-with-prescription-medication/

Cheung, Kylie, "How School Lunches Around the World Compare to America's." March2, 2016)
https://archive.attn.com/stories/6085/school-lunches-around-world-compared -to-the-united-states

Committee on Physical Activity and Physical Education in the School Environment; Food and Nutrition Board; Institute of Medicine, Educating the Student Body: Taking Physical Activity and Physical Education to School. Washington (DC): **National Academies Press** (US); 2013.

Dean, Grace, Insider, **https://www.businessinsider.com/** american-kids-were-eating-more-fast-food-before-the-pandemic-2020-8).

Elkins, Chris, "Hooked on Pharmaceuticals: Prescription Drug Abuse in America."

Drugwatch, May 17, 2019.

Epstein, David, Range: Why Generalists Triumph in a Specialized World, Riverhead Books, An imprint of Penguin Random House L.L.C., New York, NY, 2019

Felter, Claire, "A Guide to Global Covid-19 Vaccine Efforts." Council on Foreign Relations, October 2021.
https://www.cfr.org/backgrounder/guide-global-covid-19-vaccine-efforts
https://www.forbes.com/sites/benmidgley/2018/09/26/the-six-reasons-the-fitness-industry-is-booming/#16a8bb31506d.

Frances, Allen, M.D., "We Have Too Many Specialists and Too Few General Practitioners," Psychology Today,   Jan 21, 2016

---------"Patient-Centered Vs. Lab-Centered 'Personalized Medicine," *Huffington Post* Updated July 24, 2017

Freeman, Joshua, "Towards a Definition of Holism." *British Journal of General Practice, 2005* Feb 1; 55(511): 154-55.

Galliea, Josep, "Integral Thinking." Integral World, Newsletter 812: November 30, 2019 **http://www.integralworld.net**

Griffiths, Sarah, "Bingeing on fast food leaves a scar etched in your DNA which is passed down to your children, study finds." *Daily Mirror*, 7 July, 2014.

Jones, Thomas C. and Betsy M. Chalfin, *From the Family Doctor to the Current Disaster of Corporate Health Maintenance.* AuthorHouseUK, 2016.

Kapoor, Hansika and James C. Kaufman, "Meaning-Making Through Creativity during COVID-19." Frontiers in Psychology, 18 December 2020 **(https://doi.org/10.3389/fpsyg.2020.595990)**

Keating, Xiaofen Deng et al, "An Analysis of Research on Student Health-Related Fitness Knowledge in K–16 Physical Education Programs." Human Kinetics Journals, V. 28: Issue 3, 333-349.

Landhuis, Esther, "Your Immune System Is Made, Not Born." *Scientific American*

January 29, 2015

Lyall, Sarah, "We Have All Hit a Wall." The New York Times, April 3, 2021. **https://www.nytimes.com/2021/04/03/business/pandemic burnoutproductivity.**

html?campaign_id=9&emc=edit_nn_20210404&instance_id=28847&nl=the-morning&regi_id=106975020&segment_id=54857&te=1&user id=9ce00b47b37a6b7f1190627dae9e2fba

Miller, Kenneth. "Why Food Allergies Are Surging," *Leapsmag*, May 9, 2019

Myers, Candice A. and Stephanie T. Broyles, "Fast Food Patronage and Obesity Prevalence During the COVID-19 Pandemic: An Alternative **https://doi.org/10.1002/oby.22993).**

National Research Council (US); Institute of Medicine (US), U.S. Health in International Perspective: Shorter Lives, Poorer Health. Washington (DC): National Academies Press (US); 2013.

Poth, Cheryl N. et. al, "Using Convergent Sequential Design for Rapid Complex Case Study Descriptions: Example of Public Health Briefings During the Onset of the COVID-19 Pandemic." **https://doi.org/10.1101/2020.11.11.20229393**

Ritchie, Hannah and Max Roser, "Obesity," Our World in Data, 2020 **https://ourworldindata.org/obesity**

Safety Health, Dec 6, 2018. "Nearly 37 percent of Americans regularly eat fast food, study shows"

Sawyer, Bradley and Daniel McDermott, "How do mortality rates in the U.S. compare to other countries?" Peterson-KFF Health System Tracker, February 14, 2019. **https://www.healthsystemtracker.org/chart-collection/mortality-rates-u-s-compare-countries/**

Science News: 6/18/11, p. 26.

Simon, William E. Jr., "Physical education is key to longer, happier lives. Our kids and schools need more of it," USA Today, Dec 12, 2018

Snyderman, Ralph and Weil, Andrew T. "Integrative Medicine: Bringing Medicine Back to Its Roots." Archives of Internal Medicine. 2002. 62(4).

Tariq, Rahan A. and Yevgenia Sherbak, "Medication Errors," StatPearls

The New York Times Morning Brief, Friday, Jan 31, 2020.
https://www.nytimes.com/2020/01/31/briefing/president-trump-coronavirus-brexit.html?te=1&nl=morning-briefing\&emc=edit_NN_20200131&campaign_
id=9&instance_id=15628&segmentid=20853&user_id=9ce00b47b37a6b7f1190627 dae9e2fba&regi_ id= 10697502020200131

"U.S. Health in International Perspective: Shorter Lives, Poorer Health"
https://www.ncbi.nlm.nih.gov/books/NBK154469/
"U.S. Obesity Rates Reach Historic Highs," Trust for America's Health, 2019

CHAPTER I

Why Biopsychosocial Wellness or Holistic Health?

Everyone wants the answers to pain-free optimal health and wellness, but are they ready for that commitment which those answers provide? Dedication is what makes or breaks clients' or patients' ability to succeed in anything, specifically achievements and outcomes in human performance and recovery. Being in the healthcare and fitness industry for over 25 years, I still find it incredibly difficult to guarantee results for any outcome. These days at gatherings, the initial introduction of who I am or what I professionally do usually triggers people's immediate hand-grab on my neck or low back and a reminder that they have been meaning to speak to someone like me. Daily questions arise in my clinical health care practice, Accelerated Care Chiropractic, and personal life about the best tools, systems, and strategies to ensure optimal wellness.

I am a practitioner who envisioned a book that would help guide the reader for best practices from some of the best individual doctors, therapists, coaches, and trainers. I recognized that all of these people, in different ways because of their specialties, share with me a passion for bringing to their specialization the best and widest-ranging complementary practices and tools to assure total wellness for their clients. And like me, all writers of this book recognize that as holists, or "jack-of-all-trades and master of one," they know who can do better with certain other aspects of wellness than they do. The most successful healthcare professionals understand their own best qualities but are most effective when they realize that other holists may be more advantageous for a client than themselves.

There are many times I am asked why I am so different from the other practitioners in my field, and unfortunately I do not have an answer other than I love the human body and how it functions, along with the humbling thank-you I receive when a patient's problem is resolved. My continual training and learning about my craft is what keeps me, I believe, ahead of the pack. My understanding as a young personal trainer in the 1990's was that in order to help people get in shape and live a healthful lifestyle I needed to know how they think, how they eat, and what demands they put on their bodies. I started my educational career on a premed track, graduating with a Bachelor of Science in athletic training, with minors in psychology, nutrition, and education. I was well on my way into the world of medicine when a severe injury during training changed my path. I went through the medical model of pain management, searching for a "cure" until meeting a sports chiropractor at a personal training forum who changed my life. During a presentation, he evaluated me from head to toe and without any knowledge of my history asked if I had been having mid-back pain.

Never having heard of a chiropractor at that moment, I was extremely intrigued because here was a man standing in front of me with no knowledge about me, yet understanding exactly my struggles with pain. He did not know my failed treatment history of receiving countless evaluations, x-rays, MRI's, nerve conduction studies, and spinal steroid injections. Even more disheartening, all of this treatment was coming from specialists I one day wanted to be like. After he gave me some basic education on proper training and made me realize that the exercises I was doing were building muscles but were costly and counterproductive, he also showed me some basic mobilization movements that are now considered mainstream functional movement exercises; within two weeks of sticking to this routine, I found that my pain had subsided immensely. That relief did not just make me happy; it changed my mindset on the kind of doctor I wanted to be.

Throughout my chiropractic student career, I was lucky enough to have the opportunity to shadow many doctors, but one stood out from the pack, a sports chiropractor out of Brooklyn NY who had a huge patient base through the Public-School Athletic Leagues. Mostly he specialized in football and track and field injuries. It was not so much his amazing clinical or manual skills that I was impressed by but his humbling ability to not follow the latest gimmick or craze on the market. He strongly believed if patients are educated well and follow through with his guidance, most of their problems can be resolved. Jumping through the hoops of my chiropractic education required a singular belief tremendously preached in school: the body's innate ability to heal itself entirely through the alleviation of spinal segmental restrictions, also known as chiropractic subluxations. But my having had such an extensive background in human anatomy, physiology, emergency medical systems, and athletic training made me feel like an atheist sitting in church and listening to the gospels. Further, graduating from chiropractic school is like being born into the wild with no parental protection. You are strictly on your own and have to develop tough skin to handle everything that can possibly come in the door. We are not provided any system that can educate and promote our clinical excellence, such as a hospital system. Instead, many of us are compelled to open on our own and run a practice to the best of our ability by trial and error. All of my education throughout my career was in the mindset of getting my players back on their respective fields, with trial and error, until we got it right. I have strayed away from common mainstream beliefs that a patient needs to be under my care "Forever."

These beliefs have developed over the years with newfound research in the muscle skeletal world, which helps me express exactly what it is my manual skill sets allow me to do. Understanding that also makes me believe that since every person is so complexly unique, then there can't be a simple approach to their optimal health and well-being. When I first started my career as a chiropractor, I realized pretty quickly that manipulation was just a tool in my practitioner utility belt and not at all the means to a full resolve of symptoms. Patients would leave my office feeling better but always came back for more. If I were a salesman, it would be the perfect scenario to keep your customers coming back—but at what price?

As a holist, I believe I am what any healthcare practitioner ought to be: not a restricted specialist, but someone who has qualities of a humble empath, a practitioner who takes in everything and doesn't automatically reach conclusions or respond emotionally but instead takes time to know the client as an individual person. Soon, the humble empath develops a third eye, an experience-based sixth sense about each client. To arrive at health-promoting diagnoses, all health care practitioners must be non-judgmental, accepting clients' excuses bred and reinforced in their subconscious, and quietly listening to their rationalized or misinterpreted blaming. Soon, a game plan can be strategized for each individual and, as the client opens up, more will be accomplished appropriate to her or his needs. For me, being a good doctor means that the client must have an "aha" moment. The "aha" moment is when they realize what it truly takes to keep them at optimal health. For many it becomes ritualized in daily routines that turn into habitual self-motivated processes through nutrition, movement, sleep, meditation, and mentally focused recovery. Nothing in life can be genuinely appreciated without work and determination. A person's health is a forever process which changes constantly, and the only way to conquer it is to stay ahead in the game of life.

Therapy, in my opinion, is a two-way street and cannot ever be attained solely by the practitioner. In no way do I take any responsibility away from the practitioner to be a good evaluator, educator, skilled provider, and coach. Detective work has become my therapeutic motive as a wellness practitioner; the questions I ask come from experience not just with what I have been trained to ask, but with investigation taken from these other modalities. The result is that frequently I must take a different, non-standard approach.

My first session starts with reciprocal education between myself and the patient or client. Even my introduction has been thought through over the years: now I walk into a room always smiling, because a serious look can be interpreted to be too serious and at times intimidating. As I enter a room, I tend to introduce myself as Dr. Vlad, my way of starting the relationship without making things too formal; rather than emphasizing a white coat and stethoscope, I accentuate a big smile, warm heart, and a personal name attached to the teddy bear exterior that is there for them, ready to listen observantly.

As the years have developed my education, I have changed many of my procedures, specifically when they come to evaluation. I no longer use only the standard approach of taking a simple history, performing a fundamental neurological and a focal orthopedic exam, and then beginning treatment. The history is always important, but many times does not express the actual reason they are in the office. To effectively assess their prognosis, I need to know their motives and how they think in order to stimulate them toward not only a successful outcome but a long lasting one. Most of my cases I wish were as simple as a sprain or strain of one body part or region. However, a typical case may reveal not just a flare-up in one specific body part, but usually also in other regions found during the session that require attention but aren't as expressive as the primary region.

The fun begins when the patient presents herself with the problem, not knowing what could possibly have triggered her injury or pain in the first place. Where do we go if all we had was the basic questioning of what, where, when, and how? Unfortunately, most of what the patient can relay is usually too subjective, because opinions and recollections sometimes have emotional connections but are not facts. This kind of information is truly limited and can be used only in the background while objectively investigating. My objective examinations start with a theoretical construct developed by two heavy hitters in the fitness and physical therapy world, Gray Cook and Michael Boyle. Called the Joint-by-Joint approach, it represents a common association between each part of the body and its relation to the ones closest to it above and below. This theory, which focuses on alternating patterns of stability and mobility from one anatomical region to another, promotes the understanding that certain areas like your ankles, hips, shoulders, and thoracic need to express more mobility, while the feet, knees, lumbar (low back), and cervical spine (neck) need to appreciate stability. More specifically, mobility can be appreciated in a region when there is enough muscle extensibility to complete a statistically normal range of motion passively and actively under load; stability includes the timing and neuromuscular motor control of a region. Understanding this intricate balance between mobility and stability allows us to focus on things we need to help move and things we need to stabilize. Along with the Joint-by-Joint approach is the Selective Functional Movement Assessment, SFMA, a diagnostic system created to evaluate basic movement relationships with known musculoskeletal pain. It helps guide me to the most dysfunctional movement patterns that are not always expressive of pain but are usually a huge contributor to the pain-generating tissue.

Patients and I take the evaluation further for understanding what makes them tick by knowing about their habits, careers, and family interaction to translate what their average daily movement patterns and emotional well-being could be. After taking a history of what their current complaints are and prior injuries, we start with a selective functional movement assessment where we look at how they generally move, just like peeling the layers of an onion, homing in on their neuromuscular deficiencies and probable pain generators producing their symptoms. We progress from unloaded to loaded movement to begin to differentiate between structural limitations, functional limitations, or both. Palpatory skill sets are used to further define reflexively guarded muscle tissue that could be the primary cause of pain and dysfunction or dig further through the web of muscular layers, connecting junctions, and joint connections to find a secondary culprit of pain origin. Within the same palpatory process I also evaluate specific joint movement, taking note which joints lack movement and which might be overworking.

Once we have defined the patient's deficiencies, we begin the process physically, but the education starts immediately with the understanding that this will be a two-way street. You see, my job is to take the last few decades of clinically researched information, bottle it up into a digestible, easy to understand informative protocol for the client to absorb. The understanding has to be made that the biomechanical world of therapy has been constantly updating, with new theories of what is actually occurring in the body. Prior was a simpler understanding of just stretch and strengthening to recover from injury. With a newfound organ system such as the muscle skeletal fascial system and its vast sensory network, we have developed a better understanding of how our skin and fascia play a role affecting the body. Consequently, I have had to stay current with these newly developing theories and techniques, and frequently, although I understood them, I could not always fully explain them to a patient; maybe that was because each theory and technique wasn't actually a singular idea or process, its effects extensive and complicated.

As time proceeded, I began to learn that combinations of therapies yielded even more effective results. In my office I feel as if I'm the composer of a synchronous variety of modalities to produce my melody of manual input for the patient's brain to be subdued for a better appreciation of pain information. During a typical treatment session, the patient's body and mind are being stimulated with different modalities. We start with a relaxing process with heat (diathermy) to increase blood flow and increase muscle relaxation, and electric muscle stimulation to decrease muscle tone, increase circulation, and desensitize the targeted areas. Once the body is relaxed, I use not only topical creams to decrease friction on the skin, but also penetrating compounds such as capsaicin, menthol, and/or CBD to affect pain receptors by desensitizing them. I apply soft and/or deep tissue massage to continue mobilizing the tissue to promote fluid distribution, increase blood flow, and decrease muscle tone. I introduce Instrument Assisted Soft Tissue Mobilization (IASTM) to the prepped tissue to facilitate the healing process through increased fibroblast proliferation and increased collagen synthesis, maturation, and alignment to break up myofascial adhesions. To further promote tissue glide and reperfusion, I might incorporate some soft tissue flossing. After the use of all of these compressive forces I will decompress the tissue with cupping therapy, further promoting increased blood flow and decreasing pain sensitization. Once the soft tissue has been released, relaxed, and vascularized, I now have a window of opportunity to properly affect the joints that are restricted and lack movement with the use of various Joint Mobilizations and Grade 5 Manipulations (AKA Chiropractic Adjustment or Osteopathic Manipulation). Joint mobilization and manipulation promote better movement with stimulation of mechanoreceptors, reflexively relaxing muscle tissue, and breaking up fibrous adhesions within the joint, allowing it to move properly.

Once the patient and I have convinced the body to relax, I continue by instilling movement through static and dynamic flexibility to increase range of motion and promote, in a sense, a muscle memory to the new range the muscles have expressed. Typically depending on the patient's skin sensitivity, an application of kinesiology taping will be applied to promote continual therapy for a few more days by consistently feeding the skin with information to actively inhibit pain through sensory mechanoreceptor activation. All of these stimulations, when the patient leaves, carry with them a spillover effect for the next few days. Keep in mind that my practice is principally designed, or specified, to be physical, and in this exact moment is actually where the magic happens.

Once patients have experienced some relief or in many cases an unloading of stress, they begin to accept some of my future suggestions and next steps. What I have realized is that my treatment sessions are important but are most definitely not the sum of patients' whole recovery. My therapy is only a gateway for continued self-care. My clients develop a better understanding that body work is one piece and that the other pieces have to come together with how they think, what they put into their bodies, and how they move.

My professional and personal experience with doctors has taught me that wellness will be insufficient if a doctor does not have a network of contacts. Keeping my ego always checked, I understand that I too have limitations out of my eclectically informed specialty. This is also because every individual is a complex, many-pieced puzzle that often requires additional experts either to see the whole therapeutic picture, or to bring in new pieces to make that puzzle more complete and more visible, thus more holistic. I rely on a set of colleagues related to my patients' needs. These needs definitely have therapeutic layers guiding whom to refer to. First, we put out the fire when a specialization is needed for a focal and specialized approach such as orthopedics, neurology, anesthesiology, etc. But when the fire is out, we must find the reason for the fire so it doesn't happen again. The chronic or insidious reasons require a biopsychosocial intervention, and therefore solution to clients' needs will range from a functional medicine practitioner and/or nutritional consultation to subdue their inflammatory markers, to a psychological consult to address biopsychosocial limitations, and/or a personal training life coach to solidify the movements we achieved in our therapy session for improved performance. This accessibility of colleagues allows patients to have accountability to achieve their goals.

Their part starts with the understanding that their body's healing has its own process, its own timeframe, its own reality. They must begin to be more mindful of what their body is telling them—and no, ignorance is not bliss. Having a high pain threshold is no longer sexy when you try to accomplish optimal health. Pain is your best expressive sensory motivation to help you change the demand you are unknowingly placing on your body. After all the physicality that I perform within a session and the client leaves the office, with improvement, is when the true healing process actually begins.

Therapy and the body's ability to adapt and heal is the process. A misconception brought to my office, often, is that my treatment will be like a "Hollywood Chiropractic" scene. The patient will be placed on the table, and I will "Presto Chango!" their body with a forever pain- free life. Now that would be an amazing superpower, but unfortunately that is not how true therapy works. Fortunately, instead of superpowers we have prior and current wisdoms that have been passed on from a multitude of practitioners and researchers to help us guide what we can do. Many times, the hardest part is remembering to do them all. Therefore, it is truly not a commitment to me that I require of patients but a holistically multivariable commitment to themselves. This dedication is not an overnight success, as this commitment comes usually within the process and it is my job to help my clients reach an "Ah-ha" moment, when recognition comes to them and they get results they have not seen before, driven by needs that are not necessarily performed by the specialist. Any application performed on the body passively or actively has a multivariable dosage-to-recovery response time. For example, performing soft tissue mobilization on a 6-foot, 220 pound, 25 year-old professional athlete will be totally different frion working on a 5'6", 140 pound, 55 year-old working woman with comorbidities. How you recover many times is directly proportionate to what kind of environment you provide for your body. If the body is young, oxygenated, and nutrient dense, the probability of a faster recovery is certain. If the body is, in a sense, fighting within itself, the recovery time takes longer. This is why patients need to affirm a true commitment to themselves in order to provide a proper environment for healing and recovery.

Everything that I have mentioned seems to boil down to one concept: any person, when considered a complex puzzle requiring the integration of so many possible pieces, will be better managed by professional advisors than by doing it alone. The patients that have had the most productive success in their outcomes have all had realizations that their approach must be a multivariable approach just as their lives have a multivariable road. One patient comes to mind who has had what I would call an extraordinary life and has become a gracious student of his own body. Genetically he wasn't dealt such a great hand of cards, as he has had a slew of problems that came on throughout his life, none relating back to his lifestyle. With persistence of seeking out guidance from many professionals with different backgrounds, he now has the luxury of not only appreciating life but actually still having one. This is a man in his seventies who has checked his ego with his body a long time ago. He has many people he holds close to keep him biopsychosocially accountable, starting close to home with his amazing wife, and bolstered by the three professionals he sees weekly: his lifestyle performance coach, a fitness trainer of over 18 years who keeps him in check nutritionally and challenges his heart, breath, and body in general; his Pilates coach, who keeps his mind connected to his body under strenuous demands; and his manual therapist, who helps his body recover from the demands he puts on his body weekly. When things arise unexpectedly or when he decides on a new goal to achieve that might be out of the scope of practice or knowledge from his immediate advisors, he will reach into his rolodex to access his team of other practitioners for guidance, a cardiologist for his bypassed heart, a urologist for his prostate cancer, an endocrinologist for his diabetes, a podiatrist for his slightly neuropathic feet, an ophthalmologist for his blind right eye, an ear specialist for his deaf left ear. This is a man who had his "aha" moment a long time ago and now continues to appreciate his journey. That's what this book is about: a collection of health care providers from different fields helping you understand how to appreciate your physical and mental lifestyle journey.

As you will see, "what can I do or where should I start?" is sometimes a very hard question to answer. Fortunately, I've asked a few of my colleagues to help me answer these questions and much more through their own personal and professional perspective to help you define what you should do and where you could start. Our aim is for you to be able to understand the different components of health and optimal living and to help you begin your journey of creating a mindful game plan for an optimal life. Throughout this book we will help you better understand the biopsychosocial fundamentals and where to begin, with behavior modification and habit change strategies to help you implement the process of change. For you to build confidence to overcome pain, a true understanding of physical and emotional pain is a must to build a resilient body and mind. Throughout my years in practice a realization has been made that what you put into your body directly relates to how it and your mind will function—the ability to understand that there truly is a difference between living to eat and eating to live. That is why we have included a plethora of information on fundamental nutrition and diseases that easily develop from our Standard American Diet. We hope to enlighten you on how to be aware of your dietary individuality and point you in a better direction of customizing your nutrition and lifestyle based on your health concerns. Regeneration and recovery are the buzz-words mostly used in the health and fitness industry, and understanding the fundamental biopsychosocial necessities of nutrition, sleep, and stress management will guide you to better recovery from physical and mental stress. It has been known for the last few decades that the Western world has accepted many philosophies and techniques from the Eastern world, so as holists we introduce some Eastern medicine practices and protocols for authentic living. Movement, in my opinion, is the key to your body's life; as I mention to my patients, the only time you don't need to move is when you are six feet under. Yes, as grim as that sounds, it's still the truth. If you're not moving, you're dying. It can be seen very simply once an individual is casted for a broken limb. To promote bone healing, we at times must restrict movement of the affected limb and, once the cast is taken off (usually 6-8 weeks), muscle atrophy is immediately appreciated. Therefore, movement is truly one of the most important facets for optimal health, and we bring you the most common practices known from the worlds of yoga, Pilates, and strength training. When your mind conceives and perceives what needs to be done, your body will achieve it. But dreams without goals are just wishes, which is why we have also included some information for SMART goal setting, to understand personal baselines and how to progress your routines with a focus on movement and training applications.

CHAPTER II

Biopsychosocial Fundamentals of Wellness

I've always had an interest in sports and an athletic background, playing soccer first, then learning and competing in Taekwondo, kickboxing, and Muay Thai. Member of the Moroccan 1988 Olympics Taekwando team, I studied Muay Thai in Thailand between 1992-1995, during which time I won the 1992-3 Dutch Muay Thai boxing competition. Moving to the U.S., I then won the U.S. 1999 Excaliber Muay Thai Challenge gold medal and, later, another gold medal at the first U.S. national Muay Thai competition in 2001, which placed me on the national team. Beginning as an Equinox trainer in 2000, I attained the fitness company's highest ranking trainer position, Tier-X, in 2004. Since then I've received the Equinox Lifetime Achievement award in 2012, co-founded and become a member of the Equinox Olympic Committee, which for three consecutive years promoted Equinox Games, and now am General Manager of Hudson Yards' E Training Studios in Manhattan, the most elite coaching platform offered by Equinox. Additionally, I have worked at Mt. Sinai Hospital's Rehab Center for Addiction, training one-on-one with patients to promote their physical movement, coached soccer teams, individual celebrities and high-profile business people, and have certifications including the 21-credit NYU Program in Business and Coaching.

I mention my history as a competitive athlete and fitness trainer because my credentials show how much time I spent learning and experiencing new theories, techniques, and challenges about health, wellness, and longevity, and in particular the fundamental practices needed to live properly. These fundamental abilities not only have helped me to continue to improve my daily tasks, but will help me to share with you all that's needed for biopsychosocial wellness, managing properly and efficiently the body, mind, and surrounding influences in life. Wellness requires multitasking, a fluid integration of reactions to accomplish a goal without negatively affecting our objective. This biopsychosocial multitasking cannot be properly achieved without first knowing the fundamentals introduced and explained in this chapter. Everything in life has a base, a proper way of how to start it, a foundation upon which to build it. Therefore, if you lack foundations or fundamentals, the primary rules or principles, you will not succeed fully or solidly or last longer efficiently throughout the process of your life. Any changes from learning and mastering all of these biopsychosocial fundaments will come when each of you has the courage to question your own fundamental values and beliefs and then see to it that your actions lead to your best intentions.

I. The Mind:

A. Mental conditioning

No matter what you are setting out to accomplish, the very first step to getting you to where you want to go, begins with the mind. Your thinking has so much power over your ability to reach your goals, and it's very important to recognize that your thoughts, attitudes, and beliefs are both choices and skills. This is good news because just like any other skills, these can be learned and improved with practice. Mental conditioning is a process of training your mind to modify your thoughts, attitudes, and beliefs to accept thinking patterns, tendencies, and/or mental states in order to optimize positive thinking and ultimately optimize your performance. When you become aware of your thinking patterns and assess your starting point, it's from this baseline that you can intentionally set a path forward to practice in areas where you'd like to see improvements that will translate into both increased performance and quality of life.

This is true for each of the fundamentals of the mind that follow below. By focusing in these areas, you will build a strong foundation of practice in using your thinking as a powerful tool to create the mental meaning, focus, flexibility, and stamina that we all need in the journey towards our goals. At the core of each of these is practicing to keep your mindset to stay in the present moment. In other words, keeping an emphasis on only the now and returning to it again and again when you find yourself drifting away from the moment. This helps to prohibit stress and anything else destructive that we might bring to an exercise session.

B. Positivity-motivation (Positivity feeds motivation.)

A positive state of mind is one that continues to seek, find, and execute ways to win or to find a desirable outcome, regardless of the circumstances. This concept is the opposite of negativity, defeatism, and hopelessness. It is living by the philosophy of finding greater joy in small joys and to live without hesitation or holding back our most cherished personal virtues and values. Optimism and hope are vital to developing and nurturing a positive mindset that will help you to sustain the motivation and problem-solving skills needed to carry you through mastering new skills, inevitable challenges, and unpredicted set-backs.

C. Openness for mental clarity = Understanding

Communication and education are the building blocks to both understanding and a strong relationship that is based on trust. Why is this important? Because you can't trust something that you don't understand. What are you personally doing and why? What is the process and the science behind your plan? These questions should be part of ongoing conversations between the coach and the client because, without experience, the client will not necessarily know why they are doing something.

I like to ask my clients this question, "Would you rather be the sail boat or the wind?" I like it because it is a good solid question to make them stop for a second and become aware of both their thought process and where they stand. It helps to clear up their identity a bit by bringing awareness to what drives them and what they want. Sometimes, who they think they are is not actually who they really are. and what they think they want is not actually what they really want. There is no right or wrong answer; just useful insight into their mind in that moment and an opportunity to consider, "Is that really what I want? Is it working for me?"

Keeping an openness to taking a closer look at the why behind what drives you and all the elements of your plan is the path to greater mental clarity and understanding. This helps to build trust in your coach, your plan, and within yourself.

D. Acceptance of capability

Acceptance of capability is about setting realistic goals, motivation, and injury prevention. If you can accept your capabilities in the present moment, then you also are setting yourself up for feeling encouraged, building motivation, and preventing injuries that could set you back in your plan.

So what are you capable of today? How does this match with your stated goals? It is here that coaching becomes critical. Some coaches, in an effort to keep the client happy, just stay on plan. But the best coaches know that creating an exercise program and successfully executing it requires constant attention to your current capabilities and builds into it, the flexibility to adjust your incremental goals to meet you where you are today. in the present moment.   Here are just a few examples of when the conversation with your coach needs to come back to the present moment to discuss your current capabilities, what could go wrong (injury), and include a path forward toward the goal that also matches your current capabilities.

1. You come into an exercise session stating as a physical goal that you want to do 10 pull-ups, but the reality is that you don't yet have the conditioning to achieve this goal safely and would be better served with an incremental plan to build up to 10 pull-ups.
2. You've been up all night with your kids and you come to the gym on 2 hours of sleep and tell your coach that you "want to crush it today," but a lighter workout would allow you to still condition and not further exhaust your body when it really needs recovery.
3. You have the mental goal of wanting to squat 150 lbs., but you need understanding to accept that you are physically not able to squat 150 lbs. and that attempting something not meant for your body is not good for your health and well-being.

It is human nature to want to push limits, but you have to be able to say to yourself, "It's OK. I can accept the reality of where I am and will pull back for the moment so that I am able to move forward and keep progressing on the larger plan." Sometimes it is hard to accept these limitations. This is especially true for over-achievers and for people who are aging. When you approach 40-50 years of age, it can be really challenging to learn what your new limitations are. It's like walking a tight rope between your mind and body of what you used to be able to do, what you now can do, what you shouldn't do, and alternatives. Here, coaching becomes so much more important, as the focus needs to shift to injury prevention and longevity and not to continue bench pressing as much as possible and going to the beach. That's how you know that you are in good hands: when the coach helps you to take a step back in order to be able to continue to move forward to prevent new injuries and limitations so you can continue on your path toward your goals. A huge part of this relationship is trust. Trust has to come from the beginning. It is rooted in transparency of the plan and expectations, and then it takes a little time for actions and situations to build up as proof you can trust that person. You shouldn't expect to have trust on day one. Both coach and client have to show commitment and actions that demonstrate to each other that they can trust each other.

When you accept your current capabilities and have established trust with your coach, you will be receptive to their communication and recommendations, but make no mistake, you still own your decisions. For example, if you are training hard and your coach recommends that you pull back and bit and take the weekend

38

off for recovery, it is a suggestion. Your coach cannot decide for you. It is still you who needs to decide that you will take the weekend off so that you can feel that much better on Monday; on Monday, when you perform better, that's ownership.

E. Expectations/Commitment

Commitment is the state of being dedicated to a cause or activity. It is tied to ownership, but it's not the same. Commitment is tangible. For example, I can ask you, on a level from 1-10, how committed are you to your fitness program? If you answer 8, my next questions are going to be a) Why are you an 8 and not a 10? and b) How can we make it a 10? If you tell me that it's because you can only work out twice per week, this is tangible and now we have a starting point for more discussion. You can't reinforce the commitment of someone if they are not committed. It's up to them. It's also useful mention that if someone can commit to an 8, the actual output more likely will be between a 6 and an 8 because of the inevitable things in life that can pull you back at times (people get sick, injured, etc.)

It's good to be aware of this and to set expectations that not everything is going to go the way you planned. Communication between client and coach along these lines should be honest. The coach cannot simply tell the client what they want to hear, but rather the coach has to tell the client what they think is right for them in that moment. It's very important here to use the proper language with the client so they understand. This language has to be tailored, meaning all clients cannot be treated the same. You need to know how to speak to each client individually, based on the language they understand, the relationship, level of trust, knowledge, and their experience. It has to be simple, clear, honest, direct, and short—not a speech. This is a skill the coaches have to work on themselves to have the confidence and trust in themselves to know who can be pushed and who cannot—not because they can't be pushed, but because it won't work. Certainly here, experience can help.

F. Ownership

Self-ownership means being comfortable in your own shoes and owning your attitudes and actions. People with self-ownership take responsibility for their lives. They have exceptional self-confidence, which allows them to unconditionally love themselves and accept their minor imperfections. So how do you trigger self-confidence and foster ownership? A good starting point is for the client to answer the critical question of "Why are they there?" What is their goal and the reasons behind it? I ask this question because it's hard to reinforce confidence if there's no clarity around the goal. During this discussion, as a coach, I take myself out of the equation. The coach should not set the goal because, if the coach sets the goal, this kills ownership on day one, leaving nothing that the client can own after that. Now, the coach is in charge. So this is important: the client must set the goal. Here are some examples of how this could take shape and some strategies to address them:

1. They have a clear goal and know why they want it, but they are not confident. A strategy here could be to look to draw upon other parts of their life in which they are or were/ very confident so they can tap into what it feels like and be able to envision it in this new space.
2. They have a clear goal, but the goal isn't realistic. For example, someone who has never run before stating that they want to run a marathon within 6 months. This situation calls for the coach to be honest, but not discouraging, by providing a gentle reality check and laying out a plan that starts with building a base and then building upon that base in phases towards incremental goals.
3. They don't really know what they are there for, or they are just there because they see someone else doing it (social media, celebrity, friend). This situation requires more discussion and search for mental clarity. This can take a bit of time over several discussions, so it's good to approach this with patience.

With all these scenarios you can draw upon these answers to give guidance and set up the client for success by assessing their starting point and making a plan with realistic outcomes and expectations that also creates opportunities for incremental wins which build their self-confidence along the way.

Seeing the starting point of where you are and having clarity on where you want to go, along with clear steps to take to get there, is a journey to self- ownership. When you decide what you want from deep inside of you, and you work hard through obstacles to achieve what you believe you want, you own it. No one can take it away from you. And that in itself is very powerful in fitness and in life.

G. Motivation: When you have ownership, that gives you motivation.

Motivation, derived from the word motive or a need that requires satisfaction, is a reason for actions, willingness, and goals. These needs, wants, or desires may be acquired either through the influence of culture, society, and lifestyle (outside forces, which are extrinsic motivations), or may be generally innate (intrinsic motivations). Considered one of the most important reasons to move forward, motivation results from the interaction of both conscious and unconscious factors. Mastering motivation to allow sustained and deliberate practice is central to high levels of achievement, in elite sports, medicine, music, or any practiced skill. Motivation governs choices among alternative forms of voluntary activity.

For sustainable motivation, one should tap into the motivation coming from a meaningful place inside of you, to understand what drives your need. This involves reflecting on what drives you to want what you want. This is found in the moments that you sit deep with yourself and try to connect to the inside instead of outside— not the exterior drivers, but what drives you to do something inside, that really connects you with yourself. That is the true motivation. That's what will really get you to complete a task or a goal without creating obstacles or dropping the tasks that will get you there.

For example, if you want to run because your neighbors are running, but you hate running and yet I give you a program for running, what is going to happen in 3 weeks? With the passage of time, it will become increasingly challenging to sustain the extrinsic motivation to keep training. It's easier to simply lose the drive to continue at the first sight of challenge.

In contrast, if you want to run because of a need or desire that you are deeply connected with, you are more likely to sustain your motivation to push through challenges and towards your goal. If your desire to run is meaningful to you so that, for example, you are fit and capable to run behind your child while they learn to ride a bicycle, this is a connected meaning that is much more likely to sustain your intrinsic motivation through the inevitable challenges ahead.

Deep meaning will sustain your drive. Everyone has this inside motivation; some people are aware of it and some people have to work hard to discover it.

H. Meditation.

Whereas the preceding paragraphs about mental fundamentals follow a sequence of preparation, the practice of meditation can occur any time throughout your mental preparedness. Meditation trains you to give oxygen to the mind and body and to calm your biopsycho operations. The distribution of oxygen to the body helps to settle down the mind's energy and to prepare for the upcoming physical task, by again reminding a person to enter the present, the now.

Meditation helps you to discover how you feel emotionally and where in your body any tension or irregularity is felt (e.g. neck, lower back). Then, wherever stress is most intense, put yourself in a relaxing position to take stress off that area; in this position there will be no gravity. Placing the back of your head on the floor and your body in a supine position, with knees bent, will change the entire dynamic of how you feel; this is what on a very basic level yoga attempts to accomplish, helping you to find balance and to remove stress. Furthermore, beyond breathing, visualizations and sounds can be added to attain meditative benefits. Visual imaging, which can increase psychological peace, helps anyone to feel better about the past and to prepare for the future: by seeing a joyful image, such as crossing the finish line of an upcoming race or being a future grandparent playing actively with grandchildren, we can set an optimistic tone in our psyche. Hearing actual tones or sound from music, a mantra, or from any external vibration, or even silence, goes through your body to promote circulation and energy flow in an attempt to synchronize with human brain waves to de-stress the body. This purity attained through visual and tonal receptivity is accomplished partially by allowing thoughts to come and go without consciously processing or directing them. In effect, relaxed breathing with visualization and sound will help the meditator to pacify the soul.

II. The Body

A. Breathing

If you don't breathe properly, your body won't function properly, because it needs to be fed with oxygen. The only thing that doesn't change throughout your life, from your birth to your death, breathing is a fundamental part of your existence; you can't have circulation, or life, without breathing first. The first thing to become irregular when people are stressed or feel any kind of emotion is their breath.

1. Breathing at Rest: Lying on your back with your knees bent, breathe through the nose, not through the mouth. Keep your shoulders relaxed, and place your hands on the belly. Take a couple of minutes to relax.
2. 2After a couple of minutes, ask yourself where you are feeling tension: in

the belly, chest, shoulders, neck? Creating awareness of where tension is felt, with gravity taken out of the equation, you will realize the source of why you're not breathing diaphragmatically. The diaphragm opens your lungs for performance and recovery. Now, take a deep breath through your nose with hands still on the belly, and feel your belly filling with air like a balloon. As a guiding inhale/exhale ratio with this breathing, inhale for one and exhale for three. When you exhale, the opposite of the inhale should happen: the balloon deflates. This basic ratio will change when the body performs different techniques, as in yoga or when exercising.

B. Set your goals for success.

What is a "smart goal"? A smart goal:
1. must have specific metrics, be measurable, for example a distance (run one mile?), a length in time (a one-mile run under nine minutes?), a number of pounds and repetitions (ten biceps curls with 30 pounds?)
2. is attainable or achievable. Can you realistically accomplish this goal, and do you have the skill needed?
3. is guided by a time frame: have you set a date for when you want to achieve this goal? Because you will start modestly, will that allow you enough time to achieve it?
4. is informed by relevance and realism:
   a) is the goal worthwhile?
   b) is this the right time to achieve this goal?
   c) are you honest with yourself that you're capable both mentally and physically to achieve this goal?
   d) test yourself first to know if the goal is realistic, and be certain that you're prepared to work within the deadline you've set

C. Set-up and needed tools
Set-up refers to your biopsychosocial preparedness for your bodily goals, which includes all factors to guarantee your workout's success: proper sleep and nutrition; hydration before and water during the workout; guaranteed privacy or separation, without needless interruptions from environmental demands of work, family, and other external responsibilities. Have at hand whatever equipment you will need, such as mat, weights, bars.

D. Acceptance of challenges, where synergy must enter

Self-awareness of capabilities is essential. You must be able to accept your limitations and challenges. If needed, look for easier versions and readjust your goals. Focus on what you can do, not on what you can't. Remember that you are competing against yourself, not against others. Keep in mind your goals for success.

E. Practice/practice/practice;

With A through D formulated, you now are prepared to teach your body to achieve success with your goals. Improvement of all skills requires practice, whether it's playing piano, writing essays, or shooting or dribbling a basketball. With practice you develop your skill sets.

F. Self-reward

Throughout the process of attaining your goals, be sure to acknowledge your accomplishments and to pat yourself on the back. From a successful workout comes an elevated mood, so congratulate yourself that you are one step closer to your goals. Self-reward includes giving yourself a break from your routine: take off the weekend, enjoy a good walk, see a movie, get a massage. Literally bring the synergy of your biopsycho accomplishment to the social context, so that your feeling of wellness becp,es biopsychosocial.

Total ownership of the product your process has led to is the purpose of setting goals. With that comes a sense of completion and fulfillment.

III. Synergy

We can refer the blending or merging of energy between the mind and the body as synergy; it's an interaction that becomes a unity or union, a harmony or alliance. In effect, synergy is an efficiency resulting from trial and error which leads to a co-ordinated balance of expended energy while still being in the moment and able to adapt to different needs.

One of the goals of synergy is energy efficiency, which simply means using less energy to perform the same task – that is, eliminating energy waste. Energy efficiency brings a variety of benefits: reducing greenhouse gas emissions, reducing demand for energy imports, and lowering our costs on a household and economy-wide level. On a personal level, energy efficiency also can be attained, through a person's developed implementation of synergy.

A useful analysis of synergic blending within my mind and body occurred when at 51 years old I competed in the 2020 New York City Marathon. My mental and bodily training of course included all the fundamentals discussed here. Because synergy is a developmental process, its product during the marathon was how well I handled the marathon competitively. It's important to know that I had trained to compete not against other runners but against a time-goal I'd set: below four hours. My motivation therefore was a personal goal, and my preparatory fundamentals were conditioned by that.

Despite whatever goals or necessities you may have trained for, the competitive moment requires a dialogue between your mind and body from beginning to end, a synergy changing itself as changes occur. Two times while running the marathon I was challenged by a bodily/mental imbalance or lack of coordination. First was when, between miles 18 and 20, I became physically challenged due to the dead silence on the bridge from the Bronx to Manhattan, a span with no people, no distractions, and a lack of external energy literally encouraging me, only the sound of feet pounding; that was when mental energy needed to become a restorative influence. As I felt my body slowing, legs heavier, with awareness of my breathing, questions at that moment began to fill my mind about my body's abilities, and I wondered if I should quit or maybe just slow down. Then, my synergic training brought focus into the moment, setting one coordinated mental/physical goal: to get off the bridge and out of that area. And suddenly the focus on my lethargic legs and butt was removed, refocusing instead to look for the next crowd to provide me with further energy. Back to life again and aware that I was 3/4 done with the race and back in Manhattan with crowds, I knew I was going to make it. And, with that, I returned to a focus on my finishing time.

Another moment of challenge came at mile 22, when I couldn't get my body to accelerate. So, I dialogued with myself, forgot about my body, shifted the focus away from speed and started looking at people, using them as a series of targets to reach, one person after another, until the finish line. Unlike many people who "hit the wall" and stop at this point in the race—four miles to go—I was able to shift mentally, make a quick decision in the moment, and set a new goal that was attainable.

Running the NY City Marathon was an amazing learning experience! Not only about running, it also was about what you have in your core. You have run all the strength, all the superficial fitness out of yourself, and it really comes down to what's left inside you. The POWER OF THE MIND! To be able to draw deep and pull something out of yourself is one of the most tremendous things that I feel today about my experience running the NY City Marathon!

IV. Spiritual and Emotional = Social:

When working to attain biopsychosocial wellness, there's a third fundamental additional to preparedness of the body(bio) and the mind (psycho): spiritual and emotional aspects of our being (social).

A. The Spirit fundamental

Like the word wellness, spirit is fraught with multiple meanings. Wherever the sources of its meanings stem from—religion, philosophy, psychology, physics, neuroscience—we know that spirit seeks purpose and worth in our own life and in how we live it. Our spirit must partner wisely with peaceful acceptance and respect for what exists beyond our self: family, trusted friends, and the duties required by them: unconditional love, guidance, and support, whether through religious instruction or through ethical codes of behavior. Supporting one's family is attained through a person's or a couple's work, through professional income, which can create stress. Further stress can arise from inescapable social and cultural realities surrounding us, especially those found in broadcast media and in printed news, which reproduce politics and economics and add to our stress.

How we receive, interpret, and manage natural and manmade forces depends on our spirit. To know our spirit requires not only inspecting our world view, our values, and goals, but also peacefully learning to modify or eliminate our needless intolerances. Important to spiritual wellness is feeling true to oneself while being gentle with all that is not oneself.

B. The Emotional fundamental

All humans have feelings and emote. Awareness and acceptance of one's feelings is the first step toward emotional wellness; with that, we learn to see realistically our

46

emotional limitations, emotionally charged behaviors, and emotional memories. This learning provides insights into how to manage our feelings and their related behaviors, and ultimately how to take responsibility for our actions. Through our self-awareness, we develop our ability to cope, to be self-reliant, and to generate positivity and enthusiasm about self and life. We face challenges, take risks, and recognize conflict as potentially advantageous. All of this leads to maintaining satisfying relationships with other people and to establishing social commitment, trust, and respect.

Emotional wellness helps us to live and work productively and to realize the importance of seeking and valuing the support and assistance of others. We are more likely to see life as an exciting, hopeful adventure, not as a fearful, bothersome, anxiety-producing struggle when our emotional being is in balance.

Possibly you've noticed while reading this chapter that so many of the different biopsychosocial fundamentals I've discussed interconnect and overlap with one another, creating new synergies which, if properly balanced, can respond to new demands and serve our immediate needs. This is natural, because we humans are multifaceted beings, complicated organisms whose functioning is itself interconnected and overlapping.

With the fundamentals introduced and explained in this chapter, I've shared with you all that's needed to start on your path to biopsychosocial wellness, managing properly and efficiently the body, mind, and surrounding influences in life. In sum, it all can be boiled down to these three key elements of biopsychosocial health:

1. Mental conditioning, the process of training your mind to modify your thoughts, attitudes, and beliefs to accept new thinking patterns, tendencies, and/or mental states in order to optimize positive thinking and ultimately optimize your performance.
2. The body, a complex mechanism and organism, needs multiple factors to interact among each other for us to complete a task or a goal; this includes breathing, exercising, sleep, nutrition, hydration, and a synergistic relationship between the energies of the body and mind.
3. Spiritual wellness, from which we derive meaning and purpose, is a feeling of being true to oneself while being gentle with all that is not oneself.

As you journey through the remaining chapters of this book, my colleagues will talk more and in greater detail about the aspects or theories that interact in the different ways I've described. It all falls under this master umbrella of biopsychosocial wellness. I wish for you that this chapter has given you some understanding and clarity of how we human beings function and that it brings you an awareness and knowledge about yourself—about the fundamentals of your mind, body, and spirit, which make up your biopsychosocial health as you seek to approach longevity and a better quality of life.

CHAPTER III

Changing Bad Habits for Good

Along with knowing the fundamentals of biopsychosocial wellness before dedicating yourself to a more healthful life, you should know conceptually and strategically how to break bad habits and, with behavior modification, to create good ones. Within psychology, "habitual behaviors are defined as actions triggered automatically when people encounter situations in which they have consistently done them in the past. Repeating behavior in the same context reinforces mental associations between the context and behavior." Prompted by environmental settings and their specific stimuli, we become conditioned to respond in habitual ways:

> Habit is said to have formed when exposure to the context non-consciously activates the association, which in turn elicits an urge to act, influencing behavior with minimal conscious forethought. As an initially goal-directed behavior becomes habitual, control over behavior is transferred from a reasoned, reflective processing system, which elicits behavior relatively slowly based on conscious motivation, to an impulsive system, which elicits behavior rapidly and efficiently, based on learned context-behavior associations. Habitual behaviors thus become detached from conscious motivational processes (Gardner, 1).

Habitual behaviors detached from conscious motivational processes aren't necessarily detrimental or negative; in numerous contexts all of us have created and can continue to create conditioned behaviors benefiting our own and other people's life through positive reinforcement that becomes instinctual. The focus here, however, is to help you change whatever negative behaviors you have that may prohibit or be injurious to your biopsychosocial wellness.

Behavior modification and habit change mean, first, that obviously you've concluded there's some compulsion or urge, pattern or practice in your life you need to change for some reason, whether it's to do whatever your doctors advise you to do, to make your partner and kids happier, or to make yourself satisfied and peaceful about who, what, and where you are physically, psychologically, socially, and economically. Bad habits and limiting behaviors can be caused by innate human defiance, the need for social acceptance, the inability to truly understand the nature of risk, an individualistic view of the world and consequent rationalization of unhealthful habits, and a genetic predisposition to addiction (Bryner). Buried into your behavior, these causes of bad habits are triggered or cued principally either by stress or by boredom, but sources of stress and boredom are broadly various as influences, and the bad habits caused by them can be diverse. Willpower certainly will aid your determination to break bad habits, but there's no need to rely on it exclusively, just as there's no need to feel shame because of bad habits.

The first necessity for breaking bad habits and changing to beneficial new ones is to realize that everyone in the world, different by nature and nurture, has bad habits and behaviors warranting improvement or change; therefore, because nobody's perfect, you aren't alone if you want to make changes to improve. Possibly, the difficulty to make changes has intensified because we live in an increasingly non-contemplative age of immediate gratification in which many people have very high and unrealistic expectations of theories and practices about habit change and consequently aren't willing to take the time to learn more about them and to test them. In some cases, many of us don't even truly understand what our own desired outcome should be for behavioral change and eliminating bad habits.

Breaking bad habits and changing to beneficial new ones also requires a second necessity, that you accept medical science's repeatedly proven finding observed here by Dr. Mark Hyman: your zip code is more of a determining factor of your health than your genetic code. "The story of your health is much more complex than genetic programming," Hyman writes. "It is ultimately determined by the dynamic interplay of the environment washing over genes creating the 'you' of this moment." Many of us have assumed that inheriting strong, favorable genetics allows us to get away with or withstand bad habits and behaviors which, although potentially injurious to other people, aren't likely to affect us negatively. Bury and forget that belief! Hyman informs us that the October 2010 issue of Science magazine "published an important paper that reviewed the notion of the 'exposome'—the idea that the environment in which your genes live is more important than your genes themselves. What this suggests is that applying genomics to treat disease is misguided because 70-90 percent of your disease risk is related to your environment exposures and the resultant alterations in molecules that wash over your genes" (Hyman). Please read that last sentence again, as it's an underlying presupposition helping to convince you of the importance of habit change. Exposomes come from what we eat, what we're conditioned to think, how we feel, environmental toxins, the microbiome (the collective genomes of the microbes—composed of bacteria, bacteriophage, fungi, protozoa, and viruses—that live inside and on the human body), and our stress levels, exercise, and sleep. Bathed daily in these exposomes, your genome is the recipient of a host of unhealthful, even harmful influences—if you allow it to be.

Obviously implied by this scientific reality is that you, yourself, can alter "the resultant alterations in molecules that wash over [your] genes" by changing your behaviors and habits, especially those that are damaging or "bad." Unlike the warning which you're given on a pack of cigarettes, far too many exposomes negatively impacting our lives don't offer warnings or even a hint of their detrimental influences. On many levels, therefore, behavior modification and habit change require additional awareness and new recognitions that you must discover and own. In this chapter I'll give insights guiding you to help yourself understand the values and priorities underlying your behavior; those insights will enable you to create a strategic approach to setting proper behaviors and habits that allow you to reap the benefits of living a full, biopsychosocially healthful life.

One of my favorite scientific processes with which to modify bad behavioral habits and to change to good ones is The Transtheoretical Model (TTM) or Stages of Change Model. Proposed in the late 1970s, TTM was developed through studies examining differences between the experiences of smokers who quit on their own and those of smokers requiring further treatment. These studies determined that people quit smoking only if they were ready to do so. Thus, TTM focuses on the decision-making of the individual and is a model of intentional change, operating on the assumption that people do not change behaviors quickly and decisively. Rather, change in behavior, especially habitual behavior, occurs continually through a cyclical process. Because "The TTM is not a theory but a model," we should remember that "different behavioral theories and constructs can be applied to various stages of the model where they may be most effective" (The Transtheoretical Model).

The TTM posits that individuals move through six stages in their process of change, each as important as the others; however, I personally would say that the second stage, Contemplation, or the beginning of conscious involvement in habit change, is the most important and probably most difficult. Contemplation is where, in order to get started with habit changes we desire, we need to identify our values and priorities and to recognize the internal voices guiding and persuading us toward our habitual behaviors.

51

The first stage, **Precontemplation (Not Ready)**, represents people who aren't intending to take any action and/or aren't even aware that they need to make a change because they don't realize that their behavior is problematic to them and, possibly, to others. Although identified as "a stage" in the model, this isn't actually a stage or step in change so much as an indicator of what exists before change begins. The second stage, **Contemplation (Getting Ready)**, represents people who become aware that their behavior in fact is problematic and begin to explore, understand, and discuss pros and cons of their problematic habits and to investigate the values and priorities that inform those habits. At the third stage, **Preparation (Ready)**, people are biopsychosocially prepared to begin their change within the next 30 days and, when they begin, to take small steps towards their goal(s), all along believing that change will improve their lives. During the fourth stage, **Action,** people intend to keep moving forward by modifying their problem behaviors or acquiring more healthful new ones. With the fifth stage, **Maintenance**, people have sustained their behavior change for at least six months, guaranteeing there will be no relapse. And with the last, sixth stage, **Termination,** people know and feel that they have no desire to return to their bad habits and no worry about ever personalizing them again.

TTM identifies its model as cyclical because progress as we develop behavior and habit change often is momentarily interrupted or prohibited by biopsychosocial factors requiring us to retrace or reinforce previous steps that originally had moved us forward. To be used at any stage in the Change Model, TTM offers "cognitive, affective, and evaluative processes. . of change [which] have been identified . . . result[ing] in strategies that help people make and maintain change" (TTM).
I encourage you to think about each of these processes and, throughout your expedition toward change, to use any of them that best suit your needs and will promote your progress:

1. **Self-Liberation:** Your commitment to change behavior based on the belief that achievement of the healthful behavior is possible.
2. **Self-Reevaluation:** Realizing through self-reappraisal that the desired healthful behavior and habits are part of who you want to be.
3. **Dramatic Relief:** Involves emotional excitement and favorable stimulation about your current behavior and the psychological relief that can come from changing from Stage 1 Precontemplation to Stage 2 Contemplation.
4. **Consciousness Raising:** Increasing your intellectual awareness about

the wellness behaviors you want to incorporate into your life to replace your bad habits.

5. **Environmental Reevaluation:** Social reappraisal to realize how your bad behavior and habits can or do affect other people.

6. **Stimulus Control:** Re-engineering the environment to have reminders and cues that support and encourage the healthful behavior and remove those that encourage the unhealthful behavior.

7. **Social Liberation:** Making attempts to decrease the prevalence of your former problem behavior in society. This can come through "counter-conditioning."

8. **Counter-Conditioning:** Substituting healthful behaviors and thoughts for unhealthful behaviors and thoughts, and possibly participating in environmental opportunities to support your improved behaviors, which in turn will empower you through new, changed behavior.

9. **Helping Relationships:** Finding supportive relationships that encourage the desired change.

10. **Reinforcement Management:** Rewarding the positive behavior and reducing the rewards that come from negative behavior.

Use these ten biopsychosocial processes whenever you return to the TTM to locate whatever stage requires attention to your immediate needs, and whenever you want to add to the self-helping strategies you learn as you continue through this chapter.

You can further develop your management and control of ***The Power of Habit: Why We Do What We Do in Life and Business*** by understanding Charles Duhigg's "The Habit Loop," which explains how bad habits have triggers or cues that provide short-lived rewards. Nicola MacPhail argues similarly and explains how this "habit loop" can condition our behavior. In a response to a particular cue, MacPhail writes, you behave in a certain way. When that behavior or response feels good, you respond that way again the next time you encounter that cue. The more you respond that way, the less you think about it—and the more likely you are to respond again and again in the same way. This 'habit loop' of cue or trigger, response, reward is present in everyone, and as adults we perform habit loops conditioned in childhood that have informed our behavior whether or not we're aware of them. Important to know is that scientific studies suggest you're much more likely to fall into a habitual loop due to negative emotions. In fact. those emotions often become the cues or triggers to the habit's responses themselves; for example, people complain that they eat more when they're bored or tired. Others drink alcohol more or smoke when they're stressed. People procrastinate—in itself a bad habit—because they feel no joy about the task they face. MacPhail concludes by noting that much of our behavior, and our ability or inability to execute it effectively, is the result of our physiological and emotional needs and impulses. And, unfortunately, the habits that are linked to emotional cues are the hardest to crack. However, by being aware of what those cues are, you can intervene by replacing your responses.

This awareness, emphasized by MacPhail and Duhigg, is the second stage of TTM, Contemplation, and, as I said earlier, probably is the most difficult yet important part of behavior modification and habit change. To help you to promote your own self-awareness, here are five introductory questions you should ask yourself, suggested by Pete Liebman in "What Causes Bad Habits—And What Can You Do About Them?" These questions are intended to be general leads that you can follow as you initiate your inquiries into your unhealthful behavioral habits. As always, be honest with yourself as you reflect on your habitual behaviors and examine their causes and effects:

I.   Where are you when you enact or do your bad habit? Your physical environment can cue bad behaviors, such as a bar and drinking, work and junk food, living room and television.

II.   Whom are you with—or are you alone—when the bad habit occurs? Examine your social environment, whom you're around, and, if any of the surrounding behaviors seem potentially contagious, consider if they've been likely to affect your own. For example, encouragement to "let loose" or "be free" is a contagious behavior; as a cue it also might trigger additional drinking, unnecessarily increased loudness, or "unwoke" physicality.

III.   How do you feel (physically, mentally, emotionally) when you enact your bad habit? When you're tired, which is a physical cue, possibly you crave ice cream. When you need to procrastinate, a mental cue, possibly you turn to social media online. When you're stressed, an emotional cue, possibly you smoke "to relax."

IV.   What typically has happened immediately before you enact your habit? Possibly you eat junk food because just before you've argued with your spouse or child or colleague at work. Possibly you explore social media whenever you want to avoid an immediate responsibility. Possibly you smoke or drink whenever you enter a social setting.

V. Are there particular days and times of day when your bad habits are likely to occur? (Liebman)

Although it may seem that habit change is as simple as proceeding systematically through programmed stages, I think you and I know that there always will be obstacles standing in the way of our behavior modification and habit change and preventing it from being easy—regardless of whatever kinds and degrees of success we've attained in the past. Remember: TT2's model is cyclical, allowing us to return to earlier stages whenever necessary because significant behavior modification seldom progresses forward in a straight line. I discovered this truth most instructively when taking Precision Nutrition's amazingly profitable PN2 Coaching Certification as part of my diverse fitness training; its valuable biopsychosocial lessons helped not just myself as a coach, but my clients alike with an understanding of what must go into habit change and what the underlying roadblocks obstructing that change may arise from. As self-advertised, Precision Nutrition "is the industry's first comprehensive program of its kind—and the only one built specifically for health and fitness coaches to add a rare 'deep health' skill to their toolkits." This "comprehensive program" addresses not only nutrition as its focal center, but "the science and practice of better sleep, effective recovery, and more resilience to stress . . . [by] unlocking hidden stressors" (ttps://www.precisionnutrition.com/).

Beyond its certification's academics, Precision Nutrition has a masterful way of helping one understand how to begin the process toward change, illustrating the compassion and empathy needed to keep you focused even when you fall off the game plan. Since each person's values and priorities may differ, there is no "one size fits all" approach that will work with habit change. Change requires lots of digging in and research to find out each person's relationship with what needs to change, and why it needs to change.

As you read further, keep in mind the important word "relationship," used in the preceding sentence. Let's consider, as an introductory example, your relationship to the television, which I choose because most people have and watch a TV. Each of us has specific ways we interact with or relate to our TV, some of us to get information through the news, some of us to connect with people, to gather a family, to share a ritual such as eating with friends while watching a movie or a show. These relationships to the TV are great ways to use it; however, life isn't one-dimensional and we know there are other sides to those "great ways," in this case maybe watching TV out of boredom, watching TV when you need company, watching TV when you're stressed, watching TV when you're angry or sad, watching watching watching. It's fair to ask why this is a problem. The answer is because this second method of using the TV is more of a distraction and isn't done for a genuinely beneficial purpose, thus taking awareness and resolution out of our control and turning off our minds, as if that avoidance of our boredom, loneliness, stress, anger or sadness would bring us tranquility and rest. On the contrary, this is one of the main reasons why today's society has so many health issues such as depression, anxiety, and obesity, to name only a few. In my experience, many of these health issues—and often they're triggered or cued by watching TV or other tech screens—can be resolved with awareness of and compassion for one's self. In the next few pages I intend to explain this, keeping in mind the important word I mentioned earlier: relationship.

While I was listening to Pastor Michael Todd and his friend Dr. Dharius Daniels discussing Relationship Goals, they said something profound: "Your greatest pleasure and greatest pain both come from the same place, Relationships." It struck me that although they were speaking about human relationships, this same principle applies to our personal relationships within ourselves and with everything around us, on a daily basis—in sum, our biopsychosocial relationships; those include our relationship with sleep, food, stress, vices, ourselves and how we view ourselves and, given how we view ourselves and our self-worth, very possibly our families, inner circle of friends, and work colleagues.

Comprehending the nature of our relationships leads us to better understand our values and priorities and, with that understanding, to modify any behaviors or change any habits that can damage us and others in our world. In one of his uncut videos, Pastor Michael Todd further states that you cannot have relationship goals if you do not have aim, and many times people do not have aim because they are looking at the wrong target. For biopsychosocial wellness or health, this theory can be applied similarly: you can't have wellness goals if you don't have the proper targets or markers that you're aiming at to change. With so many things that one can choose to focus on, what should today's society take aim towards? This is where the art of biopsychosocial wellness plus behavioral modification gets to apply its creativity, because each person not only has different values and priorities, but also has different susceptibilities and compensatory needs.

One of my favorite terms that I learned while studying PN2 was "allostatic load," which explained exactly what had been weighing on me personally for so many years, driving some of my bad decisions and habitual behaviors that I couldn't control—but needed to control—for self-improvement. Introduced by McEwen and Stellar in 1993, allostatic load is the cumulative burden of stress from life events, more specifically "the cost of chronic exposure to fluctuating or heightened neural and neuroendocrine responses resulting from repeated or chronic environmental challenges that an individual reacts to as being particularly stressful" (Karger). Your body naturally responds to these stressors in an attempt to regain homeostasis (stable bodily conditions), but when environmental challenges exceed an individual's ability to cope, then "allostatic overload" ensues. Unfortunately, you carry this allostatic overload with you into everything you do in life, and therefore it influences many—possibly too many—of your decisions. This is why I think behavior change is about relationship management, which is how we interact with every component in our lives. If you want to do well in life, you really need to do well in relationships.

In many instances the allostatic load comes from your relationships with immediate family, possibly even extended family. It also can be society-driven: very often we look at what our current societal "norms" are, use them as reliable measurements and guides, and contrast our situations against these "standards." Understandable but nonetheless injurious, these societal norms may cause stress because of our perceived economic situation or our dissatisfaction with our employment; less defensibly, we rely on those standards to set the expectations we have for all the relationships in our lives. The unfortunate part of looking at these societal norms is that many times the snapshots of a moment that we look at, admire, and choose as our measurements and even our goals have neither historical nor future value attached to them; intangible mirages of desirability, they become meaningless when we try to actualize them. Instead of focusing on societal norms, we should focus on what we consider as being our actual flaws and then reset our values and priorities. Because "Habit protects us from anything we don't have a set way of handling" (Alsadir, 1), revocation of a bad habit requires a bigger awareness of self! And if I possibly can get better at knowing and being me, then we all possibly can get better at knowing and being us! Imagine a world in which all or most of its people were able to manage their allostatic load and had no overload driving their compromising and socially divisive behaviors.

In his book *Wellness Counseling,* Paul F. Granello defines wellness as "prevention or lifestyle-habit change"; further. he believes that "the future of professional counseling (and all helping professions) is going to be strongly related to prevention and wellness" (vii). Initiating habit change at any time in your life, because it's self-helping, is a form of prevention as well. Applied to this idea of prevention, the "Highlights" section of the article "Pathways to well-being: Untangling the causal relationships among biopsychosocial variables" presents all six potential pathways among biological (B), psychological (P), and social (S) factors. All of these preventive relationships influence wellness and can potentially contribute to subjective well-being and to objective physical health outcomes—if we're aware enough to change our negative habits requiring alteration. In summary, the article explains that

> The influential pathways that lead to subjective well-being are S→P and B→P pathways, although these pathways can be impacted by psychological factors that differ among individuals. For objective health outcomes, the P→B and S→B pathways appear to be important, where the latter pathway is mediated by psychological factors. We additionally highlight the importance of systematically understanding subjective experience, which represents an epistemologically distinct domain, and describe how subjective experience can explain individual differences in causal pathways (Karunamuni).

Indisputably, overall health is an active state in which you must make constant efforts, in your environment, to achieve and maintain wellness and, logically, to prevent unwellness. You have a distinct group of biopsychosocial factors influencing your actions to attain overall health, and, frequently, certain kinds of habit-change are required before that total wellness can occur. What follows in three sections are 18 desirable targets for improved "relationships" decreasing your allostatic overload and leading to greater wellness. Grouped separately for your convenience, these three sections actually are inseparable, listing and exploring reciprocally reinforcing biopsychosocial behaviors and indicators. This list will help you further to recognize and to contemplate—Stage Two of The Transtheoretical Model—your values and priorities as actualized in your thinking and demonstrated through your behavior.

Bio[logical]

1. Health Biomarkers

Biomarkers are measurable substances in humans and any other organism whose presence indicates disease, infection, environmental exposure, or post-treatment medical status; not symptoms, these biomarkers can be found through blood tests, x-rays, and CAT scans, and they are our best medical means of risk prediction or post-operative recovery. As an obvious example, high LDL cholesterol is a biomarker of cardiovascular risk. Investigating your health biomarkers will help you to know whatever potentially may be standing in your way for attaining wellness. Although additional studies are warranted, one study's 2003 results of eight published, randomized trials "suggest that biological information conveying harm exposure, disease risk, or impaired physical functioning may increase motivation to change" (McClure). Since 2003, many additional studies have found that physical activity, healthful eating, and emotional well-being do in fact improve if patients receive feedback about their personal biomarkers.

Begin by asking yourself if you have a family history of any type of disease. Do you have any current symptoms of disease that you have been diagnosed with? Have you been prescribed any medication(s)? Do you suffer from any symptoms of your health issues? Do you suffer from any symptoms of your medication(s)?

2. Do You Listen to Your Body?

Are you aware that your body speaks and sends messages to you constantly? Did you know that your brain, in addition to receiving information from your five senses, receives information from the internal sense receptors located in muscles, joints, and internal organs? As any of your internally coordinated functions move away from balance and optimal function, your brain learns about it. It follows that these messages are feedback which, if listened to, can help you to determine if something's wrong with you and, if so, to identify the cause or source of that wrongness and, then, to restore balance. Restoration of your internal balances may need to come from habit change or modification of some of your behaviors.

The next three bio[logical] categories—Movement, Nutrition, and Sleep—are discussed at length later in this book; therefore, if you know you'll be needing to break any bad habits or to modify your behavior in the context of these three categories, then use whatever knowledge and self-awareness you gain here and apply it to the subsequent chapters.

3. Movement

Do you exercise at all and, if so, how frequently do you exercise? What kind(s) of exercise do you do? Are you mostly inclined to lead a sedentary life? Do you have any injuries or orthopedic conditions that impede your ability to exercise? Is exercise difficult because of heart disease risk factors such as obesity, high blood pressure, high blood cholesterol, and type 2 diabetes?

Whatever your situation and present level of activity, you can change it for improvement. Remember that Rome wasn't built in a day, and keep in mind the Chinese proverb that says, "A journey of a thousand miles begins with a single step." You may fear this first step because your goal for physical movement seems too remote, the distance to it impossible to attain. Yes, taken individually, each small step you take, were you to take it, may not seem all that significant; probably it isn't. Nonetheless, it's become part of a process leading to new levels of productivity. And when you add up each day's small step over time, cumulatively those steps can show discernible progress and lead to extraordinary results.

4. Nutrition

It's remarkable that people don't connect the dots between how they feel and the foods they eat. Because food affects every body, everybody needs to understand the ways that insufficient nutrition can keep them down, hold them back, and limit their abilities to thrive and succeed as individuals or as a society.

To move forward toward better nutritional habits, first develop your self-awareness by noting the foods and liquids you eat and drink, when you eat and drink them, the frequency with .which you eat and drink in a given day, especially if snacking is involved, the quantity of food you eat at each meal, and an understanding of the quality of food you eat at each meal and over the course of the day. See the Big Picture of your food and liquid intake. Certainly it may help to consult a nutritionist to learn the qualities and acceptable quantities of your intake, but you eas
ily can find nutritional values online if you want to begin on your own.
Next, discover if you're aware of your hunger cues. Are those cues natural and biological, thus true cues, such as your stomach growling, or low energy, shakiness, headaches, and problems focusing? Or, conversely, is your hunger cued or triggered by psychological and/or social factors? Listen or sensitize yourself to these signals, so that in the future you'll recognize them for what they are and help you to decide if you're really hungry.

Last, are you aware of your satiety cues? Have you eaten slowly enough to allow your body time to let you know it's full? Even if you know you're full, do you continue to eat more because there's more on your plate? Is it possible that long-term stress, which floods your body with cortisol, a hormone that makes you want to eat more, is an ongoing state for you? If you're constantly fatigued, the likelihood of your eating more than you need also is hormonally triggered: your levels of ghrelin, a hormone that makes you want to eat, go up, while your levels of leptin, a hormone that decreases hunger and the desire to eat, go down, the result being that you feel hungry even if your body doesn't need food. Is it possible that when you feel nervous or anxious you're inclined to eat more? Do you experience peer pressure or less obvious social influencing to cause you to be excessive with drink or food during social gatherings? Have you ever experienced yourself eating simply because the food is there and easy to grab from your refrigerator or pantry? (Mikstas).

5. Sleep

As with all the other biological factors discussed here, begin by surveying your sleeping habits and your relationship with them. How many hours of sleep do you get per night? How many hours of sleep do you get per week, if for example weekday nights provide less sleep, weekend nights more? How would you rate your sleep (Very Poor to Excellent) on a scale of 1-10)? Are you a light or heavy sleeper? Are you affected by Sleep Apnea? Is your sleep disrupted frequently or infrequently? What causes the disrupted sleep?

Psycho[logical]

1. Perfectionism:

Although the pursuit of excellence can be an admirable, healthful habit (it's always important to do your best when trying to achieve an important goal), keep in mind that habitual pursuits of perfection can become negative if you set standards beyond your reach, which means they're not "smart goals." Unhealthful perfectionism exists if you're dissatisfied with anything less than perfection, preoccupied with failure or disapproval, and habitually see mistakes as evidence of unworthiness. Additionally, when your perfectionism turns negative, it can escalate your anxiety and stress, and can tear down your healthful boundaries. When you're focused solely on being perfect with no boundaries on how to get there, it's easy to get lost. Many behaviorists advise practicing mindfulness to steer your perfectionism to the positive side; mindfulness ironically isn't a clear concept, however, so let's just say that ruminating darkly about your own worth, skills, or prospects won't influence or change an inherently irrational voice; therefore, work to recognize your inner critic as nothing more than an entrenched bad mental habit, and shift your relationship with it. Create some distance from your inner voice of negative judgment.

2. Regret:

A possible consequence of perfectionism is the bad habit of regret, which, with daily practice, can turn into lifelong rumination—dark contemplation—over what might have been. Some people are woulda-coulda-shoulda regretfuls, whose habitual practice can lead to depression, anxiety, sleep problems, and difficulty concentrating. Creating those slowdowns, regret sometimes can inhibit forward movement and can even negatively affect physical health. The truth is that you can't go back in time and that you didn't do, in fact, what you woulda-coulda-shoulda done. So be it. Even if your decisions cause you pain and discomfort, they're only temporary. Don't cry over spilled milk.

I advise that you not think in absolutes: to believe that you have or had to make the right decision and that anything else is unacceptble is almost certainly setting yourself up for failure and unnecessary pressure. However, if you assess your decisions with the knowledge that you make thousands of choices each day and that human limitations prohibit you from getting them all right, then you're more likely to make a decision knowing that you can endure the consequences. Change your habit of regret from the rigidity of right and wrong, of perfect and horrible, to a flexibility that allows you greater peace somewhere between those binary opposites. You're just not going to be 100% satisfied after every decision in life, although regretfulness often makes you react as if you expect yourself to be. Know that there always will be "what ifs" and that sometimes—dare we admit it—we just don't have all the answers. Accept that you're fallible. Making a bad decision doesn't make you a bad or incompetent person; you're still the same person. So take a breath, and remember that harping regretfully on a bad decision can lead only to a bad case of the coulda-woulda-shouldas.

3. Guilt:

Guilt has a proper function in society, because recognizing causes for feeling remorseful about a wrongdoing usually prevents a person from committing that offense again. The habit of guilt often starts in childhood, when you learned to act a certain way out of fear that your family wouldn't be proud of you or that you'd be punished for "bad behavior"; as you grew older, the emotional grip of guilt may have matured too, because, as a person's ego forms in adaptation to the external world, the many "thou shalt nots" whose restrictions we impose on ourselves to be admired and accepted can bring embarrassment and shame if we find ourselves not abiding by them. Rational self-awareness helps to mediate this tension, but many people subconsciously allow guilt to well up within them and, as life develops and you age, bad habits of guilt can develop; these include the distorted magnification of problems, which in turn causes guilt; your claimed responsibility for creating or resolving problems that had little or nothing to do with you; your perceiving yourself as a bad person for committing minor offenses; and your refusing to forgive yourself.

Rational self-intervention can help you to avoid those negative kinds of excessive guilt by balancing ego with guilt, and by understanding behavioral limits that provide well-being—in effect, by processing guilt in a way that's actually productive. Because guilt comes up when there's a tension between your actions and expectations, you can examine your guilt honestly and change those expectations or change your behavior. You may feel guilty about leaving your family to go to work, for example, and then feel guilty about leaving your job to go home to your family. Left unchecked, you may find yourself in a state of perpetual guilt that prevents you from giving your full attention to any one task.

4. Failure Mindset:
Self-doubt and negative thoughts can discourage you from setting smart goals, diminish the value of your natural talents, and magnify your missteps. To minimize your self-doubt, create a list of your skills, talents, and achievements, reading the list regularly to remind yourself of both your potential value and achieved worth and, when you hear the self-doubting voices in your head that say you cannot succeed, that you have no choice, and that you should back out before the world discovers you're a fraud, remind yourself of all the reasons you're "good enough." Another way of understanding the failure mindset is if habitually you put yourself down. It's impossible to perform well when you're telling yourself, "You're stupid" or "You can't ever do anything right." Negative self-talk will discourage you from putting in your best effort, and it will drag you down fast. Stop the put-downs: talk to yourself like a trusted friend, and be compassionate. If you wouldn't use such harsh words with someone else, don't allow your inner critic to say them to you.

5. Making Excuses:
Blaming other people or external circumstances for your lack of achievement harms your performance. Saying things like "My boss is holding me back," "All this paperwork makes it impossible to do my job "Society sees me as being too

old," "Not enough time exists for me to do this," or "I'm not getting support from my spouse and friends" will only keep you stuck. Stop making excuses: focus on all the things you can do rather than on what you think you can't because of external circumstances. When you pay attention to the positive, you'll put more effort into your performance.

6. Catastrophizing the Future:

Negative predictions about your personal and professional future easily can turn into self-fulfilling prophecies. If, when going to the gym, you presume you'll be inefficient, relatively weak, and won't last long, then it's very possible that you'll become distracted by that negativity, whose energy—all thinking is energy—will indeed help to mess up your performance at the gym. If you have to give a speech at the PTA and believe that you're going to forget parts of it, then in fact you've increased the likelihood that you will. Break the habit of catastrophizing. Predicting disastrous outcomes will cause a spike in anxiety that could cause you to choke.

Psycho↔Social:

Most of the habits discussed previously, under Psycho, may not affect anyone but yourself, although certainly their impact can reach beyond you. It's likely that you'll privatize your self-help in modifying or changing those habits because you don't want them to affect anyone else's life and don't feel that they should be shared. In this psycho↔social section, however, you'll learn that some psychological habits inevitably spill out into social situations and that their damage can impact more than just yourself.

Four Horsemen of Relationships

All of us need to be aware of and to sensitize ourselves to the "Four Horsemen of Relationships" when we interact with other people. Taking a toll on whoever is involved, both the giver and receiver, the Four Horsemen are

• criticism
• contempt
• defensiveness
• stonewalling (giving or receiving the "cold shoulder").

While such habits may not seem detrimentally large-scale, they nevertheless can affect our and others' mental health and, taken to extremes, can even be classified as forms of emotional abuse (Lisitsa). Although modifying these bad habits may seem common-sensical, "Being able to identify the Four Horsemen in your conflict discussions is a necessary first step to eliminating them and replacing them with healthy, productive communication patterns" (Lisitsa). Again, important yet difficult to achieve, this identification, elimination, and replacement of these bad habits is what the second stage of TTM (the Transtheoretical Model) is about. Self-awareness is critically important if we are to effect change for self-improvement.

First, then, be honest: can you become critical, contemptuous, defensive, or a stonewaller in social or professional situations? After you've recognized that you have (≠ you are guilty of) any of these tendencies, begin to examine the contexts in which they're likely to occur. I, for example, still can be and in the past definitely was both critical and defensive, so I've taught myself to recognize the cues or triggers that condition/ed my habitual critical and defensive responses. Now, when the cues occur, immediately I think of how to reformulate—replace—those two habitual reactions; over time, I've created better conversational habits.

If you're likely to parade any of the Horsemen, don't let them trample other people.

Social

1. Stress Levels

Stress is a vast category, broad and deep, and it looms large whenever health professionals speak of wellness because its omnipresent influences of differing kinds and degrees do in fact impact on sensitive humans throughout each day, at every turn. The most major causes of stress include the death of a loved one, divorce, moving your residence, major illness, job loss, and economic insecurity, but stress in its steady streams can be caused by work, relationships, finances, health, and media overload. The Mayo Clinic tells us that "stress symptoms can affect your body, your thoughts and feelings, and your behavior. Being able to recognize common stress symptoms can help you manage them. Stress that's left unchecked can contribute to many health problems, such as high blood pressure, heart disease, obesity and diabetes" ("Stress Management").

True for all biopsychosocial factors pertaining to wellness, stress first must be recognized: you need to be aware of whatever and however stress affects you. Simple questioning can help:How stressed do you feel? What do you think causes your stress? When are you most stressed, and does knowing this help you to determine the cause? How do you deal with your stress? Keep in mind that all of us experience and process stress differently because all of us are different. Some people are worry-warts and drive themselves into stressed irrationality over mundane realities or possibilities. People obsessive about time may feel an inordinate amount of stress if held immobile in a traffic jam, or if late to a lunch with a friend. People determined to control their lives may become stressed when anything or anyone impedes that need for control. Related to that need for control, stress can come with uncertainty; all of us on planet Earth have felt stress because of Covid's unpredictability. Some people internalize large amounts of stress by watching the world's infuriating and gloomy news, or ruminating on dark subject matter. The yapping dog next door may cause you stress, or the honking horns and jackhammers on the street outside, or the way someone looked at you on the sidewalk.

Self-helping cures for stress can come in many forms, all of which involve activity: exercise; relaxation techniques, such as meditation, yoga and deep breathing exercises, tai chi or massage; keeping and exercising your sense of humor; being around non-toxic family members and friends in enjoyable social situations; reading, listening to music, and engaging in hobbies, all of which remove you from self-focused tensions.

2. Overuse of Social Media

According to The Pew Research Center in a late 2018 article, "69% of adults and 81% of teens in the U.S. use social media [undoubtedly those percentages have increased since Covid]. This puts a large amount of the population at an increased risk of feeling anxious, depressed, or ill over their social media use," a conclusion corroborated by "a recent survey of 1500 adult Facebook and Twitter users in which 62 percent of participants reported feelings of inadequacy and 60 percent reported jealousy from comparing themselves to other social media users. Thirty percent said using just these two forms of social media made them feel lonely" (Sawarkar). And a recent, 2021 study published in Psychiatric News further links the use of multiple social media platforms with an increased risk for depression and anxiety. Before you know it, with this kind of social media existence, you're second-guessing decisions you make, values you hold, and the validity of your goals because you keep comparing yourself to someone else's success; further, you subject yourself to needless emotional hurt and potential psychological damage. One possible mechanism accounting for this depression and anxiety "is that people who use many different platforms end up multitasking, such as frequently switching between applications or engaging in social media on multiple devices. Studies have found that multitasking is related to poorer attention, cognition, and mood. Other potential problems of using multiple platforms include an increased risk of anxiety in trying to keep up with the rules and culture associated with each one and more opportunity to commit a gaffe or faux pas since attention is divided" (Zagorski). But whatever factors work as causes for the conclusion that overuse of social media is a bad habit, the effects themselves confirm it. We can understand these negative effects elementally by using the psychological presupposition that most social media follows the Greater Internet Fuckwad Theory, proposed in 2004 by Mike Krahulik and Jerry Holkins, which says that when a normal person "is allowed anonymity and an audience, they lose social inhibitions and act inappropriately." In other words, "people become trolls on the internet because there is someone to pay attention, but no one to shame them" (Quora). What therefore can and does run rampant on social media are shaming, cyberbullying, and mental harassment and aggression.

3. Overuse of a Smartphone

An absence of good news in notifications, a steady stream of distressing news coverage, and fighting on social media can amplify negative effects of smartphone overuse.Bad smartphone habits include constant checking to see if you've been contacted; reading or texting while you're walking or driving; consequent inattentiveness to your surroundings, including its natural beauty and architectural magnificence; relying on your phone's GPS, which limits your own navigational abilities, spatial sensitivities, and sometimes common sense; substituting calls or texts for interpersonal human contact; even using your phone in public restrooms, as has been true the multiple times that I've seen and heard men speaking on their cells at office and gym urinals. And speaking of urinals: did you know that phone screen surfaces are dirtier than toilet seats? Yes, our smart phones now seem indispensable to our normal daily coursing of affairs and management of life's many duties. Nevertheless, it may be time for a digital detox, a modified removal of yourself from your relationship with our cell.

~~~~~~~~

All of us are creatures of habit, some of those habits biologically natural and unvarying. Our autonomic nervous system, for example, controls the function of our organs and glands, as well as our reflexes; it confers with our Circadian rhythm and winds our biological clock, which beats and ticks habitually, as does our heart. We sweat to control body temperature. Babies suck their thumb once no nipple is available.   In countless ways, we humans are hardwired to exist with certain kinds of autonomic habits, a bodily truth. Psychological hardwiring, however, is another story. Nigel Nicholson tells us that recent convergent theories from research and discoveries in genetics, neuropsychology, and paleobiology have been brought to light by the new field of evolutionary psychology, which posits that

> although human beings today inhabit a thoroughly modern world of space exploration and virtual realities, they do so with the ingrained mentality of Stone Age hunter-gatherers. Homo sapiens emerged on the Savannah Plain some 200,000 years ago, yet according to evolutionary psychology, people today still seek those traits that made survival possible then: an instinct to fight furiously when threatened, for instance, and a drive to trade information and share secrets. Human beings are, in other words, hardwired. You can take the person out of the Stone Age, evolutionary psychologists contend, but you can't take the Stone Age out of the person.

If you don't agree with the preceding quotation, then you're like many academics still involved in the ongoing nature/nurture debates concerning human behavior. And those who dispute the quotation will argue that so much of what we do with habit-breaking is an attempt to take the Stone Age out of our behavior, or at least to modify it.   That Stone Age "drive to trade information and share secrets," for example, may be what inclines many people to be gossipy; however, social ethics inclines many of those many to work to break or modify that habit.

Setting aside whatever innate drives may or may not exist in human nature—and I encourage you to set them aside, as you can go in endless circles about the essential nature of human nature—we in fact also live according to humanly manufactured routines that breed habits. The impositions of time and its schedules regiment much of our daily movement and impose regularities upon us. We behave with high levels of repeated activity within similar contexts, as putting our mobile phone onto charge when coming home from work and mixing a drink or pouring a glass of wine.   We live in standardized sequences or routines commanded by logic, such as brushing our teeth after we eat.   Some of us rely on specific steps of a certain "proper" order, first this, then that, always the same, such as habitually putting on your socks before your pants, or vice versa. Some of us eat the same foods bought at the same stores, typically sit in the same seat at the dinner table, use the same barber or hair stylist, follow the same ole, same ole. Some of us won't step on sidewalk cracks or walk under a ladder, superstitious habits.

We safely can conclude that internally and externally the clocks of our existence inform and regularize our lives, with habits whose developed frequency often supplants what we'd like to think is our freely willed behavior. The beauty of free will, however, is that its subversion can be reversed by itself, and indeed we can plan and think to eliminate bad habits by knowing what they are, becoming aware of how they affect our behavior, and working to modify the cues or triggers that have conditioned us to react or respond in detrimental habitual ways. To the extent that you have free agency in the directions of your life and the management of your behavioral inclinations, therefore, I encourage you to add as another fundamental of biopsychosocial wellness the elimination of what you know to be your worst habits inhibiting your best self.

WORKS CITED

Alsadir, Nuar. "Clown School," Granta, 31 October, 2017. https://granta.com/clown-school/

Bryner, Jeanna, "Bad Habits; Why We Can't Stop," January 11, 2008. Live Science. **https://www.livescience.com/1191-bad-habits-stop.html**

Duhigg, Charles, The Power of Habit: Why We Do What We Do in Life and Business. New York: Random House Trade Paperbacks, 2014.

Gardner, Benjamin and Amanda L. Rebar, Habit Formation and Behavior Change. King's College London: January 2019. **https://www.researchgate.net/publication/330406744_Habit_Formation_and_Behavior_Change**

Granello, Paul F. Wellness Counseling. Boston: Pearson Education Inc., 2013.

Karunamuni, Nandini, "Pathways to well-being: Untangling the causal relationships among biopsychosocial variables." Social Science & Medicine,10, February 2020.

Liebman, Pete, "What Causes Bad Habits?" *StrongerHabits.com*

Lisitsa, Ellie, "The Four Horsemen: Criticism, Contempt, Defensiveness, and Stonewalling." The Gottman Institute, April 23, 2013 **(https://www.google.com/search?q=%E2%80%9CThe+four+horse-men+of+relationships&ei=W3eqYZCJFuSbptQPtbqk8A4&ved=0ahUKEw-jQovfdtcj0AhXkjYkEHTUdCe4Q4dUDCA4&uact=5&oq=%E2%80%9CT-he+four+horsemen+of+relationships&gs_lcp=Cgdnd3Mtd2l6EAMy-BQgAEIAEMgYIABAWEB4yBggAEBYQHjIFCAAQhgM6BwgAEEc-QsAM6BQgAEJECOgUILhCABDoOCC4QgAQQsQMQxwEQowI6CA-gAEIAEELEDOgsILhCABBDHARCvATDNEpUTHQoQUJMHLrErG-JyHg89uy71MyuHABBCxAxCDATDNEpUTHQoQUJMHLrErGJy-Hg89uy71MyuHILhBDOgsILhDHARCvARCRAjoKCC4QxwEQow-IQQzoECAAQQzoICC4QsQMQkQI6BQguEJECOggIABAWEAoQH-koECEEYAFDJHliXcmCodGgBcAJ4AYABxgGIAd0akgEEMzYuNpgBA-KABAcgBCMMABAQ&sclient=gws-wiz)**

MacPhail, Nicola, "What Causes Bad Habits—And What You Can Do About Them"

McClure, Jennifer, "Are biomarkers useful treatment aids for promoting health behavior change? An empirical review." American Journal of Preventive Medicine, 2002 Apr;22(3):200-7.

Mikstas, Christine, "Why Do You Eat When You're Not Hungry?" NourishbyWebMD
https://www.webmd.com/diet/obesity/ss/slideshow-why-eat-when-not-hungry

Rosenthal, Samantha R. et al., "Negative Experiences on Facebook and Depressive Symptoms among Young Adults." *Jonson and Wales University: 2016*

Sawarkar, Ananya, "6 Things That Could Damage Your Mental Health." Psych2Go, July 23, 2021.

"Stress Management," Mayo Clinic.
https://www.mayoclinic.org/healthy-lifestyle/stress-management/in-depth/ stress-symptoms/art-20050987

Thrive Global
https://www.google.com/search?q=causes+of+bad+habits&ei=jVCmYf-HEArXmxgG89owAQ&ved=0ahUKEwixv_CUwMD0AhU1szEKHTz7Ax-YQ4dUDCA8&uact=5&oq=causes+of+bad+habits&gs_lcp=Cgdnd3Mt-d2l6EAMyBggAEAcQHjIGCAAQBxAeMgUIABCABDIGCAAQCBAe-MgUIABCGAzIFCAAQhgMyBQgAEIYDMgUIABCGAzIFCAAQhgM6B-wgAEEcQsAM6BAgAEA06CAgAEAgQDRAeOggIABAIEAcQHkoE-CEEYAFDHGVimOmD3SmgBcAJ4AYABTYgB2QSSAQIxMJgBAKA-BAcgBCMABAAQ&sclient=gws-wiz

Zagorski, Nick, "Using Many Social Media Platforms Linked With Depression, Anxiety Risk."   Psychiatric News, 17 January 2017 https://doi.org/10.1176/appi. pn.2017.1b16
https://drhyman.com/blog/2010/12/31/the-failure-of-decoding-the-human-genome-and-the-future-of-medicine
https://www.karger.com/Article/FullText/510696
https://www.precisionnutrition.com/
https://www.sciencedirect.com/search?qs=habit%20change%20and%20 biopsychosocial%20wellness

CHAPTER IV

Before Trauma Hits: Avoiding the Worst Habits

"Without commitment, you'll never start, but more importantly, without consistency, you'll never finish." - **Denzel Washington**

Me: Hi, I'm Rob. And I have bad habits, which allow me to make decisions which I regret at the end of the day or sometime in the future.

You: Hi, Rob

I invite you to examine the two top charts on my desk on any given day.

Patient A: a 75 year-old woman who had fallen while going from the bedroom to the bathroom. Her x-rays and CT scan reveal a hip and pelvis fracture, as well as bleeding in and around the brain. Her history reveals that she is on medications for osteoporosis, high cholesterol, high blood pressure, gout, arthritis, and "blood thinners" to prevent the blood clotting, which could cause a stroke.

Patient B: a 57 year-old male with an infection, cellulitis, in his lower leg. He has been diagnosed with Type 2 diabetes mellitus for over ten years, has a lifelong history of obesity, and takes medication by mouth for his diabetes.

Without my assigning blame or having a crystal ball, many of the conditions which cause us so much pain, stress, shame—and did I mention BILLIONS of dollars in medical costs and unproductive days—are somewhat self-inflicted. Let's look at the first chart a little further, which presents an older adult who fell, a very common occurrence. A fall from standing height which results in hip and pelvic fractures is commonly associated with the bone-loss disease osteoporosis, and muscle loss, known as sarcopenia. In 2019, 34,212 older adults aged 65 and older died from preventable falls, and over 3.1 million were treated in emergency departments. Over the past 10 years, the number of older adult fall deaths has increased 58%, while emergency department visits have increaed 34%. But, osteoporosis doesn't sneak up on you like a sniper. While it is true that bone loss is higher in women after menopause, in this patient menopause was likely twenty or more years ago. Was she monitoring her bone health? Did her New Year's Resolutions include strengthening her bones and muscles every year?

Muscle mass loss is an age-related condition and one of the physiologic changes involved in sarcopenia. Muscle mass loss has a cause-effect relationship with muscle strength. Loss of both muscle mass and strength increases with age and is a problem for the elderly since it can result in a poor quality of life and in physical disabilities. Muscle mass loss can be caused by various factors, including disease, decreased caloric intake, poor blood flow to the muscles, a decline in anabolic hormones, and an increase in pro-inflammatory chemicals. Weight loss is also associated with the development of muscle mass loss. In addition, studies have shown that aging is associated with a physiological loss of appetite that leads to weight loss. Loss of hormones, such as testosterone, DHEA, and growth hormone occurs with aging. People with diabetes mellitus have accelerated muscle loss. Stroke and hip fracture are highly prevalent among the elderly and usually rapidly lead to an increase in muscle loss. This appears to be due to disuse and inflammation, stroke, and/or denervation.

The prevalence of muscle mass loss is increasing and is expected to continue to rise in the years to come. 5-13% of people 65 years and older have low muscle mass; the percentage increases up to 50% in those over 80 years old. By the age of 80, an estimated 40% of the muscle mass present at age 20 is lost. Currently, sarcopenia affects more than 50 million people worldwide and is expected to affect 200 million individuals in the next 40 years.

Bone mass loss is a condition known as osteopenia. Osteopenia often progresses to osteoporosis, a condition characterized by the reduced bone mineral density and increased rate of bone loss. Bone mineral density decreases with age. Therefore, the probability of a person suffering from osteopenia or osteoporosis, and related skeletal fragility, increases with age. The causes leading to bone mass loss are multifactorial and similar to the causes of muscle mass loss. The most common cause of osteopenia is aging. Skeletal aging is known to progress faster in women than in men due to hormonal changes after menopause.

It is estimated that the number of adults over age 50 in the United States with low bone mass, including osteoporosis, is 64.4 million. By 2030, that number will further increase to 71.2 million. It is anticipated that the number of fractures will grow proportionally.

What can you do?
There are a number of strategies to prevent further bone and muscle loss. Muscle

can even be GAINED at every age tested so far under the correct supervision and coaching. But, such tests need to be done wisely, in consultation and collaboration with experienced medical professional(s) to prevent injury to bones, hypertensive and cardiac complications, and even death. All of these strategies begin with a comprehensive medical examination performed by a professional with experience and expertise; note that this might not be your regular primary care physician. Talk to your doctor or medical provider about your concerns so that you can be referred to an appropriate specialist and that your records can easily be transferred and discussed. Physicians who truly work with patients to reverse muscle loss and stop bone loss most often have completed a residency or fellowship in sports medicine, preventive medicine, physical rehabilitation, or women's health. A physical therapist or exercise physiologist should also have advanced certifications and experience in the prescription and supervision of exercise programs, specifically to reverse muscle loss and maintain bone strength. Prescriptions for restorative hormone therapy and bone loss agents may be considered based on the results and monitoring of blood tests.

Adequate nutrition, especially protein intake, is the cornerstone of reversing muscle loss and preventing bone loss. Reducing food intake in the older adult has consequences that could be important for muscle mass and strength. Reduction of energy intake corresponding to lower levels of energy consumption leads to weight loss and, ultimately, to muscle mass loss. Proteins provide the necessary energy source for muscle protein production.

Strength training using adequate and appropriate resistance has been shown to be effective to combat the loss of muscle mass. Regular weight-bearing and muscle-strengthening exercises can reduce the risk of falls and fractures. This type of exercise can increase the bone density as well as the strength by micro-architectural bone arrangement. A 6-month Tai Chi program was shown to be effective in decreasing the number of falls, the risk of falling, and the fear of falling, in addition to improving functional balance and physical performance in physically inactive persons aged 70 years or older.
Maybe our 75 year-old Patient A thought it was too late for her?

As the economy and society have changed over time, so have our habits. We are more sedentary. Less than 5% of adults participate in 30 minutes of physical activity each day, and only one in three adults receives the recommended amount of physical activity each week. Both of the patients above could have benefitted and could still benefit from an appropriately prescribed exercise program. In one study, people with Type 2 diabetes exercised for 175 minutes a week, limited their calories to 1,200 to 1,800 per day, and got weekly counseling and education on these lifestyle changes. Within a year, about 10% got off their diabetes medications or improved to the point where their blood sugar level was no longer in the diabetes range, and was instead classified as prediabetes. Results were best for those who lost the most weight or who started the program with less severe or newly diagnosed diabetes. Fifteen percent to 20% of these people were able to stop taking their diabetes medications.

Diabetes results in active years lost, earlier heart attacks, strokes, and dialysis. Our habits can prevent it and even reverse it in early stages.

Our habits, what we do every day, define us. To understand a poor food choice habit is not to just say, "I overeat," or "I eat too much sugar," or "I had pancakes at 2 a.m." One has to see there are psychological, emotional, societal, and other pressures at work in all of these habits, biopsychosocial influences impacting on wellness. Some people are "stress eaters"; that is their nature, their brain sending calming, relaxing signals only when it receives signals that the stomach is filling with food. What fills the stomach quicker: bacon, egg, and cheese on a bagel, or carrots? How did emotion play into that person's mind when they were shopping? What does the instant gratification of a pizza delivered at any time do to your brain's regulation and impulse control? These patients don't need a lecture on healthy eating; rather, stress eating is almost an unstoppable force.

I have read that a man named Isaac said that an object that is at rest will stay at rest unless a force acts upon it. Every personal trainer, physical therapist, and cardiologist will agree. Physical activity is almost as complicated as eating. There are psychological factors at play, such as the camaraderie of team-sports, especially when picked up at an early age, which can help a child fit in, develop relationships and a peer network of other "athletic" people to whom physical activity becomes second nature, and is enjoyable. The other side of the coin is the person who goes to a gym or facility and has to "work it out," where it is a task. They may be great at 100 different things, but none of them involve sweating for a half hour or more several times a week.

Brain Biology
There are a few select chemicals in the brain that are important to this discussion.

One is dopamine, known as the feel-good neurotransmitter—a chemical that ferries information between neurons. The brain releases it when we eat food that we crave or while we have sex, contributing to feelings of pleasure and satisfaction as part of the reward system. This important neurochemical boosts mood, motivation, and attention, and helps regulate movement, learning, and emotional responses. You may already be familiar with dopamine from the condition Parkinson's Disease, which is a profound loss of production of dopamine.

Much of our understanding of habits and brain chemistry, while still rudimentary, comes from observing how much dopamine is produced when a test subject does something. We know that dopamine is released when the light on your cellphone blinks or you feel/hear the vibration. Any parent of a current teenager can argue that there is a cell phone habituation/addiction, and every teen can probably argue that their parents are just as addicted.

Habits-Anonymous
Alcoholics Anonymous and organizations that have followed in its footsteps have saved countless lives by providing a support group and in some cases accountability for people. Did you know that there was no science or evidence in planning the "Twelve Steps"? There were 12 steps because there were 12 Apostles of Jesus Christ. Be that as it may, how many of us could use the support offered by a 12-step program to help develop better, healthier habits?

For many people it is the New Year's Resolution to lose that weight, get in shape, get to the gym, drop the bad habits. According to one non-scientific study, by January 12 a majority of the group reported they had broken their "resolution." Many of those resolutions regarding health have to do with trying to turn back the hands of time. We want to lose some weight we have gained over time so our knees, hips, and back don't feel so sore after a regular day that the thought of exercise makes us cringe. We want to still be attractive to our partners, or maybe we are looking forward for a new relationship.

How are our habits formed? First, you pair two things together, a stimulus (food) and a response (salivating). Stimulus (food) results in Response (salivating). Then you add an additional stimulus: Stimulus 1 (food) + Stimulus 2 (bell) results in Response (salivating). Over time you will be able to remove the original stimulus, and have just the additional stimulus elicit the response: Stimulus 2 (bell) results in Response (salivating).

Let's look at smoking:
Stimulus 1 (seeing cigarette) results in Response (light up and smoke the cigarette). Then we add:

Stimulus 1 (seeing cigarette) + Stimulus 2 (feeling bored) results in Response (light up and smoke the cigarette). Until we get:

Stimulus 2 (feeling bored) results in Response (light up and smoke the cigarette). Keeping this original research in mind, let's explore what we now know about creating or changing habits.

1. Small, specific actions are more likely to become habitual.
Writing down you want to lose 50 pounds by July is ludicrous. Or you will be able to do 50 pull-ups. Cross that off as a resolution. Let's discuss the habits that will result in….um..results! Let's start small. Assess your average day. Are you very sedentary? Is your idea of exercise walking up the steps to the train each morning? Let's change that. Let us start small, but impactful, perhaps "I am going to walk from home to the supermarket and back every day after work (if you have dogs bring them along they'll love it!). The walk to the supermarket is probably not going to result in weight loss, but you are laying the foundation for a habit. After this has gone on a while, now you have scheduled maybe a twenty minute or half-hour opening in your day to walk to the supermarket and back. With that, now you might be able, instead of walking to the supermarket, to add that you are going to watch an exercise video on Youtube for free, a low impact exercise tape. Further, now your arms and legs are moving. And after a while you can say..maybe, I'd like to try this kickboxing or higher impact video (I want to sweat some more). You started with making a relatively small commitment, but it carved out time in your life, and look at you now: every day after work your routine includes 30 mins of kickboxing, or multi-joint high impact exercise, getting you sweating and your heart rate elevated.

Perhaps you are working from home or at an office. What can you accomplish with 5 minutes an hour in an office or in your home office/school? Would your heart benefit from some increased blood flow from marching in place for just five minutes each hour? Not a race, just movement. When you move, the joints you are moving self-lubricate. Marching in place moves blood and fluid out of your lower legs, moves the big muscles in the front and back of your legs, and helps the ankles, knees, hips, and low back stay loose and healthy. After an 8-hour day, you will have marched in place for over half an hour.

Maybe you are reading that Keto diets or Paleo diets or whatever the flavor of the day is will cause weight loss. But, you love your pasta, or you live near THE BEST pizza place in all of Brooklyn. The likelihood of your maintaining that no-pizza diet is nearly zero. So what can you do? Now, again, we need to look at ourselves, this time examining our eating habits. Keep a journal, maybe take a camera pic, or keep a video diary of everything you are eating and why. Were you truly so hungry just three hours after a bowl of lasagna that you needed 8 chocolate chip cookies? Maybe you were, maybe you just saw those cookies and your brain lit up its happy hormones for you. So, maybe, can you have just a half-bowl of lasagna (or just one slice instead of two slices of pizza)? Come back tomorrow for the other slice. Can you break that one habit of having 2 slices of pizza at a meal? Trust me, your brain will be having an earthquake eruption: "THERE'S ANOTHER SLICE THERE FOR ME." But leave it for tomorrow. Over a period of time, your body and brain will get used to just one slice. After a period of time your body and brain will get used to you having only five beers of a six-pack, throwing the last two cigarettes out with the empty pack, etc.

As you start on this journey … what are your goals? Do you want to stop shopping at the Big & Tall store? Do you want to go from XXXX clothes to XXX, to XX, to XL? Is there a waist size you remember as an adult that you want to target? Maybe you haven't seen your toes in a few years? Maybe you don't want to have so much leg pain? Maybe you want to be able to bounce your grandson without breaking out in a sweat? Know first what your habits are, and then set goals that include NOTHING RADICAL!

Substantial weight loss is possible across a range of treatment modalities, but long-term sustenance of lost weight is much more challenging, and weight regain is typical. In a meta-analysis of 29 long-term weight loss studies, more than half of the lost weight was regained within two years, and by five years more than 80% of lost weight was regained. Indeed, previous failed attempts at achieving durable weight loss may have contributed to the recent decrease in the percentage of people with obesity who are trying to lose weight5 and many now believe that weight loss is a futile endeavor. It follows that "I will lose ten pounds this month after giving up pizza and alcohol" is more than likely a foolish commitment. Instead, give yourself a comprehensive review of when and why you are eating. Can you really not wait for your dinner at a restaurant without an order of potato skins or mozzarella sticks or buffalo wings? Isn't that a bad habit, appetizers before a feast at a restaurant or diner? Here we encounter loads of opportunities to make good choices. Mashed, baked, or French fries? Soup or salad? With Dressing? Something smothered in cheese perhaps? Well, maybe, but hopefully not again this month.

On medical forms it says to ask about "Sleeping Habits," because we all have our own routine. We know this can be negatively affected if we have guests, or if the kids come in and kick around, or our work schedules change, and for a period of time our brains and bodies will struggle to get back to our baseline. But, eventually, we will reach a new normal.

I'd rather read these:
Patient A: a 75 year-old came in for her annual physical. Last year's exam revealed bone loss and muscle loss. She also needed medication for her high blood pressure, gout, arthritis, and "blood thinners." She led a sedentary lifestyle, occasionally going out to meet friends or meet at the senior center. Her exam reveals that she has not lost any bone since last year, has gained 8 pounds and 5% of her muscle mass. She can do several push-ups and barely complains of arthritic pain. She joined a Tai-Chi club and does Tai-Chi online for 45 minutes twice per week. She has a serving of protein with every meal. Her blood pressure is down from 150/94 last year to 138/80 now, a dramatic improvement reducing her likelihood of suffering a stroke. She has moved away from the status of "pre-frail" to "not-frail."

Patient B: our 57 year-old male, also presenting for his checkup, has been diagnosed with Type 2 diabetes mellitus for over ten years, has a lifelong history of obesity, and takes medication by mouth for his diabetes. His average blood glucose last year was 285, his blood glucose at today's visit is 130. He has lost fifteen pounds from his visit last year, and gone from a size 44 waist to a size 38 waist in pants. His New Year's Resolution was to "sweat every day for 25 minutes," which he did, on most days. After meeting with his doctor for clearance he began walking up and down the stairs from the lobby to his second-floor apartment. First, he started only when there were commercials on during his shows, then it continued to "during halftime" of his sports shows.

Don't end up as one of those sad self-defeated charts at the beginning of this chapter. There are healthful habits you can make right now to change your future. Put this book down and walk, wheel, crawl to a destination of your choice! DO IT NOW!

CHAPTER V

Neuro-Orthopedic Pain Management

Your brain is a lawyer, and a really good one at that. Your brain will rationalize its behavior based on what it thinks is the truth or credible evidence. For example, when you feel pain, your brain will try to convince you that your shoulder is bad, or your posture is poor, or your hip is weak, presenting a case to yourself against your shoulder, posture or hip. But what if you overwrite those thoughts and present a case to counteract the pain? What if you start to think, "My shoulder is secure, my posture is good, my hip is strong"? What if you reframe your thoughts to convince yourself that you can function healthfully and without pain?

This leads to some fundamental questions about the nature of pain:

What exactly is pain?
What is the biology of pain?
Why do people feel pain?
Why does physical and emotional pain get mixed up?
How is pain managed at different stages in life?

In essence, the modern understanding of pain is that the brain decides when it occurs. For example, if you're walking across a busy highway and stub your toe, you're less likely to feel pain because there are cars moving back and forth and you have to concentrate on running to safety. But if you stub your toe with the same level of force at home in the middle of the night, you'll experience more pain. Why? Because pain is related to the context in which it occurs; perception of pain depends on the momentary balance between danger and safety. Pain exists when the lawyer-like brain finds more credible evidence of danger to the body than it does safety. Conversely, pain does not exist when the credible evidence of safety is greater than the credible evidence of danger. The brain constantly assesses all the perils going on around you, creating pain episodes according to its perception.

Luckily you are not your brain, and your brain is not you. We are much more than just our brains, and our brains can be trained, usually with the help of more information from a trusted source. Our brains can therefore adapt and change via a process known as neuroplasticity. Presented with new information and/or experiences, the brain can effectively release a body part from a pain episode.

To manage pain, instead of looking at the body as a biomedical tool in separate parts – shoulder, elbow, wrist, etc. – it is more holistic to assess the body from a biopsychosocial standpoint in which biological, psychological, and socio-environmental components intersect. As healthcare professionals we can provide evidence and educate patients to help them understand that everything, every body part, every thought and emotion, every environmental experience, is connected. And this knowledge gives the patient permission to look at pain and injury objectively, and not from a place of fear.

The biopsychosocial framework and a reminder:

"Pain involves the intricate variable interaction of biological factors (genetic, biochemical, etc.), psychological factors (mood, personality, behaviour etc.) and social factors (cultural, familial, socioeconomic, medical etc)."

INTERSECTING BIOPSYCHOSOCIAL GRAPH

When working with a new pain patient, the first step I use to evaluate them and unlock their mind-body-pain connection is to share the benefit of looking at the person as a whole. I help them understand how their systems integrate and function and assess the areas of their body and their life that are in and out of balance. Not just physical balance, but also the balance of their mental and digestive wellbeing, and how it all interrelates. As a healthcare professional, by not directly addressing the painful part of the body per se, we're helping the patient re-center their equilibrium to treat the whole system first. Depending on the age of the patient, their willingness to accept the mind-body-pain connection will vary, so we must adapt the approach accordingly

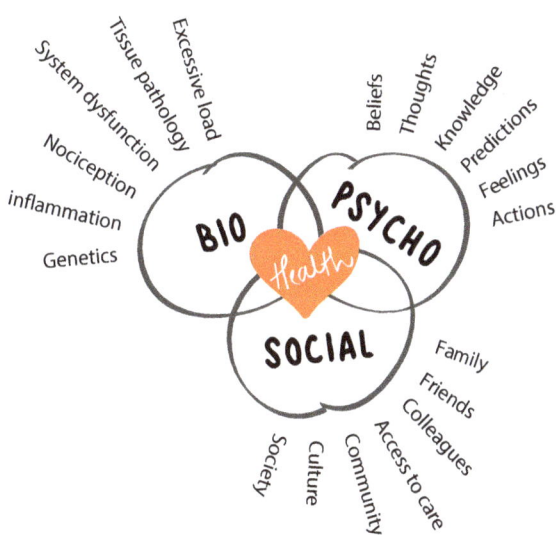

Young high school and college students are often open to new ideas. They want to learn. However, they look good, they feel good, they perform well and so are less likely to end up in the office in need of pain management. But when they do, they are easy to work with. You can educate a student.

While millennials are often similarly openminded and willing to learn, they can sometimes be a little more challenging. They know their bodies but they don't necessarily understand the mind-body-pain connection. They are confident and tend to challenge authority when something doesn't fit their paradigm of thinking. When educating millennials that there are alternate, more holistic ways to treat pain, care must be taken with both words and tone to avoid unsettling such individuals and potentially limiting their learning.

Those aged 40+ want to stay in their 40s for as long as possible; it's like they're investing in a 401(k) for the body - thus reducing healthcare costs. For the most part they've worked very hard for a long time. They are tired, perhaps single, married, or in a relationship, may have kids, and have taken on a lot of responsibility managing emotional and personal relationships. This naturally creates stress or manifests itself in the physical body as pain. Their outlet is running, walking: whatever brings most satisfaction. They want to play golf, they want to play tennis, and they're more emotionally ready to hear about abstract ideas, maybe incorporating yoga and Pilates into their otherwise hardcore sport regimes. Seeking advice from healthcare professionals, they are ready and willing to listen, learn, and invest in their future health.

Every age group struggles with the aging myth. Twenty-five-year-olds think they're 'quarter-century-old,' while 45-year-olds are consumed by 'not being 25 anymore.' Likewise, the 65+ group are still in a battle against the aging myth. Their bodies are aging but, in many cases, their minds are young. They still feel like a 40-year-old. They might also think about something their doctor has said that has resonated with them, but which can also inhibit their recovery and progress. For example, if their doctor determines the injury is "bone-on-bone," then the idea that their knee joints are rubbing together can reduce their motivation to move. People in this age group tend to rely heavily on traditional medicine, but what if traditional treatments are actually holding them back?

If someone is feeling pain, a traditional doctor usually sends them for an MRI. What if people stopped getting MRIs? A tear might not necessarily be causing the pain, and surgery might not necessarily increase the mobility needed to get them back on the golf course. Instead of getting the MRI and discovering the tear, what if they just learned about their body, how to stretch, breathe, recalibrate and move? They might still be playing golf at 75. Or older.

BALANCE

When patients have pain or have been avoiding the use of a body part because they might have a break or a tear, their body's center of gravity, or the brain's ability to trust that side of the body, is reduced. For example, if you've had pain in your left leg for six weeks, your brain no longer trusts the information coming from that leg. The result might be that your muscles tighten a little more on the left, which means less of your foot is touching the ground, possibly resulting in having less feedback from the foot telling the left side what to do. Furthermore, if your brain is not trusting the information from your left side, you might put more weight on the right, so that you don't fall over.

When we are off balance, our sensory system is heightened. All of a sudden, something that doesn't normally hurt starts to hurt, creating a hyperactive response (allodynia). Something that might hurt for a few seconds becomes startling (hyperalgesia). When we are in balance, the same stimulus doesn't elicit the same response, so we feel less pain. Instead of our system being hypersensitized and, in effect, so overprotective that it won't let you move, it will be just protective enough. When the whole nervous system is better balanced, a more accurate read of what is actually painful and what is not becomes possible.

Balance is a combination of three things:
Proprioception, our body's ability to know where it is in space
Vision, use of our eyes to see where we are and acquire visual feedback
The Vestibular System, our spatial orientation, located in the inner ear.

All three work together to retain balance and can be utilized to manage pain. Let's imagine your vestibular system, feeling off-center in the inner ear, screaming, "Hey, you're leaning to the right!" In order to maintain the body's equilibrium, this prompts your vision to take over. You might feel as if you're in balance, but your perceived center of gravity, instead of being dead center, has shifted a little to the right. People are often unaware that they are off balance, until, perhaps, they close their eyes.

Vision not only is important to balance, but is also a very important way to objectively "look at" and assess the pain in question. For example, our brains recognize big scars or a lot of blood as pertinent visual information, giving such past and present damage a lot of attention and most likely triggering a heightened pain reaction. This was demonstrated in a study published in the British Journal of Medicine in 1995 in which a person was taken to the emergency room in excruciating pain from a nail that had gone through his shoe and foot. The doctors took off the shoe and realized that the nail had actually gone between the second and third toe; it hadn't even pierced the skin! The pain the patient was experiencing was interpreted not by what he felt, but by what he saw. The visual information carried more weight and had more influence in what we call the "pain neurotag"– the group of neurons that light up when we have a pain experience.

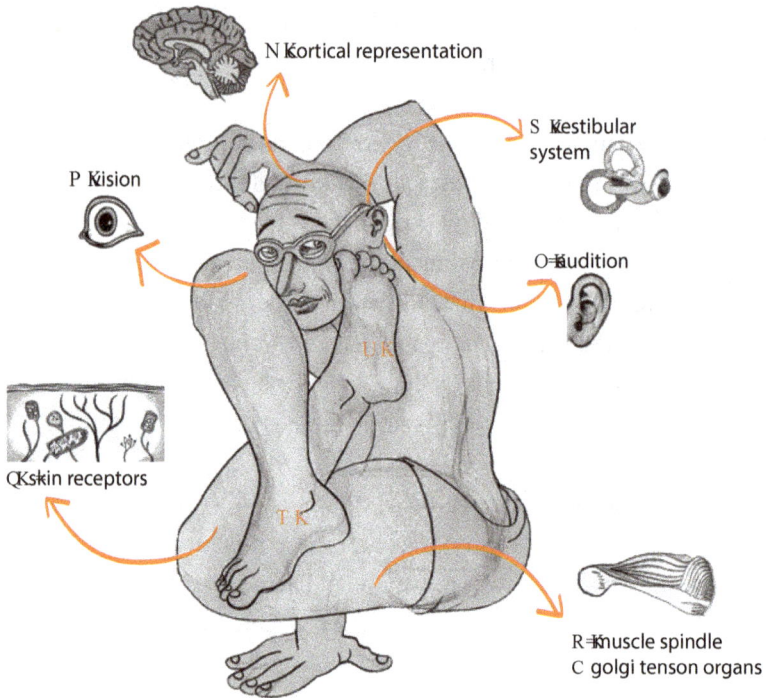

N Kortical representation
S Vestibular system
P Vision
O Audition
Q Kskin receptors
R Knuscle spindle
C golgi tenson organs

A widespread network of cortical brain areas are thought to be involved in body representation and, thus, in self-localization. However, a major role is also played by audition (2) and vision (3). In order to locate one's body part, both skin receptors (4), muscle spindles and Golgi tendon organs (5) are crucial. Together these cues contributeto create a unique and coherent percept of one's own body, well described with the concept of cortical body matrix. In particular, the innovative aspect is the body-centered representation of the body itself (instead of a body part-centered representation) such as the right leg (7) usually in the right side of the space (8) can occupy the left side of the peripersonal space simply crossing over in the space where the left leg usually is.

MENTAL WELLNESS

Anxiety is essentially the fear of the unknown and can be heightened when we feel pain in our bodies. Knowledge, combined with trust, can help re-write painful patterns, and help calm the mind and nervous system. By closing our eyes, looking inward, and doing visualization exercises, we can help mitigate a pain experience and calm the nervous system. In essence, the mind is our drug cabinet, which when calm and collected can release powerful antidepressants. Guided meditation is a great way to trick our minds into forgetting about pain. Within our brains we have a homunculus, which is basically a circuit board where each body part is represented – hands, feet, hip, spine, neck, and so on. When people who have had

a leg amputated experience phantom limb pains, it is because their leg is still represented in the brain within that "circuit board."When you have an injury, the corresponding part of the brain gets bigger; it gets inflamed and disturbs connections to other body parts, so even when you don't have pain, you are still thinking about the injury: "Is my hip going to hurt me?" Doing exercises and practices such as guided meditation can broaden attention to the

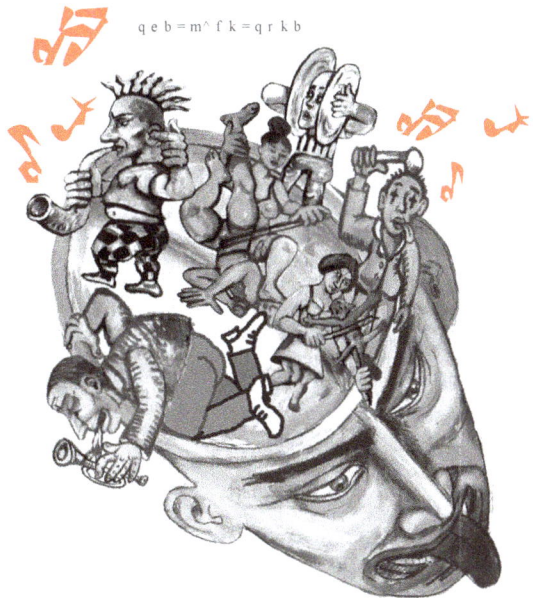

q e b = m^ f k = q r k b

other areas of the brain, effectively to the other body parts. This helps to normalize the homunculus, taking the magnifying glass off the hip. When the patient doesn't think about their hip as much, their nervous system calms down and they start to feel better.

What if I have a stress fracture and I'm running through that pain: how do I know if I'm doing too much damage? If I adopt a strategy, such as guided meditation or focusing my mind and my stride to a metronome, and the pain goes away, then I can say, "You know what? I'm engaging the rest of my body and I feel good!" Teaching people that they can control how they feel, their level of protection and their ability to move, just by changing the way they think and perceive pain, is not just mind over matter. I'm not making this up; we're actually creating biological shifts.

DIGESTIVE WELLNESS

We are what we eat. The gut microbiome is our second brain. It regulates the immune system, which is our defense system. During a stress response the immune system ignites, activating and releasing chemicals that create real inflammation. If the body perceives danger, swelling can occur without the presence of an infection (neurogenic information). It's a sign the body is readying itself for whatever might happen. Furthermore, gut health is linked to the autonomic nervous system to determine whether we are in a sympathetic "fight or flight" paranoid state of thinking (everyone is out to get me), or a parasympathetic "rest and digest" chill state (we're all connected, everybody loves us and has our best interests at heart).

When we have a healthy digestive tract, we're digesting and eliminating toxins. If those toxins are not being cleared, or we're not getting good blood flow to our gut, or we don't have healthy bacteria, studies have shown that this can lead to mental health disorders. Anxiety manifests in the sympathetic nervous system. The toxins trigger the gut to send messages up to the brain saying, "I'm in danger, I'm under threat." Under these circumstances, someone might say something to us that causes us to personalize it and jump to conclusions. But if we have a healthy microbiome, we're not getting as many danger messages. We are in a chill, relaxed state and our level of reactivity is less. If someone says something mean, we think, "Huh, they must not be having a good day." We don't take it personally. We can connect and empathize more and are less likely to be affected.

It is common in many cultures to practice gratitude to prepare the body for receiving food. Giving gratitude or thanks before each meal helps to activate the parasympathetic nervous system and enables better access to that "off switch." So too does slow, deep diaphragm breathing (in for four seconds, out for six seconds) before diving into a plate of food. In theory, we are getting into a relaxed or reduced cortisol state and enhancing serotonin and dopamine, which allows the calm, self-regulatory system to monitor more accurately—to be able to determine I have or I haven't had enough.

As a healthcare professional, gaining insight into a patient's digestive health is a window into understanding their pain and anxiety and a pathway to their healing, as well as another opportunity to educate.

RIGHT JUDGEMENT

Words matter. Different emotions, different words, different people or different things can trigger a stress response within all of us, which can result in heightened pain.

By becoming more aware of the brain's role in pain, we can counteract the misconceptions of pain with strategies that challenge us to pay more attention to other body parts. By doing so, we can change what we think and believe about pain, come to a decision about what to do, and, ultimately, calm the nervous system, alleviate anxiety, and reduce pain altogether. The patient needs to believe they can heal. Belief comes from listening and trusting their body, not from their clinician's words. I may show you an exercise and ask you to mimic my behavior, and you might be apprehensive because your doctor said not to, or "Dr. Google" advised against it.

But here is a health professional whom you've developed a relationship with, who has helped you before and you trust, giving you permission to move. This permission gives you just enough courage to take yourself through a range of motions that you wouldn't normally feel comfortable doing. And not only do you actually not feel pain, but you actually feel better!

Once we believe and trust in ourselves, we can then exercise Right Judgement: our ability to make an informed decision based on our knowledge and understanding of what we can and cannot do. This is a major step because in a state of anxiety people have a tricky time making decisions. So if we understand what is going on, and we're in a calm state, our ability to make rational decisions is enhanced. This training alleviates the panic. Clarity of mind allows a more informed choice and Right Judgement to be exercised. Should I play tennis or not play tennis?

Should I go for a hike or not go for a hike? When we have the information and we've been given permission to move, then we can make a better choice. We think, "I'm starting to feel this, I can work through it," or "Should I seek advice now?" Ultimately, we make better decisions.

PATIENT AUTONOMY

Two recent patient stories give prime examples of the teachable transition to patient autonomy.

Patient A just turned 80-years-old. Never planning to retire, he was married to his desk until Coronavirus hit and he was forced to stay home. Like most people his age, fear of the virus, coupled with the universal fear of getting older, forced him to limit activity outside the home; a sedentary lifestyle can speed the aging process. But most older people can do a lot more than they think—and Patient A was no exception.

He adapted to his "new normal" by participating in Zoom training sessions three times a week. Without having any physical interaction, he has lost 20lbs and is now able run a mile without pain around the lower loop of Central Park. He does his stretches, keeps active while safely distancing himself from others, and maintains a positive outlook on life. As a newly minted octogenarian, he is in better shape now than in his seventies. This is an example of someone who has essentially gotten younger, and who is open to being even better at 90 instead of thinking, "I've just turned 80, I'm on the downhill slope." The sky's the limit!

Patient B is in the 40+ age group, generally healthy and active. When quarantine hit, she decided to challenge herself to 30 days of yoga and fell in love with it. Thirty days turned into 60, and then zero when her back and hip started to really bother her. She was also hiking in Central Park almost daily but was in too much pain to continue. Disheartened, she reached out to me for help. Her dialogue went something like this: "I love yoga. I did it 60 days in a row. It's supposed to be good for me, but it hurt me. I knew it was too much. I knew I should've taken a break, but I didn't. I love it so much, but now I can't do anything."

Her mind and body were suffering, but she didn't know what to do. She was beating herself up. Yoga, a positive, became more of a negative. She was spiraling downward. To her surprise, the first thing I did was give her permission to keep moving, to keep at the yoga and walking. By gaining permission from someone

88

she trusted, she had the little bit of courage she needed to feel like she could take the proper steps back to health and normalcy. Then, I had her do a balance exercise to assess her vestibular system. With her eyes closed, I had her march on the spot, and to her surprise she turned 90 degrees without realizing it, indicating that her balance system was a little off. To counteract that I had her do some cognitive tasks including math and spelling. Since the neurons involved in a pain experience have other functions, the cognitive tasks light up the brain and basically hijack or override the pain, as if switching on a bright light, to help reset the balance system.

We then did a guided meditation, drawing her attention away from the back and hip and evenly towards different parts of the body. We next did a seated breathing exercise targeted at stretching and strengthening her hip flexor muscles and posture. By breathing into the diaphragm, more oxygen floods into the tissues, which in turn feel safer and less painful. We downloaded a metronome app on her phone for her to listen to when she walks, ensuring that her stride and placement of the foot on the ground was even and level, giving her an external focus, which can also help reset the brain. Patient B recorded all of these instructions and referred to them daily; the pain went away. When the pain occasionally crept back up, just a quick check in with these tools was all that she needed to alleviate the discomfort and get back on track.

Patient B's new dialogue went something like this: "I'm starting to feel that pain again, so I'm not going to do yoga every day this week; instead I'm going to do it four days. Or I'm going to do some stretching when I'm walking, or, instead of doing a full yoga practice tonight, I'm going to do only a few sun salutations. I will pay attention to my feet and breathe more, so I'm not putting myself at risk. I am in control."   She is now exercising her Right Judgment. As she, and all of us, become more mindful, our senses become more reliable and allow us to identify and address pain objectively before it becomes unbearable.

REFRAME THE PAIN

As healthcare professionals, our job is to build people's self-confidence and belief in themselves, and it is our responsibility to do so by educating patients in as honest a way as possible. Depending on the patient's age, physicality, mental and digestive wellness, and pain need, we use different language and different techniques to provide them with the knowledge and tools to assess their pain and manage it. We're not just providing physical therapy, but a combination of mental and physical therapy to treat the body as a whole.

I love the wisdom of the popular saying: Give a man a fish and you feed him for a day; teach a man to fish and you feed him for a lifetime. By reframing the patient's approach to pain, essentially we are teaching them to 'fish,' that is, how to care for their health without being reliant on others. It's then the person in pain's responsibility to acknowledge and work towards their goals if they want to maximize the effectiveness of their intervention and get the greatest return on their health investment.

If you feel pain, you have pain, but there are many ways to guide your system out of it. Knowing, understanding, wisdom: it can be that simple. Gaining knowledge is not learning; it's just acquiring knowledge. Learning is the active process. Once you've done the work, once you see and feel the positive results, you have experienced learning and seen change. You now have the wisdom to present your case and reframe your pain, releasing it, letting it go. You can confidently make decisions based on what's best for you, because now you are the expert on your own pain.

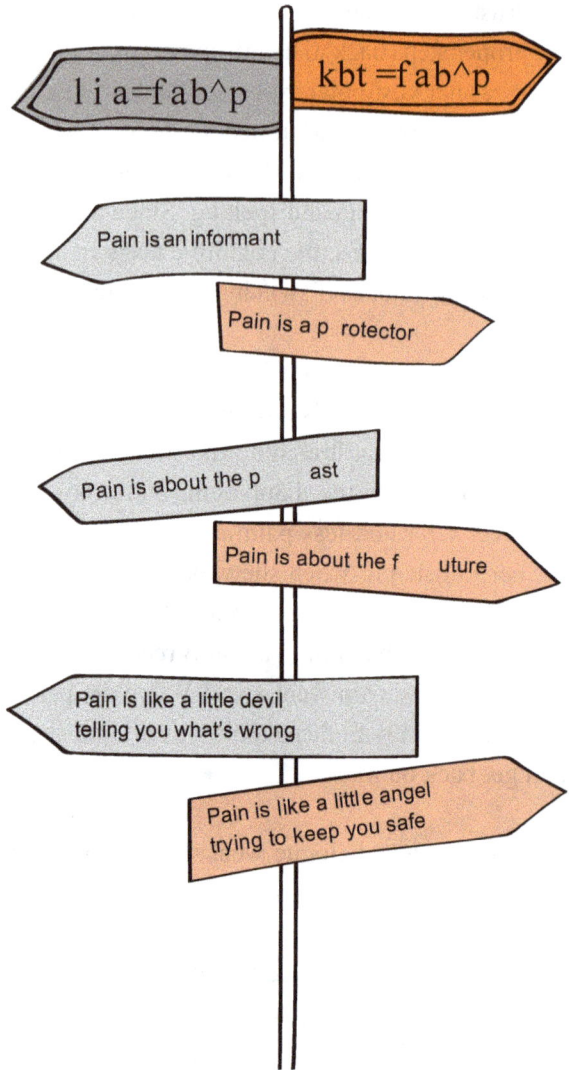

l i a=f a b^p

kbt =f a b^p

Pain is an informant

Pain is a p rotector

Pain is about the p   ast

Pain is about the f   uture

Pain is like a little devil telling you what's wrong

Pain is like a little angel trying to keep you safe

CHAPTER VI

Chronic Pain

What Is Chronic Pain And How Does It Differ From Acute Pain?
Put simply, chronic pain is pain that exists after the expected time of healing for an injury or ailment. While there is some disagreement on this, generally it works for our understanding.
We are familiar with acute pain, which is short-lived, and is often associated with an injury like amuscle strain, tear, or even a broken bone. These types of injuries heal in a fairly predictableamount of time, but if the pain persists past that time, the pain can be considered chronic. Mostexperts agree the majority of ailments in the body improve within a maximum of 6 months.

If you're experiencing ongoing pain after 6 months, it's a safe assumption you're nowexperiencing chronic pain. In this chapter, we will focus on chronic pain. The outcome is to giveyou a better basis from which to understand this type of pain. This better understanding can help you change the way you frame or think about pain, therefore changing how you respond to it, and potentially improving the results you achieve with various therapies. Learning about pain itself IS therapeutic!

How do people get stuck in the vicious cycle of chronic pain?
Approximately 20% of people will develop chronic pain, even if they do not experience an initial injury to their body! This is a staggering statistic, and one that sparks a lot of curiosity since it challenges the most common views on the nature of pain. While there are many factors that can contribute to the development of chronic pain, including genetics, and it's likely a perfect-storm type of scenario, there are a few observations that experts have noted with both the development and perpetuation of it.

Overemphasis on visual imaging
It is fairly well established that visual imaging such as MRI and X-ray don't tell the whole story when it comes to uncovering the root causes of pain. "Structural evidence of a lumbar disc hernia in a patient with appropriate symptoms is present more than 90% of the time. Unfortunately, even when using advanced imaging techniques such as myelography, CAT scans, or magnetic resonance imaging, the same positive findings are also present in 28% to 50% of asymptomatic individuals" (Leibenson, 76).Given this, you can imagine how common the diagnosis may

purely be based on a visual scan, which may or may not align with the symptoms the person is experiencing. Not only leading to the wrong recommendation of therapeutic options or surgical procedures, it can also introduce unnecessary fear or concern in the pain sufferer, generating a serious concern over their situation.

Excessive focus on structural diagnosis and subsequent treatment failure.

This is associated with what was mentioned previously, but also takes into account the myriad of structural or movement diagnoses that are often found repeated online and/or in social media. This can include postural imbalance, muscles imbalance, faulty movement, weak core, etc. While some of these areas may include elements that can contribute to the overall pain experience, they are not the only factor by far. Excessively focusing on these areas often leads to missing more important factors that can be directly contributing to the development of the chronicity of the pain.

Every time a new diagnosis is received, and subsequently, the treatment fails to meet the expectations the person has, this leads to increased likelihood of developing a chronic pain issue.

Overlooking precipitating factors such as anxiety and/or depression
"Lindsay and Wyckoff found that up to 85% of patients with chronic pain fit the diagnostic criteria for clinical depression. Interestingly, it has also been found that 39% of patients with chronic pain have a history of depression that precedes the onset of pain" (Leibenson, 557). Anxiety and depression are very common amongst individuals who suffer from chronic pain. They can be associated with the increased likelihood of developing chronic pain, and certainly can be a product of experiencing chronic pain as well.

Influences like workplace injury and job satisfaction
Research has shown that pain treatment outcomes can be negatively impacted depending on the relationship of the individual to their work. People who are injured on the job are often faced with at least some disincentive for improvement, for they typically receive worker's compensation benefits, including medical coverage and financial benefits in the form of supplementary income, while avoiding the rigors of actually working for such benefits (Occupational Hearing Loss, 17). In some studies, researchers have concluded that compensa-tion is related to increased reports of pain and reduced treatment efficacy. The results

of meta-analyses suggest that this relationship is likely causal, and Rholing et al. statistically demonstrated that if compensation were eliminated as a variable, the experience of chronic pain would decrease by an average of 24% (Occupational Hearing Loss, 18). It's clear there are multiple factors that can certainly contribute to the development and perpetuation of chronic pain that must be uncovered.

Knowing Your Pain and Why It Matters

Approaching all pain the same way is a mistake. Using the wrong tool for the job will almost always end with a poor result. The type of pain someone has must be identified as closely as possible to know where to focus attention and what types of therapeutic elements or treatments will likely be most effective. Norman Doidge, M.D., eloquently writes about two people's success in chapter one of his new book, The Brain's Way of Healing: Remarkable Discoveries and Recoveries from the Frontiers of Neuroplasticity. Because the brain can reshape neural pathways devoted to chronic pain, pain occupies a mysterious place in medical terminology and diagnosis. Getting our heads wrapped around pain can be challenging. For the sake of brevity, it helps to put pain into a few simple categories.

There are three main categories of pain, and here we discuss the first two of them prior to the third. Knowing the type of pain helps us understand the best way to approach it. Most common ongoing aches and pains people experience fall into these categories. Most of us are familiar with the kind that arises from damaged tissue. Sprain an ankle, tear a muscle, that's nociceptive pain you are feeling. Damage in tissues triggers a response to send nociceptive input to the spinal cord and brain about the state of the tissues. It's important to note that nociception is not pain, just information. Nociception and pain are not equivalent, and there are no "pain fibers" or "pain receptors" specifically dedicated to relaying pain signals in the brain or body. Our nerve systems constantly send data to the brain for consideration about innumerable stimulating things like hunger, thirst, revulsion, desire, and pain. Pain, like all of the other sensations we feel, is, technically speaking, a brain-generated experience. Acute pain that is "in our body" like a broken ankle is meaningful and functional. Without the nervous system response and the brain's interpretation, we'd keep right on going and injure ourselves further.

The more sophisticated type of pain that occurs from damage to the system that reports and interprets injury itself to the nervous system is called neuropathic pain. If the peripheral nervous system is damaged or malfunctioning, called neuropathic pain, the brain is getting the wrong information, and pain changes accordingly.

While the nervous system is adapting to and reshaping the messages that we usually call pain, we experience different aspects. Neuropathic pains include phantom limb, neuralgia, carpal tunnel syndrome, and similar conditions. With nociceptive pain, the brain is getting the right information, but in neuropathic pain, the nervous system is damaged or malfunctioning. The brain is interpreting that information differently.

The most straightforward way to understand the difference is to imagine that you dropped your computer. You might have some dents and dings and a cracked screen, or your motherboard might have been damaged, and the machine will not work or will work poorly. So, you see, it's not just the tissues, nerves, or brain by themselves, but the interaction between these elements that can affect the pain experience.

There are different categories of chronic pain, and while it's possible to fit neatly into one or another, most people are split between these two categories to some degree. The more accurately you can determine where you stand, the more likely you can figure out the best way to address it. In the next paragraph, we discuss the third category and get at the root of more complex chronic pain conditions.

The third type of pain is called central sensitization. As we've discussed, the therapeutic establishment has been preoccupied with the structural and biomechanical causes of pain. Therapists are limited in their ability to treat some types of chronic cases successfully. By necessity, more therapists today are learning to treat their clients by incorporating an expanded model of pain that includes neurological and social definitions. It may be useful to frame our definition of pain as less of a negative. Pain is not a bad thing—pain is our primary alarm system. Just as you might assume that your house is being broken into when the home alarm goes off, pain necessitates our attention. We have to get out of bed, walk around the house, and see if it's an intruder or if the wind blew open the back door because someone forgot to lock it. The alarm did its job; it is up to us to pay attention and respond appropriately. To carry the analogy further—if we become overwrought with despair every time we hear a noise, we'd drive our spouses crazy. Conversely, if we don't investigate the door that won't close properly, perhaps we risk a home invasion. The same goes for pain: when we are consciously afraid of pain, or misunderstand pain, or otherwise try to ignore this natural, protective alarm system, we invite confusion.

The cycle of overreacting to the alarm system or misinterpreting the way it works is precisely how a patient becomes more sensitive. When a patient experiences more pain with less provocation, this is called "central sensitization." This term refers to changes to the central nervous system (CNS)—in particular, the brain and the spinal cord. Sensitized patients are more sensitive not only to things that may hurt but also to ordinary touch and pressure. Their pain also "echoes." These signals fade more slowly than they do in other people. In more severe cases, extreme oversensitivity is obvious. The role of sensitization in several common diseases has been proved and well documented, and it can also persist and worsen in the absence of disease and without apparent provocation. The neurological cascade of physical and mental experience is a complication of pain, also referred to as "chronicity." Central sensitization is the most common denominator in all difficult pain problems. It's nearly a universal factor that puts the "chronic" in chronic pain. Regardless of how it got started, central sensitization is the cause of its chronicity. The existence of central sensitization is quite well established, and yet there is a gap that exists in our scientific knowledge. There are no clear criteria for diagnosing central sensitization.

There is no easy laboratory test or checklist that can confirm it. It could be present in nearly any severe case of chronic pain. However, the pain could still be coming from a continuing problem in the tissue, with or without central sensitization. When central sensitization is suspected to be a strong contributor to a person's pain, therapists must adjust their methods. Central sensitization can easily be made worse by careless, deliberately rough, "no-pain, no-gain" treatment. When physical therapists, massage therapists, and chiropractors treat a chronic pain patient too intensely, they trigger the alarm system and make the person more sensitive, usually leading to more pain. Patients going through the "therapy grinder" often find themselves in the hands of overly intense therapists who are not familiar with central sensitization. Patients waste time, money, and precious energy on expensive and ineffective therapies only to find themselves crippled by pain and, sadly, depressed.

Care for chronic pain starts with normalizing the nervous system. Vigorous therapy can exacerbate a less serious problem and disturb the whole system easily. Early in treatment, patients with stubborn pain problems may start to feel that they are experiencing "too much" pain —more than seems to "make sense." It's not an easy question to answer. When we hurt, our pain needs a voice. Like the patient with oversensitive hearing (hyperacusis) trying to figure out if sounds are too loud or just sound that way, pain can overwhelm the brain's ability to process it accurately. Essentially, when the nervous system is overly sensitized, and pain levels seem much higher than they may be, we need to be cautious when applying therapies that are painful to implement, such as deep pressure massage and even rigorous exercise. Tissue pathology that does not explain chronic pain is overwhelming (e.g., in back pain, neck pain, and knee osteoarthritis). Purely biomechanical explanations for pain are not helpful, so it's best to make sure any professional you see is aware of central sensitization. This is a solid criterion for choosing a therapist. If your doctor or therapist doesn't know what central sensitization is, it's likely best to take your pain elsewhere.

Keep in mind that you might go through quite a few professionals before finding one who shows "sensitivity to sensitivity." Keep in mind that even though medications that work on the central nervous system are the most promising treatment for severe pain system dysfunction, only a physician trained in the care of chronic pain can prescribe them. The best place to look for such a doctor is in a pain clinic. If you have persistent and severe pain, start looking for one today.

A note: regardless of whether or not central sensitization is happening in your body now, it always makes sense to be kind to your central nervous system. Make your life "safer" and less stressful. Gentler. Easier. Pain is not an "all in the head" problem, but a "strongly affected by the head" problem, such as an ulcer caused by a genuine bacterial illness and then severely aggravated by stress. When your CNS is "freaked out" and overinterpreting every signal from the tissues as more painful, it's best to step back and let the body rest and reorient itself. The ability of the brain to form and reorganize certain synaptic connections, especially in response to learning or experience following injury, is known as neuroplasticity. The brain intuitively modulates excitability and neuronal activity when we are injured or distressed. Central sensitization is a modulatory process in the brain akin to a persistent state of high reactivity. In this state, the pain threshold is lower, and individuals may still feel pain after an injury has already healed.

In cases of nerve injury, both mechanical and chemical, the first alarm of peripheral sensitization is perceived by the brain as a constant, and it morphs into central sensitization. At this point, the initial pain signal is experienced as "louder." Central and peripheral sensitization may be responsible for various forms of pain that cannot be explained by a biomechanical model. The specific type of anxiety triggered by central and peripheral sensitization has two main characteristics—

hyperalgesia and allodynia. Hyperalgesia is an exaggerated perception of pain after a stimulus that is mildly painful, such as slight pinpricks. Allodynia refers to experiencing pain with a stimulus that is not usually painful, as in simple touch or gentle pressure; however, individuals experiencing unexpected or random shifts in pain sensation are not making up their symptoms. The same goes for those who sometimes experience improvements after taking medications, from physical movement, or from therapeutic massage. Diagnosis of central or peripheral sensitization is problematic. There is no laboratory test for this. How do we assess whether central sensitization is an actual diagnosis or a sort of syndrome that comes along with certain kinds of chronic pain in some but not all patients? This is a difficult question to answer, and in time, hopefully we will learn more about this, but one thing is certain in the meantime: A multidisciplinary, biopsychosocial-based TEAM approach is best when it comes to working with chronic pain to cover as much territory as possible.

The Biopsychosocial Model And Its Application To Chronic Pain
Until recently, the medical establishment tended to lean on a purely biomechanical description of pain that often fails to treat the whole person effectively. This leads to chronic pain sufferers, often experiencing a dizzying array of explanations for their condition. When we focus too much on biomechanical aspects of pain, we run the risk of ignoring the social and psychological issues of discomfort. This can feed into nervous system sensitivity and provoke further pain.

We know, for instance, that multiple inputs interact and contribute to a person's experience of pain. You will recall that pain falls into two primary categories. We discussed nociceptive and neuropathic pain. The former is associated with a specific injury, and the latter is a condition or disease in the nervous system. Adding a third category—central sensitization—provides a fuller explanation for more complicated pain cases. Most practitioners agree that it is best to focus on the whole person, not just on the area where the pain is. Person-centered therapy is unique. For it to be successful, it requires a thorough screening. Practitioners screen for biological, psychological, and sociological (biopsychosocial) factors and other health issues. If this is done well, we can identify the biopsychosocial factors that influence pain and disability.

It's necessary to communicate clearly with the individual to identify potential biopsychosocial drivers of pain. These include beliefs about pain, emotional coping responses, social context, and physical and other lifestyle factors. Chronic pain sufferers need to know how to confront how much their pain impacts their lives as a whole, the ability to work, interact socially, and positively integrate with society. This style changes the dynamics of the health practitioner-client relationship to "patient-centered communication." Naturally, if someone is suffering from chronic pain, they want to know that their health care provider cares about them by building rapport and connection to understand them rather than just treating them as a statistic, which unfortunately is the collective experience many people have in the current medical system.

Slowing down and taking the time to fully understand the scope of the person's issues, how it's affecting their lives, and getting details on the presentation of the pain can help build an alliance between the therapist and client. Research shows how powerful this alliance is when it comes to therapeutic success. An initial screen might include the following types of questions:

1. What is your pain story?
2. What do you think is the cause of your pain?
3. What do you do when pain increases?
4. Please tell me how your symptoms affected your ability to engage with functional and physical activity.
5. Do your symptoms worry you?
6. Why do you think you should not bend/lift/run?
7. What is your home/work/social life like?
8. What are your goals?

The answers to these questions can then guide an examination that explores the client's concerns, functional limitations, and physical capacity linked to their goals. I have found this dialogue to be of critical importance to many people. Often, clients will report that a considerable part of their improvement occurs when they feel their specific circumstances are addressed, rather than being given a generic approach based on their diagnosis, or condition. Thus, we are addressing the person, not the pain or biology itself.

This model was initially developed in 1977 by George Engel and is referred to as the Biopsychosocial Model (BPS). Since the biological aspects of pain are often over-emphasized, let's consider the psychosocial aspects of the BPS model. Psychosocial elements are profoundly impactful on an individual's health and, as we will discuss, their pain. A great deal of research has been done in this area, especially as it relates to issues such as back pain, which affects a large percentage of the population. When we become more aware of the impact of these elements, it becomes easier to understand why chronic pain sufferers may not respond to traditional nociceptive-based interventions. In the psychological aspect, there are some prevalent emotions that coincide with chronic pain. "Depression, anger, anxiety, and somatization (i.e., high pain sensitivity) are four broad emotional categories that have frequently been cited in the literature as being prevalent in the lives of patients with chronic pain." It's unclear in some cases if these elements are stemming from chronic pain, or preceded it, but consider this: "Lindsay and Wyckoff found that up to 85% of patients with chronic pain fit the diagnostic criteria for clinical depression. Interestingly, it has also been found that 39% of patients with chronic pain have a history of depression that precedes the onset of pain" (Morris, 557).

This is exceptionally high when you consider that the CDC says about 9% of Americans report feeling depressed on occasion, and about 3.4% suffer from major depression. Anger can be present in a number of different ways: the individual may be angry at their employer or some individual precisely for what they believe to be the cause of their pain; they could also be angry at their healthcare provider or their insurance company for the quality of the care they have been receiving; additionally, the individual could simply have a history of being a type of person that tends to be more angry or aggravated. No matter the cause, the presence of heightened levels of anger have been shown in some cases to lead to poorer pain therapy outcomes. Anxiety tends to exacerbate pain via activation of the sympathetic nervous system. This leads to increased muscle tone, fatigue, and thus more pain. Anxiety seems to go with the territory when it comes to chronic pain, and understandably when exposed to the biomedical model. It's easy to see how someone can become fearful of their "tissue issues" and become stuck in a seemingly endless loop of failed treatments, avoidance of activities, deconditioning, more fear, loss of hope, and thus more pain.

Waddell et al. identified a set of five "nonorganic signs" (the so-called Waddell signs) that can indicate a patient is being strongly influenced by factors other than the nociception generated by damaged tissue. Marital and relationship stress can be a significant factor in the chronic pain client as well. The ways in which spouses, family, friends, coworkers, and strangers respond to a person with chronic pain will have a tremendous impact on that individual through processes such as reinforcement and punishment. The role of relationships in chronic pain is very complicated. Pain may be serving the individual in their ability to have diminished functions in household and/or childcare duties, or income production. It can also be the opposite: their perception of their inability to perform in these roles may be exacerbating their stress and increasing pain. The role of the therapist is not to address these various psychosocial factors directly, but it is appropriate to educate the client on them, as well as validate to the client that these issues may exist, are genuine, and are indeed crucial in the overall therapeutic approach to resolving their pain experience. In both educating the client and validating their experience as usual as far as pain goes, we can effectively assist in reducing fear and anxiety, and thus improve the likelihood of a successful outcome in their pain therapy program.

Using a multi-disciplinary approach to address all aspects of the Biopsychosocial model No one can be an expert on everything, and each area can be addressed to start, but identifying which factors may need a deep dive requires the knowledge of an expert familiar with doing so. Careful consideration must be made not to overwhelm the person and their financial situation, and actual needs.

Key Areas To Address For Easing Chronic Pain
It's easy to get overwhelmed at the vast array of therapeutic options available for chronic pain. This is one of the more challenging issues facing the pain sufferer. The good news is, however, we can take a step back and "chunk" the options into larger categories based on what research shows us is successful. Working down into details within each category can always be done if needed.

1. Pain neuroscience education
New research shows the more you know about pain and how it works, the more likely you are to not only make improvements with various therapies, but also experience reduced pain and develop better coping skills. The majority of individuals suffering from chronic pain have not learned from their health care providers what generates their pain. This lack of understanding keeps people searching for structural-mechanical causes of pain, and pursuing therapies that align with those beliefs. The volume of searches online for topics related to specific muscle problems, postural distortions, and other explanations for physical aches and pains such as fascial restriction is staggering. For example, it's a little known fact that generally all tissues in the body heal in a maximum of 6 months. When pain persists past this point, the issue lies within the brain and nervous system, rather than the tissues. This means there are often multiple factors that are contributing to the pain experience beyond structural elements and, if left

unaddressed, will likely lead to treatment failure. As discussed previously, having many conflicting diagnoses and subsequent treatment failures leads to staying stuck in the vicious chronic pain cycle. Pain neuroscience education is an established approach designed to educate chronic pain sufferers about their pain to help them move better, exercise with a greater degree of tolerance, experience less suffering, and regain their hope.

2. Sleep

Sleep is essential for life, and every organism with a nervous system requires this type of resting phase. Moreover, it is noted that other types of organisms without a brain do have a circadian rhythm as well. This only highlights the importance of sleep in the physiology of living beings. It is further noted that sleep deprivation is associated with many diseases, including mental health problems, impairment in the immune system, and metabolic dysfunction, including obesity and type 2 diabetes.

The connection between chronic pain and sleep deprivation has been established for a long time. For instance, back in 1979, it was noted in a scientific study that rats that were subjected to sleep deprivation had a significantly lower pain threshold, which means they are more susceptible to pain. More recent studies in humans have confirmed the validity of these findings and that they are a risk factor in people suffering recurrent migraine attacks. Similarly, the current evidence on the matter describes a higher pain perception in various settings, including fibromyalgia, joint dysfunction, and muscle soreness. Not getting enough sleep at night predisposes people to chronic pain and increases the severity of the symptoms and the recurrence of the attacks because it is associated with hyperalgesic changes. In other words, when you don't sleep properly, your body starts feeling pain differently. Besides clinical trials on migraines, there is plenty of supporting evidence to show a definite link between sleep fragmentation or deprivation and chronic pain. We can see the scientific evidence in various medical settings:

- Arthritis and joint pain: According to a clinical trial published in 2016, sleep fragmentation induces an increased sensitization to joint pain. The study compared patients with knee arthritis with a healthy sleep pattern with others who did not sleep properly. After this comparison, the authors concluded that treating sleep is fundamental to improving chronic pain in patients with arthritis.
- Fibromyalgia: This is a condition that features chronic pain, and it is often

- difficult to trace and diagnose.
- Insomnia is strongly associated with anxiety (not as a result of pain but as an aggravating factor).
- Low back pain: It is a common problem, and most people have at least one episode throughout their lifetime. However, it was found that 53% of people with chronic symptoms of low back pain have sleep problems compared to 3% of pain-free patients who reported insomnia.
- Other musculoskeletal problems: One of the first associations between sleep deprivation and the pain centers on the issue of musculoskeletal symptoms.Sleep-deprived patients report an increase in muscle tenderness and more frequent musculoskeletal symptoms. Moreover, recent findings pointed out that the perception of musculoskeletal pain in these patients is increased by 24%.

People who do not sleep properly have a higher sensitivity to pain. According to the evidence published in the journal Psychosomatic Medicine, when pain sensitivity is increased, it is possible to measure this organic change, and there's no additional alteration in perceptions that may contribute to bias. There were no studies on brain perception of pain during periods of sleep deprivation until recently. For instance, healthy young people who do not sleep properly have higher activity in brain areas that trigger pain (the primary somatosensory cortex) and reduced activity in brain areas that coordinate movement and modulate the perception of pain (the insular cortex and the striatum). After the above-mentioned study, practitioners could trace the exact reason why sleep deprivation modulates pain. Sleep deprivation and higher sensitivity to pain increase the sensitivity of the neural network, primarily focusing on neurons that trigger anxiety. At the same time, the body becomes unable to modulate or mute pain sensation and perceives more sharply these sensory impulses. Moreover, the study found that even mild sleep deprivation affects pain perception. Similarly, it should be a wakeup call for anyone who has a continually disrupted sleep pattern and feels any type of pain symptom the day after.

Insomnia hurts, and there's much we can do about it. One of the most severe chronic pain diseases is fibromyalgia, and according to a clinical trial, applying a few sleep hygiene tips has been found to improve the symptoms in these patients. Recommendations include sleeping every day at the same hour; not using the same room to sleep, eat, and study; turning off screens before going to sleep; and avoiding coffee, alcohol, tobacco, and dense, greasy foods. There are many ways to improve our quality of sleep and reduce our perception of chronic pain. What we have to do is raise our awareness of the importance of sleep and follow easy recommendations.

3. Movement

Pain education is critical before engaging in an exercise program. Competent practitioners should possess knowledge about how to set proper expectations and be able to adjust what is being done based on how the patient responds.

When it comes to strength training and chronic pain, the most basic purpose of strength training is to strengthen the larger muscle groups of the body in the basic movement patterns (push, pull, squat, bench, lunge, and twist). These fundamental large muscle groups can, if conditioned, properly help in rehabilitation.

Strength training exercises improve conditioning, build confidence in your ability to do things like bend and lift, and prepare you for physical activities. In time, patients can reduce soreness and strain, enabling them to become less sensitive and more resilient. We call this "building a bigger cup."

Research shows that beginners gain significant benefits from lower resistance, higher repetitions, and a smaller amount of sets. For example, two sets of 20 repetitions of an exercise a few times a week can provide significant benefits. Research shows the benefits of a general exercise prescription vs. individual "core" or postural exercises to be almost identical. However, I find that tailoring exercises specific to the individual's needs is ideal. For example, if someone is afraid to bend forward in fear of making a bulging disc worse, then specific exercises aimed at feeling stronger and more confident at hip hinging are going to work better.

Many people in chronic pain may have difficulty with super-specific "stabilization" exercises for smaller muscles. There is a reason for this. The motor cortex may be utilized in the pain neuro-matrix, thus leaving them decreased importance in excellent motor control. Why?

Because the system is in "threat"! Altered cortisol representation (smudging) may also be involved. If any of this is the case, it's not a problem. Simply allow for a more generalized approach or exercise until things calm down and, if necessary, revisit these movements again later. The level of fitness of the person determines what is "ideal" for that person. A low-intensity exercise (like a 135-lb Romanian deadlift) will be very intense for a person who has never set foot in a gym with chronic lower back pain. (Using a pair of 10-lb dumbbells for a Romanian deadlift would be recommended.) Experienced gym-goers or athletes may not need to regress movement all the way down to isolation exercises to make progress. They may just need modifications to their current exercise program. Beginners will likely need coaching on basic exercises. Squats, deadlifts, pushups, rows, and prerequisites are relatively "isolated" drills to learn proper motor control and awareness of muscles and movements.

A gradual and mentorial approach to training can help reduce the fear of movement and build confidence as long as progressive movement and fitness principles are applied. I like to assign activities based on the opposite pattern identified (movement/posture). If a posture and movement defined are associated with the pain experience, I would address the muscles/actions in the antagonistic pattern. I then assess for differences in pain experience and awareness, depending on the exercise.

What does the research say about movement? There are few things in the health field as versatile as exercise. It is commonly recommended and sometimes prescribed as part of the therapy for various health conditions. Even though we assume this type of recommendation for people with excess weight and even cardiovascular issues, it is also beneficial for people that suffer from chronic pain. First, before diving into this topic, we need to separate exercise into two main types: aerobic and anaerobic. Aerobic exercise is also known as cardiovascular (cardio), and anaerobic exercise is known as resistance training, weight training, or strength training. Below, we'll evaluate what the research shows when it comes to the effective use of anaerobic training to relieve chronic pain. Do pain symptoms improve with resistance training?

While many studies show that resistance training generally improves pain symptoms, others show it might not be all that useful. This discrepancy exists because of the type of pain that is being experienced and, of course, the WAY the training is being performed affects a patient's reporting.

If you have a properly designed program, and you're doing everything correctly, you'll be likely to get improvement from some types of chronic pain. A recent analysis of resistance training and chronic lower back pain demonstrates that aerobic exercise and resistance training are both beneficial. A significant reduction of pain intensity was experienced in both groups.

However, resistance exercise displayed an added benefit, the psychological well-being of the individual, which is essential to modulate the perception of pain. It's also interesting to note that there are many variants of resistance training, and each of them has proved to reduce pain in a different way. For instance, we can divide resistance training into static and dynamic muscle contractions. Static muscle contraction, which includes isometric exercise (muscle contraction with no movement), is associated with a moderate-to-large modulation of pain, and specific studies have found that maintaining contraction at a low weight for a longer time recruits and exhausts more muscle fibers, leading to a more significant exercise-induced hypoalgesia. On the other hand, dynamic resistance, which is performed mostly by shortening and lengthening the muscles, has been found to have similar effects, but usually in the short term.

When and how is strength training appropriate for chronic pain? Resistance training can be utilized for various types of chronic pain, including fibromyalgia, which is known to be a reasonably challenging condition. Fibromyalgia is a painful condition that is highly variable between people that have it, and it's associated ultimately with a dysfunction of the nervous system and increased susceptibility to the pain experience. Most of the information out there shows that controlling pain in fibromyalgia is an extremely challenging venture. Even so, "old-school" resistance training is still an effective way to reduce the sensation of pain and tenderness and maintain or increase muscle strength in these individuals.

According to a Cochrane review, aerobic exercise is superior to moderate-intensity resistance training, so it appears to be a good idea to combine them. One of the more common applications of resistance training in chronic pain is associated with things like repetitive strain injuries. For example, a randomized control trial focused on strength training to treat working populations that had repetitive strain injuries, some of which had a work disability. They underwent 10 weeks of strength training against the usual ergonomic care that is recommended to address this kind of pain. Strength training showed significant improvements in hand/wrist pain and reduced time to fatigue by an impressive 97%. Achieving these improvements in chronic pain with resistance exercise is not so difficult. We can choose critical exercises per muscle group, including one or two sets for each exercise. Then select the appropriate weight to perform a correct technique without a problem, and rest between sets for a few minutes. Each repetition should be performed at medium speed, and doing this twice every week for each muscle group is usually enough for good. Current recommendations of physical activity for health by the World Health Organization include 150 minutes of moderate physical activity (aerobic exercise) a week combined with muscle-strengthening activities 2 days a week or more (6).

Common obstacles and risks of resistance training
Generally, to be effective, resistance training needs to be done two to three times per week. This sounds easy, but there are some obstacles to be aware of.

- You may not feel immediate improvements. Even though there's a connection between
- resistance training and pain sensitivity, it does not produce rapid shifts in pain perception.
- Massage or relaxation training work in tandem with resistance training.
- Real improvements in this area take time: on average, 10 to 12 weeks.
- Change your lifestyle and habits.
- Resistance training requires time commitment and persistence. If you're not committed or cannot stick to it, you aren't likely to get the outcome you are seeking. Resistance training may not be the thing that everyone needs for their type of chronic pain, or it may not fit into theirneeds at a particular time.Here are a few more things to be aware of:
- Strength-training injuries: Be careful hitting the weights without anyprofessional help; no mastery of exercise plan may not only reduce the benefits but also get you injured. Getting injured in the process of trying to relieve pain is a common issue, and this is why you should seek help from a professional.
- Imprecise exercise protocols for the type of pain: Certain types of chronic pain won't respond well to aggressive resistance training. Some, like fibromyalgia, need to be very carefully monitored because the training program may continually need to be adjusted based on how the person is feeling. Frozen shoulder is another issue that may not respond well to strength training at all, and, in fact, it may make it much worse.

Resistance training (anaerobic exercise) certainly has its place in the therapeutic regime of the chronic pain sufferer. It is highly effective, but it must be applied to the right kind of pain issue, in the right way, and progress over time as the person adapts to the program. Exercise is often recommended for many different health conditions, especially those related to the cardiovascular system. Still, it's certainly not the only area where it may be precious. Living a sedentary lifestyle is a fairly significant risk factor for health issues, and it is not only limited to stroke and heart disease. Although many people are apprehensive of being more active when they have pain, studies show that physical activity improves symptoms of chronic pain in the short and long term. There are two primary forms of physical activity (aerobic and anaerobic), and each of them is associated with an improvement in chronic pain.

We're going to focus on aerobic exercise (often referred to as "cardio") and how pain mechanisms can be inhibited by this simple form of movement.

What happens when you do aerobic exercise? During aerobic exercise, the most significant changes involve the respiration and cardiovascular systems. Your muscles play an essential part, and the stroke volume of your heart increases to make up for the increased requirement of oxygen and nutrients. The function of your capillaries is enhanced, and the parts of your cells that produce energy, called mitochondria, increase in both number and efficiency.

Additionally, there are many nervous system and hormonal adaptations that occur after aerobic exercise. These changes improve both strength and stamina and have the ability to reduce insulin resistance and other metabolic problems. Aerobic exercise can also play a role in improving flexibility, balance, and coordination and also positively impact muscle/postural asymmetry. All of these improvements can be associated with various pain inhibitory mechanisms that we discuss below.

How does aerobic exercise inhibit pain? The exact mechanism by which physical activity improves chronic pain symptoms is not entirely understood. Unfortunately, the vast majority of clinical trials do not make a clear distinction between aerobic and anaerobic physical activity when examining the effects of exercise on pain perception. Studies are composed of interventions, therapeutic recommendations, and patient education. The variety of sources makes it challenging to set aside and evaluate the differences between aerobic and anaerobic exercise separately.
A distinction based on short- and long-term effects of aerobic exercise:

Short-term pain inhibition from aerobic exercise
Reduction of pain perception, called hypoalgesia, has been reported after physical activity in healthy individuals, people with chronic pain, and people with experimentally induced pain. The two mechanisms involved in the short-

term numbing effect are the release of endorphins and a modulation in the pain pathways in the central nervous system.

According to studies, after high-intensity aerobic exercise, there's a hypoalgesic (numbing) effect lasting approximately 30 minutes. This effect is longer compared to that after resistance-training exercise (anaerobic exercise), which lasts only a few minutes. Studies seem to show that more exercise or higher intensity is related to more hyperalgesia. The suggestion is that to generate a considerable effect, we should engage in high-intensity physical activity for more than 10 minutes or moderate to high physical activity for 30 minutes or more. Now, of course, you can imagine this wouldn't work in many scenarios. For example, some clinical trials have reported an INCREASED pain response instead of pain inhibition in cases of individuals with severe chronic pain. People with fibromyalgia, for example, do not have immediate pain inhibition after physical activity. However, of course, they can still benefit from exercise in the long run.

Long-term pain inhibition from aerobic exercise
The long-term pain inhibitory effects of aerobic exercise are reported only in individuals who maintained a regular program of activity. Long-term activity modulates the endocannabinoid system. These natural cannabis-like molecules produced by the human body reduce inflammation by improving circulation and normalize the transmission of glutamate and pyruvate in the brain and muscle tissue. By altering the release of inflammatory substances and improving circulation, it is possible to reduce swelling and other symptoms that may be associated with some chronic pain issues. Our endocannabinoid system has a strong inhibitory effect that is often targeted by pain medications. The same is also modulated by aerobic activity upon releasing endorphins. Glutamate and pyruvate are essential for sensory perception in the muscle tissue, the transmission of which is key to the central nervous system. By reducing these substances, physical activity may modulate pain perception in the long run.

The psychological effect of exercise
We can't talk about pain perception without including the cerebral function. It is well established that depression, anxiety, and similar mental health problems increase pain perception.

Individuals who engage in aerobic exercise usually report a significant improvement in mood and psychological symptoms, which may have a positive effect on the chronic pain experience. There are not, however, enough studies to evaluate these changes in a large number of people suffering from chronic pain.

So, does aerobic exercise help? Yes! In a nutshell, aerobic exercise is known to reduce pain perception immediately after exercise and in the long run. For long-lasting results, it is necessary to engage in sustained activity. In most cases of chronic pain, patients would also benefit from combining some aerobic exercise with anaerobic exercise. By joining the strengthening nature of anaerobic exercise and the physiological changes mentioned in this chapter, it is possible to reduce pain symptoms and improve the quality of life for chronic pain sufferers.

4. Goal setting

Pain relief should not be the only target of a therapeutic program. While obviously an important one, some types of chronic pain conditions do not simply go away completely. Instead, one must learn how to live alongside it. As sensitivity to pain is high already in those with chronic pain, continuing to solely focus on the changes in pain sensitivity by itself often leads to greater frustration, worry, fear, anxiety and therefore more pain.

Improved function on the other hand leads to improvement in quality of life and improved coping. One of the most debilitating aspects of chronic pain is the effect it has on an individual's ability to be active, work, and play. When pain can be reduced, these activities can often be modified and returned to, leading to positive impact on all elements of the biopsychosocial system. This in turn leads to sending more messages of safety to the nervous system, which often results in less pain. For some, the road to where they want to be may be long, which can be overwhelming without setting smaller, attainable goals that inspire, motivate, and reward accomplishments. Dealing with a lot of common life stressors on top of dealing with pain can be very overwhelming. This can sap your energy and wear you down as life's demands stack up. Setting priorities and simple goals to do a little at a time can add up over time and reduce the sensitivity of your alarm system, and therefore pain.

While these are the largest and arguably the most important categories that are needed to address chronic pain, they certainly aren't the only helpful ones. The importance of addressing nutrition, application of manual therapies, and mindfulness techniques such as meditation, hypnotherapy, or even psychological counseling should not be overlooked as important therapeutic interventions to employ.

I hope this chapter has shed some light on how to approach your chronic pain with an updated, scientific rationale, and make educated and informed decisions based on what the current research suggests. Numerous additional areas are currently being studied, such as the role of inflammation and nutritional strategies to reduce sensitivity in chronic pain. These approaches are very promising, with many healthcare providers achieving successful outcomes currently. We anxiously await their findings in order to expand our knowledge and provide even more resources to chronic pain sufferers.

Works Cited

Augle, K. M., & Riley 3rd, J. L. (2014). Self-reported physical activity predicts pain inhibitory and facilitatory function. Medicine and science in sports and exercise, 46(3), 622.

Bender, T., Nagy, G., Barna, I., Tefner, I., Kádas, É., & Géher, P. (2007). The effect of physical therapy on beta-endorphin levels. European journal of applied physiology, 100(4), 371-382.

Gerdle, B., Ernberg, M., Mannerkorpi, K., Larsson, B., Kosek, E., Christidis, N., & Ghafouri, B. (2016). Increased interstitial concentrations of glutamate and pyruvate in vastus lateralis of women with fibromyalgia syndrome are normalized after an exercise intervention–a case-control study. PloS one, 11(10), e0162010.

Ghafouri, N., Ghafouri, B., Fowler, C. J., Larsson, B., Turkina, M. V., Karlsson, L., & Gerdle, B. (2014). Effects of two different specific neck exercise interventions on palmitoylethanolamide and stearoylethanolamide concentrations in the interstitium of the trapezius muscle in women with chronic neck shoulder pain. Pain Medicine, 15(8), 1379-1389.

Kawi, J., Lukkahatai, N., Inouye, J., Thomason, D., & Connelly, K. (2016). Effects of exercise on select biomarkers and associated outcomes in chronic pain conditions: systematic review. Biological research for nursing, 18(2), 147-159.

Kisner, Colby, Borstad. Title: Therapeutic Exercise: Foundations and Techniques. F.A. Davis Company, 2018.

Koltyn, K. F. (2002). Exercise-induced hypoalgesia and intensity of exercise. Sports medicine, 32(8), 477-487.

Liebenson,. Craig, Rehabilitation of the Spine : a Practitioner's Manual. Philadelphia :Lippincott Williams & Wilkins, 2003.

Morris, Craig. Title: Low Back Syndromes: Integrated Clinical. McGraw-Hill Medical/Jaypee Brothers Medical Publishers, 2005.

Naugle, K. M., Fillingim, R. B., & Riley III, J. L. (2012). A meta- analytic review of the hypoalgesic effects of exercise. The Journal of pain, 13(12), 1139-1150.

Nijs, J., Kosek, E., Van Oosterwijck, J., & Meeus, M. (2012). Dysfunctional endogenous analgesia during exercise in patients with chronic pain: to exercise or not to exercise?. Pain physician, 15(3S), ES205-ES213.

Occupational Hearing Loss · Workers Compensation. https:// www.napolilaw. com/practice-areas/workers-compensation/ occupational-hearing-loss/

Sajedi, H., & Bas, M. (2016). The evaluation of the aerobic exercise effects on pain tolerance. Sport Science, 9, 7-11.

Visnic, Sam. Why Didn't My Doctor Tell Me That? 2020. Visnic Center For Integrated Health Inc. and Sam Visnic.

https://content.iospress.com/articles/journal-of-back-and-musculoskeletal-rehabilitation/bmr170920

https://www.sciencedirect.com/science/article/abs/pii/ S1526590012008085

https://www.cochranelibrary.com/cdsr/doi/10.1002/14651858.CD010884/ abstract

https://www.hindawi.com/journals/bmri/2016/4137918/abs/

https://www.ncbi.nlm.nih.gov/books/NBK305057/

CHAPTER VII

Welcome to my chapter discussing the biopsychosocial aspects of the foundations of health with a focus on stress management, restorative sleep, and balanced nutrition. My name is Dr. Lanae Mullane, a naturopathic doctor (ND) practicing in California. I completed my training at Bastyr University, nestled in the beautiful Saint Edward State Park in Kenmore, Washington. After graduating, I was just the second ND to complete a residency alongside a rheumatologist.

My philosophy of medicine is rooted in the idea that it takes a village to treat a patient and that each healthcare provider plays a vital role in that patient's outcome and healthcare journey. Throughout my residency and career history, I have chosen to work within integrative health clinics with medical doctors, doctors of osteopathic medicine, and registered dieticians. Providing care in these settings allows for the strengths of each form of medicine to shine through to give a genuinely whole-person approach to treating patients.

Currently, I work as the Director of Nutrition for Vejo. Our company uses a portable, pod-based blender utilizing farm-fresh freeze-dried fruit and vegetable biodegradable blends in formulas to help people live happier and healthier lives. I am also the medical director of a wellness-based clinic called Vejo+ that focuses on optimizing health with evidence-based treatments through laboratory testing, nutraceutical recommendations, and personalized lifestyle and behavioral changes. All Vejo+ members start with an in-depth look at their fundamentals of health because creating a solid foundation is vital in developing resilience.

What is Naturopathic Medicine?

Naturopathic medicine is a distinct healthcare profession rooted in the wisdom of nature that still follows modern scientific standards of care. Naturopathic doctors are trained in rigorous doctoral-level medical education at one of seven accredited naturopathic medical school programs in North America. NDs use evidence-informed therapies focusing on an individualized, whole-person approach to support the body's innate ability to heal while working to identify the root cause of illness. The basis of the practice of naturopathic medicine is established in the six naturopathic principles.

The Six Naturopathic Principles:

1. **First, Do No Harm (Primum non nocere):** Choosing the least invasive and least toxic therapies, referring to an appropriate provider when a patient's presentation is outside of scope.

2. **The Healing Power of Nature (Vis medicatrix naturae):** Creating a healthy environment as the foundation to human health by utilizing substances that originate in nature to support the body's innate wisdom to heal itself.

3. **Identify and Treat the Causes (Tolle causam):** Identifying, addressing, and removing the underlying cause of illness.

4. **Doctor as Teacher (Docere):** Supporting and empowering patients in their health management through education.

5. **Treat the Whole Person (Tolle totum):** Treating the patient, not the disease, by identifying the interconnectedness of our body to our environment and lifestyle as an integrated whole of total health.

6. **Prevention (Praevenic):** Focusing on overall wellness and disease prevention utilizing these six principles to identify potential areas of imbalance to educate patients on how to get and stay well.

A common misconception is that NDs are homeopaths. Homeopathy is the treatment of ailments using minute doses of natural substances that in a healthy person would produce symptoms of the disease. While NDs have some training in the modality of homeopathy, not all NDs use it in their practice. NDs are united more by the dynamic philosophy of the Naturopathic Principles and Therapeutic Order than a specific modality of medicine. Naturopathic treatments can include botanical medicine, nutrition, hydrotherapy, pharmaceuticals, minor surgery, and lifestyle and behavioral changes.

Building Resilience Through the Fundamentals of Health
Creating the foundation for one's health has always been a staple in naturopathic philosophy. Considering recent world events, paying attention to wellness has become even more vital. Building resilience through focusing on the fundamentals helps our body withstand, adapt to, and recover quickly from adversity and

unfavorable situations that challenge our health. Some may be born resilient, but our bodies can also improve our innate resilience. Concerning health, this idea can be achieved by optimizing three critical aspects of wellness: stress management, restorative sleep, and balanced nutrition. By focusing on the fundamentals, we create healthy soil for our bodies to flourish and thrive I will be breaking down the three aspects of foundational wellness by discussing the biology, psychosocial, and contextual features of naturopathy alongside integrative approaches that can influence one's health resilience.

Stress Management

Biological: How stress affects our body
The stress response is a standard and adaptive coping mechanism that humans have relied on for millions of years for protection (e.g., running from a bear in the wild). The stress response was designed exceptionally well for acute stressors that resolve quickly. Unfortunately, in our modern society, daily life events can lead to chronic or continuous mild stress exposures. The physiological stress response—higher heart rate, shallow and rapid breathing, increased release of adrenaline, noradrenaline, and cortisol—can occur whether you are running from a bear or sitting in the morning rush hour. As complex as the body is, it is not necessarily able to discern the differences between stressors.

Within the body, the neuroendocrine adaptation component of the stress response system is known as the hypothalamic-pituitary-adrenal axis (HPA axis). Once the body perceives the presence of a stressor, a cascade of biological events occurs, starting in an area of the brain called the hypothalamus. The hypothalamus maintains homeostasis by responding to various signals from the internal and external environment, including hunger, blood pressure, thermoregulation, and hormones. The hypothalamus releases corticotropin-releasing hormone (CRH) to the pituitary gland, sending a message via adrenocorticotropic hormone (ACTH) through the blood to the adrenal glands, which sit on top of both kidneys. The adrenal glands secrete cortisol, the "stress hormone," which controls a vast array of physiological processes, such as metabolic (raising blood sugar), immune (weakening immune response), ion transport (preventing sodium loss and accelerating potassium excretion from a cell), and memory (overwhelming the hippocampus, causing atrophy). The circulating cortisol activates a "negative feedback loop" in which the hypothalamus ceases production of CRH, which stops the pituitary from creating ACTH, thus returning the body to homeostasis.

You may also feel the physiologic effects of stress in the gastrointestinal tract: Have you ever had a "gut feeling"? That has to do with the gut-brain axis. The gut is sometimes called the "second brain" or the enteric nervous system, consisting of millions of nerve cells that line the gastrointestinal tract from the mouth to the rectum. The brain has direct effects on the digestive tract, including the stomach and intestines. The mere thought of eating food can release digestive enzymes in saliva, the stomach, and the pancreas before you even place a bite in your mouth. Issues in the gut can send signals to the brain, just as issues in the brain can signal the digestive tract; the gut and the brain are closely interconnected: Are digestive issues the cause or the result of stress and anxiety? What's more, the lining of the digestive tract also contains a majority of your body's serotonin receptors, and serotonin is a chemical needed for nerve cells and brain function and also plays a critical role in mood and cognition.

In addition to cortisol and gastrointestinal health, prolonged exposure to chronic stress can have negative impacts on numerous other areas of health, including disrupting the digestive, immune, sleep, reproductive, and cardiovascular systems and leading to heart disease, weight changes, high blood pressure, anxiety, depression, and diabetes.

Psychosocial: Daily adverse experiences and our ability to cope
The impacts of stress and adversity can be physiological, as noted above, and psychological, affecting people's social behavior. Stress can have a powerful influence on one's ability to show empathy and financial generosity, and can promote aggressive behavior or perpetuate violence. Exposures to stress as early as pre-conception, prenatal, or infancy can contribute to variable health outcomes, from chronic metabolic diseases to developmental delays. Adverse childhood experiences (ACEs) have been shown to create excessive activation of the stress response, leading to long-term mental and physical repercussions. Research is now trying to understand better how experiences transmitted through generational trauma can alter DNA (called cross-generational epigenetics).

Since 2007, the American Psychological Association (APA) has issued a yearly survey, Stress in AmericaTM, to people in the United States to identify the leading causes and impacts of stress. Throughout the thirteen surveys conducted, the contributors of external stress were influenced by economic decline, political conflict, racial disparities, and discrimination. The impact of the COVID pandemic highlighted increased stress in 2020. Most adults in the U.S. report experiencing daily discrimination based on age, race, disability, gender, sexual orientation, and gender identity.[1] The results of these discriminations can lead to heightened vigilance and changes in behavior, which can initiate the stress cascade contributing to poorer health outcomes.

Contextual: Impact of environment on stress

Our environment can have a profound impact on both physiological and psychosocial contributions to stress. Commuting in Los Angeles for years, I can personally acknowledge the increase in blood pressure and shortness of breath when sitting in bumper-to-bumper traffic. Having also lived in Seattle for school, I have experienced the lack of sun and its influence on the seasonal affective disorder. Our surroundings—whether loud noises, lack of personal space, food unavailability, or chemical exposures—affect our daily stress response.

Exposures to environmental toxins can also act as facilitators of chronic disease. We are likely exposed to hundreds of these daily without even realizing it. This exposure contributes to physiologic stress in the body (and the planet). Environmental toxins are also referred to as endocrine-disrupting chemicals (EDC) or hormone-disrupting chemicals. EDCs are external chemicals that interfere with any aspect of hormonal action and have been found in breast milk, blood, and urine. The endocrine system includes glands and receptors in tissues and organs that respond to hormones. Small exposures over time accumulate to measurable levels in the human body. They can contribute to adverse health outcomes like cancer, reproductive complications, and cardiovascular and metabolic diseases through oxidative stress, autonomic imbalance, vascular dysfunction, systemic inflammation, and HPA activation.

Some of the more notorious environmental toxins that people are exposed to are:

- Glyphosates are found in weed killers.
- Polychlorinated biphenyls (PCBs) are found in oil-based paint, insulation, electrical equipment, and caulking material.
- Bisphenol A (BPA) is found in hard/rigid plastics, metal food cans, thermal receipts.
- Phthalates are found in toys, detergents, lubricating oils, food packaging, pharmaceuticals, and vinyl floors.
- Parabens are antimicrobial preservatives found in personal care products.

Stress Management: An integrative approach to stress

No one is immune to stress; however, it is possible to change our body's response to it. The process may not be easy and will likely take some practice, yet one of the fastest, most cost-effective stress-reducing techniques is utilizing the power of the breath. Breathing is controlled by the autonomic nervous system, which allows a person to continue to breathe while sleeping or unconscious; it simultaneously will enable one to control the rate of breath consciously. Although breathing is something people have been doing since birth, we are not always the most efficient. Poor posture, shallow breathing, and breath-holding are common occurrences that we are conditioned to in our busy lives and our more sedentary computer work environments. Conscious breathing is an essential step in the reduction of stress.

Supporting an optimal breathing environment begins before the inhale. Start with your feet flat on the floor with the body in an upright position and shoulders relaxed. To remove "accessory" muscles that contribute to more shallow chest breathing, place hands on both sides near the lowest ribs. Inhale through the nose, pause, and exhale through the mouth. Allow the exhale to be longer than the inhale, as the exhale stimulates the parasympathetic nervous system via stimulation of the vagus nerve on the diaphragm, telling the brain to relax. When doing breathing exercises, to reduce the risk of feeling light-headed, place more emphasis on the rate of the breath versus the volume. Pursing the lips as if drinking through a straw when exhaling can help slow down the rate. Repeat at least four times.

Once behavioral tools are in place, a medical professional may want to do salivary cortisol testing, followed by herbal nutraceuticals to support cortisol homeostasis. A form of nutraceutical, adaptogens have been used for centuries worldwide to modulate cortisol balance by structurally resembling adrenal hormones. Some of the more commonly used adaptogenic herbs are ashwagandha (Withania somnifera), astragalus (Astragalus membranaceus), Rhodiola (Rhodiola rosea), and eleuthero (Eleutherococcus senticosus).

Another way to reduce environmental stress is to limit exposure to EDCs in toxic chemicals. Avoid plastics with recycling #3 and #7, food wrapped in plastic packaging, heating food in plastic containers, and canned foods. When possible, consume foods that are fresh, frozen, or organic. Use glass or stainless steel containers and hand-wash plastic containers. Go paperless and say no to thermal receipts. Cleanse your home and body with natural cleaning products. For more helpful resources, the Environmental Working Group has created a repository of products rated from least to most toxic.

Chronic stress comes in many shapes and forms, from physiological to emotional to environmental, all carrying potential negative health implications. Your ability to control some stressors may be unlikely, but your ability to control how your body responds to that stress is more likely. As a society, acknowledging the detrimental impacts of stress by supporting healthier work environments/requirements, dismantling racial disparities, providing access to healthcare, creating more inclusive spaces, reducing environmental toxins, and offering more mental health support would help minimize exposure to stressors. On an individual level, try to incorporate stress management techniques into your daily routine to increase the usefulness of your tools; this way, you can combat stressors as they arise. Find a stress management technique that works for you, whether that is breathing techniques, movement, talking to friends, utilizing the expertise of a therapist, being out in nature, or scheduling a bi-monthly massage. Whatever you choose, strive to make it a ritual in your self-care practice.

Sleep

Biological: How sleep affects our body
Sleep is one of the most important components to establishing a foundation of health. An inability to achieve restorative sleep leads to profound stress in the body, contributing to poor health outcomes such as chronic illness, mood disorders, hormone dysregulation, immune dysfunction, and insulin resistance. In children and young adults, sleep is when the human growth hormone is released to help with development. Sleep helps create new synapses in the brain. And yet, a growing number of people battle with nonrestorative sleep or sleep that does not result in a feeling of being rested. Research for optimal quantities of hours of sleep for overall health is still being developed. Still, the current consensus for an adult is seven to nine hours, with younger populations needing more. Lack of sleep is known to affect memory, performance, and lifespan negatively. A CDC survey reported that adults who received less than the recommended seven hours of sleep were more likely to report ten chronic health conditions, including depression, arthritis, and diabetes.[2]

To reach restorative sleep, we need to address both sleep quality and quantity. Sleep quality refers to uninterrupted sleep that reaches each stage of the sleep cycle: awake, light sleep, deep sleep, and REM sleep. These stages may also be referred to as NREM (non-rapid eye movement) and REM (rapid eye movement). Generally, the body will transition through each cycle stage sequentially four to five times over 90 minutes, with earlier sleep tending to favor deep sleep, while later in the night selecting more REM sleep.

Sleep itself plays a vital role in the regulation of hormones. As the sun sets and the light dims, your body naturally produces the hormone melatonin. Melatonin does not make you sleep but does contribute to a sensation of heavy eyelids and quiet wakefulness that prepares the body for sleep. Jet lag, change in time zones, or working night shifts can impact the body's melatonin production. Sleep is also crucial for regulating cortisol and testosterone; poor sleep quality or insufficient sleep can disrupt endocrine production. As discussed previously, cortisol is the body's stress hormone produced by the adrenal glands. Disruption of cortisol can lead to issues with the digestive, immune, sleep, reproductive, and cardiovascular systems. In cisgender men, most testosterone is released during sleep, and sleep deprivation is associated with producing lower amounts of testosterone, essential for reproduction, libido, muscle mass, and bone density.

In menstruating females, menstrual cycles have been linked to disruptions in circadian rhythms with reported inferior sleep quality during the premenstrual week. Women in the perimenopausal stage are the most likely to struggle with insomnia.

The sleep-immune connection is clear: There is no doubt that an illness can lead to an increased feeling of being tired, and a good night's sleep is commonly recommended when feeling under the weather. Sleep influences the immune system through proteins called cytokines, which not only support a restful night's sleep but also increase when there is an infection or inflammation. A lack of sleep can lower the body's production of these cytokines and weaken the body's defense system. This response can increase susceptibility to cold and flu infections, as well as affect how fast someone may recover once sick.

Psychosocial: Societal influences on sleep behavior
While diagnosable sleep disorders such as insomnia, narcolepsy, sleep apnea, and restless leg syndrome are sleep disruptors, they are not the only contributors to poor sleep. Numerous societal norms contribute to an unrestful night's sleep. Alcohol, caffeine, and sleep medications are some of the top culprits in today's society.

Alcohol is often used to help people unwind from a long day, celebrate the end of a workday, or mitigate stressful life situations due to its sedative effects that can induce a sense of relaxation. A couple of glasses of alcohol may cause a feeling of relaxation, but as the alcohol metabolizes, the relaxing effect wears off. This response disrupts the deep sleep and REM sleep cycles, leading to sleep that is not deep or long in duration; this contributes to extensive adverse effects and increases daytime sleepiness.

Caffeine can trigger our sympathetic "flight, fight, or freeze" response, leading to an increase in epinephrine, also known as adrenaline. This response is the same autonomic nervous system response that our body perceives a situation as problematic or dangerous. Caffeine can cause an increase in heart rate, disruption in sleep, digestive disturbance, irritability, and agitation, all of which can increase your level of perceived stress and anxiety. Genetics may also play a role in how well the body handles caffeine. Variations in the CYP1A2 gene can determine if someone is a fast or slow metabolizer of caffeine. Slow metabolizers take longer for their bodies to process caffeine, contributing to possible adverse effects like insomnia and anxiety. Caffeine is classified as a stimulant drug with the exact mechanism of action as an adenosine receptor antagonist. Adenosine is a somnogenic substance, so caffeine consumption blocks the adenosine receptor, decreasing the sensation of sleepiness.

Medications prescribed or sold over-the-counter for sleep are a blanket approach and do not necessarily address personalized causes of sleep disruption. Current sleeping pills do not allow for standard patterns of restorative sleep, and most sleeping pills have a mechanism of action that focuses on GABA receptors of the brain to slow down the nervous system. Although these pills can allow a person to fall asleep, inducing a sensation of drowsiness, they can inhibit deeper brain waves during REM sleep, which is beneficial for problem-solving, learning, and memory. Disruptions in the REM sleep cycle may lead to grogginess the following morning. Overlooking the root cause of the sleep disruption can lead to an unhealthy dependence on sleeping pills.

Contextual: Impact of the environment on sleep
The use of portable electronic devices has been normalized in today's society, and it has become commonplace to have a screen in the bedroom. The increase in screen time has contributed to increased non-restorative sleep in children, adolescents, and adults. Screen entertainment can disrupt sleep causing a delay

in bedtime, and therefore, shortened sleep duration. The type of media watched before bed, like stimulating video games, news stories, television shows, movies, and social media, have been shown to increase arousal before bed. This is linked to delayed bedtime, an increased heart rate, and disruption to the REM sleep cycle. Similarly, light exposure from screens when the sun goes down has negatively impacted sleep quality and quantity. The evening light exposure maximizes a state of alertness, delaying the onset of sleep while also showing other side effects, such as postponing melatonin production and disrupting the circadian clock and REM sleep cycle.[3]

Shift work schedules, increasingly high-pressure job requirements, and a socioeconomic environment that increases the need for multiple jobs have also been shown to affect sleep negatively. Numerous workers' schedules do not fit into the traditional nine-to-five workday. Many are subject to rotating, longer hours, night, or on-call demands, leading to a disturbance in the natural circadian rhythm. Circadian refers to a cycle of roughly 24 hours that helps the body regulate essential systemic functions, including hunger, hormone levels, body temperature, alertness, and sleepiness. This "internal clock" is influenced by exposure to sunlight, creating a sense of day vs. night cycle. Shift workers have to go against this natural rhythm to stay awake, possibly leading to a loss of hours of sleep within 24 hours, contributing to the adverse effects of sleep deviation and an increased risk of insomnia.

Achieving Restorative Sleep: An integrative approach to sleep
As fundamental as sleep is to overall health, achieving restorative sleep can be challenging. When working with patients with disordered sleep, after ruling out pathology, the first area we address is called sleep hygiene. These are the different practices or rituals that support an environment for restorative night sleep, as well as full daytime alertness. This starts with keeping the bedroom for sleep and intimacy only as removing distractions allows your mind to acknowledge that your bed is a place for rest. Setting the thermostat cooler around 60-67o F can help make it easier to fall and stay asleep.

Setting a consistent bedtime is also important. As complex as the human body is, when it comes to sleep, the body prefers to keep it simple with routine. Maintaining a regular sleep-wake schedule (which includes weekdays and weekends), the body will support the internal clock by making it easier to fall asleep and wake up. Another important sleep hygiene tip is to turn off or set aside all electronic media devices about an hour before bed to calm the nervous system and reduce blue light exposures that can lower the body's production of melatonin.

If falling asleep is difficult, progressive muscle relaxation, or PMR, may be helpful. This distraction technique was introduced in the 1930s by a physician named Edmund Jacobson and involved rotating between contraction and relaxation of major muscle groups throughout the body. There are numerous ways to practice PMR, and here is an example that patients have found successful. The body should be situated in a comfortable position in a quiet environment. Starting with the toes, contract by curling the toes, then slowly release, counting to 30 seconds. Repeat three times. Move to the feet by flexing and slowly relaxing over 30 seconds. Repeat three times. Continue up the calves to the thighs to the glutes, to the hands, arms, neck, shoulders, jaw, and forehead. If a wandering thought enters your mind, start back at the toes. Most find it difficult to get past the thighs before falling asleep.

For some, falling asleep is the easy part, but staying asleep is more complicated. If awakened during the night and unable to fall asleep after roughly 15 minutes, get out of bed. The bed should only be used for sleep and intimacy. Tossing and turning for long periods can lead to an increased sensation of anxiety. The recommendation is to get out of bed and sit in a chair, listen to soft music, or turn on low light to read until you feel drowsy, then go back to bed. A possible culprit causing people to wake during the night may be a dip in blood sugar levels. This dip does not necessarily need to be large enough to be considered a hypoglycemic event but is enough to alert the body to wake. This is more common in people who eat dinner early—consuming a small handful of healthy fat or protein, like nuts, 30 minutes to an hour before bed can be enough to stabilize the blood sugar and keep a person asleep.

As I noted, caffeine is classified as a stimulant substance that can contribute to difficulty falling asleep. However, the FDA considers 400 mg of caffeine (three to four cups of coffee) per day to be safe, limiting caffeine intake to no more than one to two cups of coffee before noon can make sleeping easier. For some, switching to a lower caffeine drink such as matcha or green tea or eliminating caffeine ultimately may be necessary.

Herbs can be a gentle approach to add to your sleep routine. Herbal teas with nervine botanicals promote relaxation for natural sleep. They include chamomile

(Matricaria chamomilla), hops (Humulus lupulus), lavender (Lavendula Officinalis), lemon balm (Melissa officinalis), passionflower (Passiflora incarnata), skullcap (Scutellaria laterifolia), and valerian (Valeriana officinalis). The ritual of preparing and sipping on warm herbal tea can also be a relaxing addition to one's sleep hygiene routine. To avoid waking to urinate at night, have a cup or two an hour before bed.

Nutraceuticals may be needed as a slightly higher intervention than behavioral changes for the treatment of poor sleep. Magnesium is involved in over 300 different biochemical reactions in the body, including acting as a natural antagonist of N-Methyl-D-aspartic acid (NMDA) and an agonist of Gamma-aminobutyric acid (GABA), as well as playing a role in the regulation of central nervous system excitability, all of which are important in sleep regulation. Although magnesium is found in nuts, seeds, whole grains, and leafy greens, diets higher in more processed foods and soil nutrient depletion may be contributing to increased cases of magnesium deficiency. Plus, the form of magnesium matters. Cheaper forms of magnesium, like magnesium oxide, are poorly absorbed, contributing to a more laxative effect. The recommended form of magnesium for sleep is magnesium glycinate (a chelate of magnesium with the amino acid glycine). This is a bioavailable form that has been shown to improve sleep quality.

Other favorable supplements used to support sleep include 5-HTP, GABA, and melatonin. Serotonin is a precursor of the hormone melatonin and has been implicated in the regulation of sleep. 5-Hydroxytryptophan (5-HTP) is an intermediate metabolite of the essential amino acid L-tryptophan in the production of serotonin. Short-term, oral supplementing with 5-HTP is well absorbed and bypasses the conversion of L-tryptophan into 5-HTP with the aid of tryptophan hydroxylase enzyme. 5-HTP is contraindicated when taking SSRI antidepressants and MAO inhibitors which increase serotonin levels. Gamma-aminobutyric acid (GABA) is an amino acid and inhibitory neurotransmitter. The natural form of GABA can lower stress-related beta waves and increase alpha waves in the brain to create a sensation of physical relaxation and enhanced sleep.

The most popular sleep supplement is melatonin, most commonly used for jet lag, shift work, and primary sleep disorders. The typical dosage of melatonin ranges from 1 mg to 5 mg. A meta-analysis showed that melatonin improved sleep by reducing sleep-onset latency, improving sleep quality, and increasing total sleep time compared to placebo.[4] In contrast to hypnotic sleep medications, the study also found no indications of the development of tolerance with the use of melatonin.[4] Nearly a third of our life is spent sleeping, making sleep one of the body's most important foundations of health. Creating a relaxing environment conducive for the body and mind for sleep, removing potential stimulus triggers during the day, and being consistent with a routine will help set you up for a successful, refreshing night's sleep that supports the immune system, hormones, memory, energy, and overall wellness.

Nutrition

Biological: How nutrition affects the body
When discussing the importance of nutrition and food on our foundation of health, it is essential to understand the relationship between how food is digested and how nutrients are utilized in the body. The terms "gut," digestive tract, or gastrointestinal system refers to the hollow organs of the mouth, esophagus, stomach, small intestine, large intestine, and anus. Although these hollow organs are found inside the body, they are considered "outside" since ingested contents need to be absorbed "inside" the body. If they are not interested, the contents will be excreted. The gastrointestinal system also includes the solid organs of the pancreas, liver, and gallbladder.

In the digestive tract is a complex ecosystem called the microbiome. There are trillions of microorganisms made up of mainly anaerobic (existing in the absence of oxygen) bacteria and fungi, viruses, and parasites. Over 1000 different microbial bacteria species have been identified to reside in the intestinal microbiome.[5] The microbiome starts with exposure to microorganisms as a baby leaves the birth canal and with the introduction of breast milk. Environmental, medication, genetics, and dietary exposures throughout life will alter the microbiome to support health or increase the risk of disease. The microbiota contributes to digestion by synthesizing vitamins and amino acids, communicating with the intestinal cells, and strengthening the immune system. The fluctuating microbiome can be influenced by a diversified diet, adequate dietary fiber, or consumption of processed foods.

In addition to altering our microbiota, food is vital as a foundation for our overall health. The focus on the impact of food on health and disease prevention has always fostered an interest. Over 2000 years ago, Hippocrates espoused us to "Let food be thy medicine and medicine be thy food." A diet depleted of certain nutrients or with an excess of sodium has been linked to increased high blood pressure, cholesterol, type 2 diabetes, certain cancers, and deficits in brain development.

"Functional foods" have risen in popularity recently, and they go beyond providing basic nutrition. They contain potentially positive health benefits and are correlated with a reduction in disease risk. The most commonly used example of functional food is oats. The FDA approved the cholesterol-lowering health claim that oats can reduce the risk of coronary artery disease due to the beta-glucan soluble fiber.

Nutrition impacts each of the body's systems, with nutrition and the endocrine system particularly intricately intertwined. In addition to the endocrine system's role in growth, blood pressure, sleep, and reproduction, this organ system also regulates appetite, metabolism, and nutrient storage, absorption, and use. A protein deficiency can affect the release of gonadal hormones preventing reproduction, low body fat in cisgender females can stop menstruation, and malnourished children produce less growth hormone. Probably the most famous connection between nutrition and the endocrine system is the link between overnutrition of quickly absorbed sugars and empty calories to the development of type 2 diabetes. The body produces insulin from the pancreas to maintain balanced blood sugar, but increased demands for more insulin to keep the blood sugar balanced can eventually lead to insulin resistance, diabetes, and metabolic health problems.

Food quality and quantity are known factors to affect health, but an emerging area of research is exploring the importance of a person's genetic makeup. Nutrigenomics, a portmanteau of nutritional genomics, is an area of science that looks at how food affects our genes. This focus of study aids in the personalization of medicine and health by examining how an individual's genetic makeup affects the body's response to nutrients or bioactive compounds found in the food that they consume. Nutrigenomic research has shown some promising information on biomarkers of metabolic syndrome, nutrient intake, and genetic polymorphisms concerning micronutrient metabolism and absorption. The use of nutrigenomics in a clinical setting to provide applicable, reliable, and predictable dietary recommendations for improved health is still in the early stages of nutrition research, but the potential is exciting.

Psychosocial: Mental health and its influence on nutrition
Mental health should be addressed in a whole-person approach, with nutrition being only one aspect utilized as an adjunctive treatment. As mentioned when discussing the psychosocial element of stress, the enteric nervous system—the gut-brain axis—can influence mood as the gut and the brain are closely connected. The brain has direct effects on the digestive tract, including on the stomach and intestines.

Most bacteria in the digestive tract can produce the neurotransmitters dopamine and serotonin sent to receptors in the brain to influence mood and behavior. While it is important to note that dietary changes alone may not necessarily cure mental health conditions, changes in dietary patterns may help reduce symptoms, increase energy, and support our ability to adapt better to the stress that may contribute to anxiety or depression.

One such diet, the Mediterranean Diet, has been associated with lower cardiovascular risk, and research has shown positive results in this diet's reducing depression- and anxiety-related symptoms. The PREDI-DEP study showed evidence for the effectiveness of using the Mediterranean Diet to prevent the recurrence of depression and improving the quality of life in patients with past reported episodes of depression.[6] The Mediterranean Diet is based on the eating habits of the traditional cuisine of countries bordering the Mediterranean Sea and consists of a high intake of vegetables, fruits, whole grains, beans, nuts, seeds, and olive oil. The diet recommends choosing poultry and fish over less lean protein sources like red meat, and healthy fats over saturated and trans fats.

The Gut-and-Psychology Syndrome (GAPS) Diet addresses the gut-brain connection, utilizing a dietary plan derived from the Specific Carbohydrate Diet. This dietary plan was created for those suffering from intestinal and neurological conditions due to an imbalance of the microbiota in the digestive tract. GAPS aims to remove foods that can be challenging for the body to digest and may cause disruption to the gut bacteria and replace them with nutrient-dense food options to support a healthy intestinal permeability. This diet can be difficult, and proponents recommended users get support from a doctor or nutritionist trained in GAPS diet protocol.

Specific foods and drinks have been associated with contributing to worsening anxiety and depression. Caffeine can cause an increase in heart rate, disruption in sleep, digestive disturbance, irritability, and agitation; all can increase one's level of perceived stress and anxiety. Alcohol is often used to mitigate stressful life situations due to its sedative-like effects that can cause a sense of relaxation. Although alcohol may reduce anxiety temporarily, it also has the possibility of increasing anxiety within a few hours after consumption that can last into the following day. After the euphoric effects of alcohol fade, the levels of the neurotransmitter serotonin also decrease. This can lead to feelings of anxiousness and depression. Indulging in sugary comfort foods—whether to cope with painful emotions or stress—has been shown to temporarily reduce the activity of our stress response through the HPA axis. Yet, this temporary alleviation of stress can lead to perpetuating emotional eating habits. Consuming sugary foods can also lead to a spike and quick drop in blood sugar that can cause uneasiness, changes in mood, and feelings similar to a panic attack. This can turn into a cycle of gravitating to something sweet every time you need a boost in mood or energy, leading to a rollercoaster of highs and lows that can contribute to anxiety.

Contextual: Impact of environment on what we eat

The environment plays a significant role in the quality and quantity of nutrients found in our food. The use of monoculture agriculture, a single crop in a specific area, negatively impacts our food and environmental ecological systems. Monoculture goes against nature by cultivating a lack of diversity: removing plant species that would provide nutrients to the soil leads to fewer microorganisms and fewer insect species, leading to the possibility that a single population could overwhelm the crops. This then leads to the increased use of synthetic herbicides, insecticides, and fertilizers. Microorganisms cannot process the inorganic material into organic matter, leading to poisons leaching into the soil and potentially polluting groundwater.

Likewise, ease of access to a variety of nutrient-rich foods is a significant public health issue. The USDA's Economic Research Service identified 6,500 food deserts in the United States.[7] Food deserts are areas where the population has limited access to a variety of healthy and affordable food. Locations with a higher percentage of minority populations and higher poverty rates are more likely to experience food deserts. These areas also tend to have limited access to health care, transportation, and recreational areas.

Cultural influences on food choices are commonly overlooked. The Mediterranean and even vegetarian diets have been heavily researched but have left numerous other ethnically diverse diets, such as Native American, African, and Persian. Nutrition experts are looking to change the dialogue. Dr. Kera Nyemb-Diop, who holds a Ph.D. in nutrition science and a master's in food science, works with black women to "decolonize your plate" to nurture the body and let go of food guilt and shame. She believes that food fuels not only the body but also one's heritage and traditions. She sheds light on the lack of research on culturally diverse diets and the trend of labeling traditional black food as "unhealthy."

Balanced Nutrition: An integrative approach to food

Approaching patients with personalized dietary modification interventions has been the most effective way to alter behavior, contributing to long-term success and improved health outcomes. Considering cultural background, medical history, daily output, economic access, relationship to food, goals, dietary sensitivities, and preferences means that a universal dietary recommendation is unlikely to yield sustainable results. Although working with a trained healthcare provider is recommended for guidance and support, individuals can make changes independently.

For those not struggling with specific gastrointestinal complaints but desiring a better understanding of simple changes for nutrition guidance, the Healthy Eating Plate recommendations provided by Harvard's School of Public Health is a good starting point.[8] The Healthy Eating Plate focuses on what's on your plate. One half should consist of assorted colorful vegetables and some fruit, one-fourth of whole grains (e.g., quinoa, brown rice, oats, barley, and whole wheat), one-fourth of protein (e.g., beans, nuts, and fish and poultry; limiting red meat and no processed meats), healthy fats in moderation (olive oil, ghee, coconut oil, avocado, nuts, and seeds), and finishing the plate with water, tea, or coffee. If tolerated, dairy consumption is limited to, at most, two servings daily. The main point is to create a balanced plate with quality ingredients. The use of spices and herbs is not indicated in the recommendations but is encouraged.

For those with gastrointestinal complaints (e.g., bloating, diarrhea, constipation, and gas), skin disorders, fatigue, allergies, and autoimmune conditions where an underlying condition has been diagnosed or ruled out, the Elimination/Re-challenge Program may be recommended. The Elimination/Re-challenge Program is used to identify possible underlying foods contributing to a patient's unwanted symptoms. This is the gold standard for identifying food sensitivities. To begin the Elimination part of the program, an individual removes the most common dietary allergies: dairy, gluten, eggs, soy, nuts, peanuts, shellfish, corn, alcohol, and caffeine for 21 days. The symptom(s) should show an improvement within that time. In specific scenarios, it may be necessary to remove a broader range of foods, including nightshades, legumes, citrus foods, or food colorings. Once the 21 days have been completed, the patient moves from the Elimination phase to the Re-challenge stage, in which a single food group is re-introduced every three days with two to three servings of that particular food item per day. After the three days, the patient will return to the Elimination phase for two days to ensure no delayed sensitivity reactions. If a person does not react, they can move onto the next food group, repeating the process until each food group has been re-introduced. If a patient notices an increase in symptoms when consuming a food group, they should document it and remove that food group from their diet for some time. It is important to note that foods that are identified to contribute to a reaction may be restricted for some time but should be re-challenged once gut health is addressed. For identifying possible life-threatening allergic reactions, a blood test or skin prick test is recommended.

For those looking to reduce body fat, maintain muscle mass, improve insulin sensitivity, support cardiovascular health, or promote longevity, intermittent fasting can be a helpful tool. Where most dietary interventions focus on what food is eaten, intermittent fasting is more concerned about when food is consumed. This way of eating is not new. Before agriculture, humans were hunters and gatherers who evolved to survive prolonged periods without eating. Increases in portion sizes, access to technology 24/7, and continual snacking opportunities contribute to excess caloric intake and less activity, leading to an increased risk of type 2 diabetes, heart disease, or other preventable illnesses. Intermittent fasting works by extending the period of time the body has to utilize the calories consumed from the last meal to use fat for fuel. Several intermittent fasting techniques can be used to fit personal preferences. The most popular and likely most effortless to stick to is the 16/8 fast, where one fasts for 16 hours a day and eats within eight hours. Another fasting method is the 5:2 fasting approach that involves regularly eating five days and reducing caloric intake to 500-600 calories per day on two non-consecutive days a week. A 24-hour fast one day a week is a third method that may be a little more difficult to complete. During the fasting phase, most of the time will be spent asleep, but water, tea, and coffee are permitted. Although this diet style focuses on the timing of meals, that doesn't mean it is free during the feeding phase. This method is not sustainable for those with a history of disordered eating, pregnant or breastfeeding women, or anyone under 18.

Nutrition is a continuously evolving science that can make initiating change confusing and overwhelming. Falling back on the basics of a balanced whole-foods approach with minimally processed foods continues to hold steady for positive health outcomes. Yet, the need is clear for research and guidelines around diversifying diets that are more culturally inclusive and which may therefore positively affect the health outcomes of oppressed populations. Our culture, education, medical history, unique personal preferences, socioeconomic status, and geographic location all influence our dietary choices and need to be considered when deciding what goes on one's plate.

Creating resilience through the fundamentals of health will lay a solid foundation to build one's health journey. Although the fundamentals of stress management, restorative sleep, and balanced nutrition are universally important, finding the proper technique that resonates within to achieve optimal amounts of each is a personal journey. The aim is to create autonomy and power for the individual to actively participate in their wellness. Practice and repetition will allow those techniques to become easily accessible tools in your education on how your body works and be mindful of how your body navigates the world. Listen to your body. Take notes. And, above all else, have compassion for yourself and others.

To learn more from Dr. Mullane, visit her website at lanaemullane.com

Work Cited

American Psychological Association. (2016, March 10). Stress in America: The impact of discrimination. **https://www.apa.org/news/press/releases/stress/2015/impact-of-discrimination.pdf.**

Centers for Disease Control and Prevention. (2017, May 2). CDC - data and statistics - sleep and sleep disorders. Centers for Disease Control and Prevention. https://www.cdc.gov/sleep/data_statistics.html.

Chang AM, Aeschbach D, Duffy JF, Czeisler CA. (2015). Evening use of light-emitting eReaders negatively affects sleep, circadian timing, and next-morning alertness. Proc Natl Acad Sci USA. 112(4):1232-1237. doi:10.1073/pnas.1418490112

Dutko, P., Ver Ploeg, M., & Farrigan, T. (2012, August). Characteristics and Influential Factors of Food Deserts.

Ferracioli-Oda E, Qawasmi A, Bloch MH. (2013). Meta-analysis: melatonin for the treatment of primary sleep disorders. PLoS One. 8(5):e63773. doi:10.1371/journal.pone.0063773

Rajilić-Stojanović M, de Vos WM. (2014). The first 1000 cultured species of the human gastrointestinal microbiota. FEMS Microbiol Rev. 38(5):996-1047. doi:10.1111/1574-6976.12075

Sánchez-Villegas A, Cabrera-Suárez B, Molero P, et al. (2019). Preventing the recurrence of depression with a Mediterranean diet supplemented with extra-virgin olive oil. The PREDI-DEP trial: study protocol. BMC Psychiatry. 19(1):63. doi:10.1186/s12888-019-2036-4 **https://www.ers.usda.gov/webdocs/publications/45014/30940_err140.pdf.**

The Nutrition Source. (2021, March 16). Healthy Eating Plate. **https://www.hsph.harvard.edu/nutritionsource/healthy-eating-plate.**

CHAPTER VIII

Personalized Nutrition
Ending the Hunt for the Right Diet

The field of nutrition has reached transformative horizons, motivating and empowering individuals to effectively manage their health. The increase in chronic disease has society, at large, seeking solutions outside of mainstream healthcare. There is a growing dissatisfaction with the standard of care, and it is catalyzing a new movement in the healthcare industry. The era of 'diagnose and treat' is being replaced with an enthusiastic pursuit of health promotion and wellness.

The notion that food can be used as medicine has gained enough traction to become embraced beyond the circles of complementary and alternative medicine. The research associating nutrition and dietary habits with disease prevention is mounting daily. Even renowned medical institutions accept that chronic conditions like cardiovascular disease, dementia, and diabetes can be attenuated and even staved off through diet and lifestyle interventions.

The benefits of nutrition go beyond disease prevention. As Jeffrey Bland has famously said, "Food is information." The nutrients in food provide instructions to your cells—either moving you toward or away from homeostasis. Have you ever eaten too much, or consumed a meal that doesn't agree with you? The malaise you experience is a sign your system is out of balance. Foods and nutrients acutely affect how your body functions, and how you feel both mentally and physically. This concept is empowering yet also comes with a certain responsibility. Once you learn that you can influence your health, you also realize your daily choices matter. This poses a quandary. In order to make good choices, you need to know what constitutes a healthy diet.

Through the decades we've seen new dietary trends surface, only to change as quickly as the seasons.Government agencies encourage us to eat a balanced diet using MyPlate. Medical doctors recommend we cut the fat, cholesterol, or carbs from our diets. Nutrition influencers promote popular diets. Each diet comes with claims to help you feel better, lose weight, and live longer. Yet there is no consensus and barely a common thread between dietary recommendations. Without unifying principles, you might feel as if you have more questions than answers. The information in this chapter is designed to provide a framework to reduce confusion, and to help you identify a way of eating that supports good health.

The Universal Diet Doesn't Exist
The idea that there is one diet that's right for everyone is a myth. Nutritional needs are as unique as the individual, and there are numerous factors that influence your needs:

- Age
- Gender
- Health conditions
- Medications
- Physical activity level
- Food intolerances
- Genetics
- Environmental stressors like industrial chemicals
- Geography
- Cultural and social factors
- Psychological stress
- Pregnancy and lactation

This list is by no means all-inclusive, but it does provide a glimpse into variables that influence your nutritional needs. At this point, it goes without saying: a universal diet cannot comprehensively address these numerous variables.

Even if you buy into the premise that there isn't one right diet for everyone, you might wonder if there is a prefab diet that is right for you. Surely, you or someone you know has benefited from a popular diet. Indeed, trialing different diets can lead you toward a way of eating that helps you feel better. It can also serve as a first step toward personalizing a diet that optimizes your health and prepares you to make adjustments, when needed. Due to the ever-evolving nature of our physiology, and the factors that influence function, our nutritional needs can change like the wind. Personalized nutrition allows you flexibility and freedom to make changes when your current diet no longer serves you.

What is Personalized Nutrition?
Personalized nutrition accounts for an individual's biopsychosocial construct and evaluates inter-individual differences related to the metabolism and response of nutrients. Expressed more simply, personalized nutrition is adapting diet to individual needs.

Is there any evidence that personalized diets are superior to public health diets, for instance Dietary Approaches to Stop Hypertension (DASH Diet)? You might wonder if it's worth exploring personalized nutrition when you could just follow an evidence-based diet or a diet with a successful track record. Not only is there evidence to support personalized nutrition, but the emerging research is revolutionizing the nutrition field.

A 2015 randomized control study showed personalized diets can modify postprandial elevations in blood glucose and the associated metabolic consequences The 800-person cohort was found to have high variability in the response to identical meals, suggesting that universal dietary recommendations may have limited utility. The study used a machine-learning algorithm that integrated blood parameters, dietary habits, anthropometrics (systematic measurement of the human body's physical properties), physical activity, and gut microbiota. The algorithm accurately predicts personalized postprandial glycemic responses to real-life meals (Zeevi, 2015). Consider the implications! If blood glucose can be predicted using personalized data, reductionist tools like the glycemic index become antiquated.

Turning away from glucose control and toward lipid management, a 2010 study concluded that whole grain wheat sourdough bread influences cholesterol and triglycerides depending on genotype. In participants with the APO E3/E3 genotype, there was a significant increase in LDL cholesterol, triglycerides, and elevated ratios of HDL to triglycerides when consuming sourdough bread. Even more compelling is the fact that participants' blood sugar control was taken into consideration, an established risk factor. Genotype had even more influence on lipids than elevated blood sugar (Tucker, 2010). Clearly, both examples denote individual differences in response to the same foods. With many other studies revealing the same concept, we can now shift toward a more nuanced and meaningful nutritional paradigm. Even though personalized nutrition is in its infancy, enough information is available to make more informed decisions about how to eat for health.

Designing Your Personalized Diet in Six Steps

Step One: Building the Foundation

Every human being has basic needs for macronutrients, micronutrients, and energy/ calories. A diverse, whole-food diet is necessary to meet these needs. Whole foods should form the foundation of your diet. There is a symbiotic relationship between the nutrients contained in whole foods that work together to promote health. Take, for example, an apple. One medium apple contains about 6 mg of vitamin C; however, the other antioxidants contained in the apple, such as flavonoids and catechins, produce as much antioxidant activity as 1,500 mg of vitamin C alone.

Almonds are another great example of nutrient synergy. The flavonoids found in almond skins synergize with vitamin E found in the almond meat and more than double the antioxidant power than either of the nutrients separately (Mateljan, 2007). Nature simply cannot be replicated in the lab!

While whole-foods provide the ideal foundation for a healthy diet, there is also a place for processed foods. The primary benefit of processed foods in our harried culture is convenience and time savings. A diet composed entirely of homemade meals might seem tedious at a time when ready-to-eat food is abundantly available. Why make your own yogurt, steak sauce, or tortillas, when you can simply purchase them? A semi-homemade diet can be nutritious and support good health, but there is a caveat. You want to select products that are minimally processed. Minimally processed foods do not have refined ingredients, but rather combined ingredients; for example, take minimally processed granola. When you read the ingredient list you will see a list of whole foods such as nuts, seeds, whole grains, and unrefined sweeteners like raw honey. If the ingredient list contains derivatives of whole foods or non-food ingredients, it fails the criteria for minimally processed.

A diverse diet may be just as important as consuming whole foods. The more varied your diet, the greater your chances of consuming adequate micronutrients, phytonutrients, and plant compounds with prebiotic effects. Until recently, our choices of food were dependent on seasonal availability–a natural way of diversifying and rotating the foods we eat. Evidence also suggests that a diverse diet promotes a healthy immune system, and prevents the development of food allergies (especially when started early in life) (D'Auria, 2020).

Diverse, Whole-foods Diet Checklist
> **1.** Take a look inside your pantry and refrigerator. Is your diet made up of at least 80% whole-foods or minimally processed foods?
> **2.** Are you rotating and diversifying your diet on a daily or weekly basis? Are you eating seasonally?

Step Two: Ancestral Diets
A diverse, whole-food diet alone can bring about significant improvements in

health; however, there is another layer that deserves attention. Before modern farming and food manufacturing, human beings consumed foods native to their geographic location. The revolutionary work of a dentist named Weston Price revealed the importance not only of eating locally, but eating according to ancestry, too.

Dr. Price was perplexed by the deteriorating state of his patients' oral health and facial structures. Crowded, crooked teeth, overbites, pinched nostrils, narrowed faces, and undefined cheekbones proved common. His curiosity led him to travel to remote parts of the world about 60 years ago to investigate whether the problems he was observing in his patients were a collective problem. What he found were tribes and villages where virtually every individual exhibited robust health. Tooth decay was rare, dental crowding and occlusions non-existent. The natives were invariably good natured and characterized by impressive physical development with virtually no signs of disease. He photographed the tribes and recorded his observations in the landmark book, Nutrition & Physical Degeneration (Price, 2003).

A particularly interesting finding in Price's research was the disparity in diets of indigenous populations. In fact, their diets varied as much as popular trends today. In the Swiss village where Price began his diverse investigations, the inhabitants lived on rich dairy products, rye bread, occasional meat, bone broth soups, and the few vegetables they could cultivate during summer months. In Alaska, the Eskimo diet was composed largely of fish and marine animals, including seal oil and blubber. Tribes in Canada, the Everglades, the Amazon, Australia and Africa consumed game animals, organ meats, glands, blood, marrow, a variety of grains, tubers, and seasonal vegetables and fruits. Price's findings provide revelatory clues about the significance of ancestry and eating foods native to one's geographical location as it relates to good health and prevention of disease. The only problem is most of us are transplanted from our origin of ancestry and do not come from a homogeneous gene pool. This immediately raises the question, how could you possibly apply this information?

To refine your diet based on ancestral principles, you want to prioritize consumption of locally grown food, and minimize foods that were not a part of any ancestral diet. Foods that have been grown and raised locally are more nutritious, whereas imported foods lose nutrients rapidly during transportation. There are many studies demonstrating the micronutrient depletion that occurs postharvest. One study found a significant decrease in ascorbic acid, total chlorophyll content, and carotenoids found in lettuce heads within days of harvest. The ascorbic acid lost from lettuce by the time it arrived on the retail shelf was 48% by day three, and 68.9% by day four (Managa, 2018). One of the attractions of eating nutritious foods is to obtain micronutrients and phytonutrients. If the food you're buying has lost vital nutrients during transportation, you're missing out on the very compounds you're intending to consume. There are several ways to begin introducing local foods into your diet:

- Local farmer's market
- CSA (Community-supported agriculture), subscribing to/paying for a share of local harvests
- Purchasing local produce at your supermarket
- Growing some of your own food. Herb gardens and microgreen quilts are a great place to start!

In addition to eating locally, you can also move closer to an ancestral diet by limiting consumption of food products that didn't exist before industrial food manufacturing. Adulterated foods tend to lack nutrients and the synergistic complexity of whole foods. They also possess properties that can interfere with normal function. Refined sugar, solvent-extracted cooking oils, fractionated grains, and artificial ingredients were never a part of our early ancestor diets. Those same ingredients are also absent in the diets of populations living in Blue Zones, our best epidemiological evidence for achieving health and longevity.

Ancestral Diet Checklist
1. On a weekly basis are you visiting your local farmer's market, ordering from a CSA, or gathering food from your garden?
2. Does your diet resemble the diet of your great grandparents?

Step Three: Biopsychosocial Influence
At this point it might seem as if healthy eating can be accomplished through moderation, and choosing seasonal, locally grown foods. Healthy eating, however, is much more than eating the right foods, at the right time of year, and from the right location. If healthy eating was as simple as following the guidelines in steps one and two, everyone would be doing it! Personalized nutrition extends beyond food and accounts for psychosocial elements. It addresses variables that influence your dietary choices and the way these variables alter your responses to food.

There is a dynamic confluence among your diet, inner world, and social sphere that deserves just as much attention as the foods you eat.

Let's first start with some of the factors that affect your dietary choices. Throughout the day, we experience shifts in our mental-emotional state, and encounter circumstances that affect us in varying degrees. We are not always cognizant of the contributing factors.

- Eating (or not eating) for emotional reasons
- Low energy and motivation to prioritize healthy eating
- Reliance on take-out or processed foods due to time limitations
- Lack of culinary skills or lack of interest in learning how to cook
- Dietary habits of those within your household or peer group
- Changes to your routine, such as travel
- Exceptions to your routine, such as special occasions
- Business or social meals
- The influence of news and social media

Without presumption of these psychosocial influences, you would be missing the forest through the trees. Simply becoming aware of this concept allows you to think more expansively about dietary adherence. The primary reason most people fail to adopt healthy eating patterns is because they rely on willpower, not realizing compliance is much more than self-discipline. As a biopsychosocial being, you are more like the ecology of an ocean than the mechanics of a computer. When you realize how complex and non-linear behavior change is, you are able to adjust your expectations and set more realistic goals.

Psychosocial influence is not limited to dietary adherence; it also impacts our biology. One of the ways this occurs is through the gut-brain axis (GBA): "The GBA consists of bidirectional communication between your central nervous system and your enteric nervous system, linking emotional and cognitive centers of the brain with peripheral intestinal functions" (Carabotti, 2015). This means your psychology affects your gut and your gut affects your psychology.

Have you ever felt nervous and experienced butterflies in your stomach? This is a brain-gut interaction that occurs as a result of a stress response. Blood vessels to the gut constrict and digestive muscles contract leading to a fluttering sensation. Now consider eating a meal when you are experiencing restricted blood flow and muscle contractions. Ultimately, your gastrointestinal system is forced to function within a physiological state that's unfavorable for digestion. This can lead to obvious symptoms of indigestion or asymptomatic shifts in your microbiome and gut function.

The parasympathetic nervous system is the side of your nervous system that facilitates normal digestion. It is responsible for rest-and-digest functions. The more relaxed and content you are, the better your digestion and overall health. Life stressors are a normal part of living, but there are ways to feel more at ease and to prime your digestion for meal time.

- Take a moment before eating to think of someone or something you appreciate.
- Slow your respiration rate by taking a few diaphragmatic breaths.
- Eat slowly and chew your food until it is the consistency of baby food.
- When possible, dine with people who lift your spirits.

Biopsychosocial Checklist
1. Are you aware of the psychosocial factors that influence your dietary choices? If so, are you addressing or accounting for those variables?
2. Do you regularly practice good meal hygiene to optimize digestion and gut function?

Step Four: Biochemical Individuality
Now that you have foundational principles for creating a personalized diet, it's appropriate to segue into a more nuanced approach to nutrition. Biochemical individuality is the concept that the nutritional and biochemical constitution of each person is unique and that dietary needs vary from person to person.

In 1956, the late world-renowned biochemist Roger Williams, Ph.D., published his book **Biochemical Individuality (Williams, 1975),** in which he describes anatomical and physiological differences among people and how the variations relate to individual responses to the environment. Williams was one of the first to recognize how biochemical individuality related to differing nutritional needs for good health. Williams gives an example in his book illustrating the genetic impact associated with potassium, a mineral tightly regulated in the blood. The most convincing evidence that there is substantial variation in the potassium needs of human individuals is the existence of familial periodic paralysis which is accompanied by low potassium levels. In afflicted individuals, the potassium level prior to seizure is 2.6 to 3.0 meq per liter and relief of the condition comes promptly after administration of 2 to 5 grams of potassium chloride. The disease is thought to be due to inherited needs for higher amounts of potassium, possibly due to differences in enzyme systems and excretion rates.

Differing nutrient levels, and nutrient needs, are not unique to potassium. The same evidence exists for nearly every micronutrient, macronutrient, amino acid, and fatty acid. Since nutrient needs vary from person to person, the diet that promotes good health in one individual will be different from the diet that promotes good health in another. You may have experienced this phenomenon yourself. Perhaps a friend of yours changed their diet and experienced symptom reduction or weight loss, but when trying the same diet, you didn't have the same response. This is completely normal, and now, you can understand why. Initially, this concept may cause more confusion. You're probably wondering how you could possibly figure out how to eat based on your unique biochemical individuality.

This topic is vast and it could take an entire lifetime to unravel the complex interplay between diet and inter-individual differences; however, there is a road map to help guide you. By gathering biometrics and using biofeedback, you can begin customizing your diet based on your unique needs.

Biochemical Individuality: Clinical Labs
Your physician or healthcare provider can and should run comprehensive clinical labs every year. Clinical lab data allow you to evaluate the effects of your current diet and lifestyle, identify genetic predispositions, and gain information to guide personalized nutrition recommendations.
Your comprehensive labs should include:
- Complete Blood Count (CBC)
- Comprehensive Metabolic Panel (CMP)
- Advanced lipid testing
- Glucose metabolism markers
- Sex hormones
- Thyroid hormones and thyroid antibodies
- Adrenal hormones
- Uric acid
- Homocysteine
- Prolactin
- Vitamin D

- Iron and ferritin
- hsCRP

Each of these markers provides clues about your health, and each has nutritional implications.Nutritional interventions can either have a direct impact on biomarkers or play a supportive role in balancing your biochemistry. Let's take a look at a few examples.

Homocysteine is an independent risk factor for cardiovascular disease. When homocysteine is elevated, it indicates impaired methylation and/or recycling. There are several reasons for these impairments, but simply taking nutrients like L-5-methyltetrahydrofolate (folate), methylcobalamin (vitamin B12), and pyridoxal-5-phosphate (vitamin B6), allows homocysteine to be properly converted or recycled. These nutrients directly lower homocysteine and help reduce your risk for heart disease.

Uric acid is another example of a biomarker that can be directly affected by diet. Uric acid is a metabolic waste product of purines (the building blocks of RNA and DNA). Elevated uric acid is most commonly associated with gout, but is also a risk factor for metabolic syndrome. Uric acid can be lowered by consuming adequate water and reducing alcohol, purine-rich foods, and fructose. In addition to lowering uric acid, there are nutritional factors that improve uric acid metabolism, such as vitamin C, cherries, and dietary fiber. Whether uric acid is elevated for dietary reasons or inflammatory reasons (e.g. infection or injury), nutritional interventions play a role in normalizing levels.

Now, let's examine the way nutrition plays a supportive role in adrenal health. Cortisol is an adrenal hormone with many functions. One of its primary roles is to activate the stress response. When you experience stress, whether real or perceived, your adrenal glands release cortisol to prepare you for fight or flight–a well-orchestrated physiological cascade. Unfortunately, chronic stress disrupts normal adrenal function leading to many symptoms, one of those being loss of glycemic control. This is because one of cortisol's roles is to raise blood sugar. When cortisol is constantly elevated, there are changes that reduce hormone availability and efficacy, and dips in blood sugar start to occur. By supporting your blood sugar with regularly spaced meals, you can reduce some of the demand on your adrenal glands.

Infrequent meals and fasting are analogous to whipping a tired horse. Cortisol will eventually get the job done, but it comes with a cost and exacerbates the existing dysfunction.

Clinical labs provide a tremendous amount of information that can guide personalized nutrition recommendations. Given the technical nature of clinical labs, it would be wise to work with a healthcare provider who has experience in clinical nutrition. There are also plenty of educational resources available that help decode the relationship between nutrition and biomarkers.

Biochemical Individuality: Genetic Testing
Genomic profiling is now a reality, and many individuals have already taken advantage of the technology. Genomic profiling is a comprehensive and informative analysis of tens of thousands of genes providing information on ancestry, medication tolerance, disease risk, and much more—including how to eat. Over the years there have been several gene-diet interactions established.

- Lactose Tolerance. Decreased activity of the LCT gene inhibits production of lactase, an enzyme that breaks down lactose. Individuals with decreased LCT activity who consume lactose- containing foods like milk, yogurt, cheese, and ice cream typically experience digestive symptoms like gas, bloating, abdominal cramping, and diarrhea.
- Caffeine Metabolism. Possessing even one copy of the CYP1A2*1F gene reduces caffeine metabolism. Slow caffeine metabolizers who consume caffeine are at greater risk for heart conditions and myocardial infarction. Caffeine consumption in slow metabolizers is also associated with infertility and miscarriages.
- Lipid Metabolism. The APOE gene affects how you metabolize and transport fats and cholesterol throughout your body. Individuals with a certain variation of the APOE gene, known as APOE4, tend to have higher levels of LDL and increased risk for metabolic syndrome and Alzheimer's when consuming a diet high in saturated fat and refined carbohydrates.
- Micronutrient Utilization. One of the most well-known gene-diet interactions is with the MTHFR gene. Individuals with a variation in this gene are unable to efficiently utilize folic acid and require supplementation with a methylated form of folate. Without proper supplementation, individuals with this variation are at increased risk for heart disease,

cancer, mood disorders, and having children with neural tube defects.

As you can see, your genes influence the way you metabolize and respond to nutrients and dietary compounds. Epigenetics is a process by which external factors change the expression of your genes. This is one of the reasons a personalized diet and lifestyle approach is essential.

The choices you make influence the expression of your genes, either offering protection or increasing risk for disease. This is empowering information when applied correctly.

When considering genetic profiling, it's important to select a test that provides actionable recommendations. Genetic testing is only as useful as your ability to decrease risk. Testing genes with limited gene-nutrient research has little relevance and no utility. This is an area of nutrition that can create more confusion than clarity. Working with a professional who has expertise interpreting and applying nutrigenomics within the context of your overall health is worth the investment.

Biochemical Individuality: Microbiome
At the heart of biochemical individuality is the microbiome, an entire ecosystem of microorganisms residing on and within our bodies. Your microbiome is as unique as your fingerprint, but infinitely more complex. You have trillions of microorganisms harmoniously coexisting and communicating with the cells and genes of your body, orchestrating essential biological functions.

Gut microbes influence gastrointestinal, immune, and metabolic health. They also influence neurobehavioral traits (Valdes, 2018). The most abundant microbes are present in the colon. Commensal bacteria (indigenous bacteria) have many health-promoting functions. Some of those functions include the following:

- Provide a physical barrier in the GI tract to protect the epithelium
- Prevent foreign invaders from entering circulation
- Produce substances to destroy viruses, fungus, and pathogenic bacteria
- Neutralize metabolic byproducts and toxic substances
- Inactivate histamine, chelate heavy metals, and absorb carcinogens
- Synthesize B vitamins and vitamin K
- Produce short chain fatty acids

Once you realize the magnitude by which commensal bacteria influence health, it becomes possible to understand the relationship between microbiome and disease. Deranged gut bacteria are associated with many multifactorial diseases, including IBD, autoimmune diseases, eczema, autism, psychiatric disorders, periodontal disease, atherosclerosis, allergies, colon cancer, and obesity.

Robust health hinges on a balanced and diverse microbial terrain. This is where eating a diverse, whole-foods diet shines. Whole foods contain compounds like prebiotics, polyphenols, probiotics, and omega 3 fatty acids. These compounds have been shown to influence microbial diversity.

- Prebiotics are found in foods like garlic, onion, leeks, asparagus, chicory, Jerusalem artichoke, green bananas, and edamame.
- Polyphenols are found in foods like green tea, cinnamon, cloves, citrus, berries, pomegranate, grapes, flaxseeds, and oats.
- Probiotics are found in fermented and cultured foods like sauerkraut, kimchi, yogurt, kefir, miso, and natto.
- Omega 3 fatty acids are found in foods like salmon, trout, herring, anchovies, sardines, flaxseeds, algae, and chia seeds.

If you are unaccustomed to eating prebiotic and probiotics foods, it's important you incorporate these foods into your diet gradually to prevent gastrointestinal stress. Prebiotic foods in particular have potent effects and your microbiome needs time to acclimate to their effects. Ironically, prebiotic and probiotic foods can worsen symptoms in individuals who have digestive conditions like IBS and small intestine bacterial overgrowth (SIBO). These conditions have a common thread of dysbiosis and require special diets until the underlying cause is addressed.

Personalized nutrition cannot be overstated when addressing dysbiotic conditions. Two individuals with the same condition, SIBO for instance, tend to respond differently to a low fermentation diet (a condition-specific diet). This is because condition-specific models error on the side of generalization, i.e. what works for a group will work for the individual.

As a clinical nutritionist, I spend most of my time working with clients who have functional gastrointestinal disorders. The limitations of condition-specific models are obvious when dealing with refractory conditions. Complex health conditions tend to be recalcitrant for all the reasons listed in the biochemical individuality section. A case-based paradigm, in contrast, broadens the tool kit. Solving complicated problems requires critical thinking, finesse, innovation, and above all, attention to biochemical individuality.

Biochemical Individuality Checklist

3. Do you have an annual check-up with a healthcare provider to evaluate clinical labs? If so, are you making changes to improve values outside the reference range?
4. Are you incorporating foods with prebiotics, probiotics, polyphenol, and omega 3 fatty acids to help nourish your microbiome?
5. Bonus: Have you done genetic testing to identify gene-nutrient risk factors like MTHFR?

Step Five: Family History

With a basic understanding of gene-nutrient interactions and biopsychosocial influence, it becomes possible to put family history into proper context. Family history is arguably the most important tool for stratifying disease risk. The majority of chronic conditions are the result of a complex interplay between numerous genetic variants and environmental factors. Family history is a significant predictor of future disease because of the overlapping factors between you and your family, such as genetic variants, shared environment, familial dietary habits, and common behaviors.

It is worth noting that family history should not be considered outside the context of epigenetics? Reducing disease-risk to family history alone becomes deterministic rather than modifiable. The development of disease is a multifactorial process with many interventional avenues for prevention. If early heart disease runs in your family, you could be tempted to believe it's an inheritable disease. Research, on the other hand, shows that heart disease is the result of numerous factors that extend beyond genetic predisposition. Taking an ecological viewpoint versus a deterministic viewpoint would allow you to see familial patterns that increase or decrease risk for heart disease.

- Does your family eat enough fiber, polyphenolic compounds, omega 3 fatty acids, magnesium-rich foods?
- Are their vitamin K2 levels optimal?
- How often does your family eat homemade meals?
- Do their waist-to-hip measurements fall within the healthy range?
- Is alcohol consumption within the CDC's guidelines?

- Do they have other conditions associated with inflammation?
- How well does your family manage stress?
- What is your family's physical activity level? Do they meet the exercise requirements for heart health?

The first step in reducing disease risk is to do an inventory of the diseases prevalent in your family: great grandparents, grandparents, parents, aunts, uncles, and siblings. Once you have this information you can begin to assess your risk using clinical lab tests and biometric tests like blood pressure and waist-to-hip circumference.

The second step is analyzing your clinical labs and biometric tests. Say for instance you have elevated LDL-P, triglycerides, and homocysteine. Each of these markers increases risk for heart disease and each can be modified to a certain degree using nutritional interventions.

Once assessing clinical labs and biometric tests, you can go a step further and use genetic tests to gain more information and direction. If you have one or two APOE E4 alleles, your risk for heart disease increases. Because the E4 allele is associated with impaired lipid metabolism, you can leverage the information to minimize dietary risk factors associated with deranged lipids.

Retest your values after 12 weeks of diet modification to determine how much the intervention modified your biomarkers. Your results will either confirm you're on the right track or let you know the plan needs to be adjusted.

Family History Checklist
- Have you done an inventory of your family's health history?
- Are you aware of diet, lifestyle, or behavioral patterns associated with increased risk for disease?

Step Six: Biofeedback

One of the most valuable tools in personalized nutrition is biofeedback. Biofeedback is the way your body communicates with you to promote self-preservation. Utilizing biofeedback allows you to leverage your body's innate wisdom and modify your behavior to protect your health. There are objective and subjective forms of biofeedback. Vital signs and biometrics are forms of objective biofeedback. Elevated heart rate and respiration rate, for instance, indicate sympathetic arousal.

Symptoms, or changes in well-being, are subjective forms of biofeedback. If you experience indigestion every time you eat jalapeno peppers, the symptom indicates a food incompatibility. Your body doesn't just alert you to potential danger, it also reveals what it needs. If you spend time with friends and your craving for ice cream vanishes, it's an indicator you need more connection time. If you start meditating and experience an improvement in sleep, it's an indicator you need more relaxation or restoration.

Using biofeedback may seem like common sense, yet people do not embrace it for a number of reasons. Those with busy and demanding lives tend to disassociate from symptoms. Noticing symptoms and correlations interferes with productivity. It seems more efficient to ignore symptoms and press on. There is also a category of people who don't trust their body's feedback or would rather defer to someone they think knows better. External validation seems more reliable than their intuition.

Another reason people dismiss biofeedback is because there is a payoff to certain behaviors. Giving up favorite foods or alcohol, for instance, doesn't seem worth the sacrifice.

Health is built on pattern detection. Paying attention to variables that impact your health or well-being makes it possible to intervene. Generally the sooner you take action, the greater your odds of preventing unnecessary health challenges. The same goes for factors that enhance well-being. Consistently attending to your biopsychosocial needs improves your healthspan.Biofeedback is highly useful when assessing whether you're on the right track with your diet. When you're eating in a way that balances your body chemistry, you should feel stable after meals. If you experience fatigue, cravings, indigestion, appetite issues, or any other symptom, it's a sign you need to make adjustments. One way to identify the right fuel for your engine is by experimenting with two contrasting meals.

Let's say you eat Greek yogurt and granola for breakfast, and an hour after the meal you experience sugar cravings and hunger. The next morning, try a meal with a totally different macronutrient composition, like eggs and smoked salmon. If you are free of cravings and your hunger is under control until lunch, you've identified the right fuel. The meal that maintains homeostasis is generally the meal that supports your health.

Your body's feedback should be the supreme authority when evaluating whether your diet is working for you. It can be difficult to accept this at a time when there is excessive external pressure to eat a certain way. We are inundated with headlines that influence our perspective on healthy eating. If the research shows broccoli helps prevent cancer, but you feel bloated and gaseous after eating it, it's in your best interest to stop eating it. Only you know whether dietary changes are making you feel better or worse. Research and experts can provide insight and guidance, but it's ultimately up to you to determine whether you're on the right path.

Personalized nutrition is a framework that allows you to adjust your diet according to your individual needs and responses to food. Cultivating a diet that's right for you can be basic, e.g. using biofeedback to make adjustments to a diverse, whole-foods diet. It can also be multilayered, e.g. utilizing genetic profiling and comprehensive clinical labs to refine your diet. In some ways personalized nutrition is like a game of chess. By making strategic moves, you gain leverage over risk factors and favorably influence the trajectory of your health and your quality of life.

Works Cited

Carabotti, M., Scirocco, A., Maselli, M. A., & Severi, C. (2015). The gut-brain axis: interactions between enteric microbiota, central and enteric nervous systems. Annals of gastroenterology, 28(2), 203–209.

D'Auria, E., Peroni, D. G., Sartorio, M., Verduci, E., Zuccotti, G. V., & Venter, C. (2020). The Role of Diet Diversity and Diet Indices on Allergy Outcomes.

Frontiers in pediatrics, 8, 545. https://doi.org/10.3389/fped.2020.00545

Kosower, N., Rein, M., Zilberman-Schapira, G., Dohnalová, L., Pevsner-Fischer, M., Bikovsky,R., ... Segal, E. (2015). Personalized Nutrition by Prediction of Glycemic Responses. Cell, 163(5), 1079–1094. **https://doi.org/10.1016/j.cell.2015.11.001**

Lador, D., Avnit-Sagi, T., Lotan-Pompan, M., Suez, J., Mahdi, J. A., Matot, E., Malka, G.,Tucker AJ, Mackay KA, Robinson LE, Graham TE, Bakovic M, Duncan AM. "The effect of whole grain wheat sourdough bread consumption on serum lipids in healthy normoglycemic/normoinsulinemic and hyperglycemic/ hyperinsulinemic adults depends on presence of the APOE E3/E3 genotype: a randomized controlled trial." Nutr Metab (Lond). 2010 May 5; 7:37. doi: 10.1186/1743-7075-7-37. PMID: 20444273; PMCID: PMC2877680.

Managa, M. G., Tinyani, P. P., Senyolo, G. M., Soundy, P., Sultanbawa, Y., & Sivakumar, D. (2018). Impact of transportation, storage, and retail shelf conditions on lettuce quality and phytonutrients losses in the supply chain. Food science & nutrition, 6(6), 1527–1536. **https://doi.org/10.1002/fsn3.685**

Mateljan, George (2007). World's Healthiest Foods. The George Mateljan Foundation. Price, W. A., & Price-Pottenger Nutrition Foundation. (2003). Nutrition and physical degeneration. La Mesa, CA: Price-Pottenger Nutrition Foundation

Williams, R. J. (1975). Biochemical individuality. University of Texas Press.

Valdes, A. M., Walter, J., Segal, E., & Spector, T. D. (2018). Role of the gut microbiota in nutrition and health. BMJ (Clinical research ed.), 361, k2179. **https://doi.org/10.1136/bmj.k2179.**

Zeevi, D., Korem, T., Zmora, N., Israeli, D., Rothschild, D., Weinberger, A., Ben-Yacov, O.,

"Personalized Nutrition by Prediction of Glycemic Responses." Cell, V. 163, Issue 5, November 2015, 1079-1094.

CHAPTER IX

Universal Touch: Untangling Patterns, Awakening Awareness

"And the day came when the risk it took to remain tight in a bud was more painful than the risk it took to blossom." -Anaïs Nin

Most of what we think about life comes from a set of assumptions we have been taught, which we often don't examine or even question. Medical paradigms are what determine how we think about our bodies. Over the years, our medical paradigm in the West has been shifting and advancing. We have learned more about mind-body connections giving rise to new methods of treatment and healing.

The emphasis of this book is the interconnectedness of all systems and modalities used to treat and heal the body. While my focus is massage therapy, no one system, treatment or modality can fully address each pain, restriction, weakness or strength in the body.

My main goal of this chapter is to help the reader understand not only how the living body works, but how human biology can be linked to broader considerations of how a human exists within, interacts with their environment, and experiences existence in emotional, spiritual as well as physical terms and to understand the applications, benefits and mechanisms of bodywork.

As a licensed massage therapist, trained in both Eastern and Western traditions, I use all modalities from Swedish, medical massage, deep tissue, manual lymphatic drainage (MLD), ART(Active Release Technique), myofascial release, myofascial unwinding, cranio-sacral, Shiatsu, Watsu, Thai massage, Mayan abdominal massage to reflexology in my practice. While all of these modalities are invaluable, each one has its unique function in treatment. I will in this chapter focus on those which through my experience and training I feel most connect the mind and body using a whole system approach, I am not promoting one technique over another nor even positing a mechanism for how any one technique works. What is of utmost importance is understanding that the heart of all treatment lies in our ability to listen, to perceive, to see more than in our application of technique. Comprehend the bigger picture of your own or your client's structural relationships, then apply whatever technique you have learned toward resolving that pattern. We are all different, yet we are all alike. Everyone on this earth is a work in progress, from the finely tuned athlete to the physically challenged. We all possess the ability to exceed our limits once we recognize what they are and learn to embrace the process as much as the result. To have been given the privilege of assisting one in their process has been for me the most rewarding gift.

THE TIES THAT BIND

The human body is the most enchanting and fascinating of all creations. It is an intricate web of fascia wrapping around millions and millions of cells making up all the systems of the body, each functioning in its own unique way to keep us in this complex dance we call homeostasis. The skin, the skeleton, joints and muscles, the heart and circulatory system, the lymphatic system, the lungs, the gut, the kidneys and bladder, the nervous system, the special senses and the reproductive system cannot and do not function alone. Even though each cell has its individual life function, there is always coherence. We are an integrated whole, not a sum of our parts.

In the West, the prevailing traditional paradigm that you and I were taught is the Cartesian/Newtonian model of reality, and it is over three hundred years old. This model of classic physics which is the basis of our current paradigm "proposes to analyze the phenomena from the analogy of a machine," where knowing the operation of the isolated parts is able to understand the whole formed by those parts.

Newton and Descartes both believed there was a fundamental divide between mind and matter; that is, between mental and physical processes. In the field of medical science, this paradigm has reduced human illness to the "biochemistry of disease," completely losing sight of the fact that disease or dysfunction is part of a whole system including the mind and the natural environment we live in. Essentially, what they are saying is that brain function, and emotions of fear, sorrow, anger, joy are nothing more than chemical reactions (Kurtz, R.). This separatist mechanistic approach to life, which is brilliant in its own way, lacks a connection between the mind, body and spirit, between a person and their environment, overlooking the fact that there is an intelligence running through the body connecting all.

The mainstream mechanistic view is that the brain is responsible for what we in the West call the "mind." As useful as it has been, it has objectified rather than humanized our relationship to our insides. As we incorporate more quantum physics into biology, more has been discovered about what makes us tick. The mind is understood to be not only in the brain, but everywhere in a network of flow of communication in the tissues of the body as well as the brain.

ROOTS

My introduction to massage techniques and understanding of the body as an integrated whole began in an Eastern tradition while I was living abroad in Asia. It was in Korea that I was first introduced to a book called the "Dongui Bogam," a Korean book compiled by the royal physician Heo Jun and first published in 1613 during the Joseon Dynasty of Korea. The book has been listed as one of the national treasures of South Korea and is registered with UNESCO. The title literally means **"a priceless book about medicine of an Eastern country."** Its innovative disease classification system is based on essence, Qi (energy), and spirit, and its emphasis is on the importance of disease prevention through the promotion of health regimens. Introducing a unique and pragmatic form of medicine, the Dongui Bogam regards the human body as a universe and understands body function, health maintenance, and the treatment of disease according to comprehensive and systematic approaches. It also states that humans are emotional creatures. We communicate and make relationships by expressing our feelings; when not properly released, these emotions are linked to illness and restrictions in the body. The book begins with the following elusive paragraph that fascinated me:

> Mankind is the most precious of all living things in the Universe. The round head resembles heaven, and the flat foot resembles earth; man has four limbs as the universe has four seasons, man has five viscera as the universe has five phases; man has six bowels as the universe has six extremes, man has eight joints as the universe has eight winds, man has nine orifices as the universe has nine stars, and man has twelve meridians as the universe has twelve hours. Man has twenty-four acupoints as the universe has twenty-four qi. Also, man has 365 joints as the universe has 365 divisions; man has two eyes as the universe has the sun and the moon, man sleeps and wakes as the universe has day and night; man has happiness and anger as the universe has thunder and lightning, and man has tears and nasal discharge as the universe has rain and dew; man has cold and heat as the universe has yin and willpower, and man has blood vessels as the universe has spring water; man has hair growing as the universe has grass and trees; and man has teeth as the universe has metal and rocks.

This fascinating logic emphasizes that both nature and humans are created and function together —a much different view from that of the Cartesian/Newtonian model I was taught in the West. We all have our own beliefs and theory on the mental and the physical or mind and body, and mind and brain. I understand these beliefs are not without controversy or skepticism. Through my own training, teachings, and experience I have found not only that is there is a powerful connection between the mind and body, but also that we are an infinite part of our environment. We depend on it as much as we influence it. To stay healthy, one must maintain harmony within the body and adapt to the changes going on outside of it.

Teachings in the Yellow Emperor's Classic of Medicine give a holistic picture of human life. It does not separate external changes—geographic, climatic, or seasonal, for instance—from internal changes such as emotions and our responses to them. It tells how our way of life and environment affect our health. For example, "When damp invades the body, the head will feel heavy and distended, as if highly bandaged. The large muscles and tendons will contract, and the small muscles and tendons will become flaccid, resulting in a loss of mobility, spasms, and atrophy" (Ni, 9).

It wasn't until 1977 in the West that George Engel was the first to suggest that to understand a person's medical condition it is not simply the biological factors to consider, but also the psychological and social factors. This is known as the Biopsychosocial Model and is most commonly used in chronic pain, with the view that pain is a psychophysiological pattern that cannot be categorized into biological, psychological, or social factors alone (Engel, G.).

CHRONICLE OF MASSAGE

Let's begin to understand what we have come to know today as massage with its history. Most ancient cultures practiced some form of healing touch. Healing with the hands is considered to be the oldest form of medicine. The word massage itself comes from the Arabic verb "masah," meaning to "to rub." Massage has a long history dating back to 3000 BC (or earlier) where it originated in India and was considered a sacred system of healing. It was used not only to heal injuries, relieve pain, and promote relaxation, but also to cure and treat illnesses. The Hindus in Ayurveda believe that disease is caused when people are out of sync with their environment. Massage is believed to restore the body's natural and physical balance so that it can heal naturally.

As cultures and history evolved, the healing methods of massage traveled all over the world, with all cultures putting their own spin on it. It then went on to become known by two names: Tui-Na (push-pull), and Anmo-Anma (press-rub). These methods of Chinese and Japanese origins were performed by kneading or rubbing down the entire body with the hands while using gentle pressure and traction. In the West, Hippocrates of Cos (460-377BC) was the first physician to describe specifically the medical benefits of anointing (using oil) and massage. He called his art "anatripsis," which means to rub up. He held the belief that the body must be treated as a whole and not just as a series of parts. Massage then came to the Romans from the Greeks. Julius Cesar (100-44BC) used massage daily to relieve his neuralgia and prevent epileptic seizures. The Romans believed a healthy mind is a healthy body.

The popularity of massage declined in the West until the 17th century, when discoveries in pharmacology and medical technology advanced. Per Henrik Ling (1676-1839), a Swedish doctor who brought it out of retirement, is credited with Swedish massage, although he did not invent it. The form of massage in the West today we are most familiar with, it involves stroking, pressing, squeezing, and striking. While Ling's methods are still used today, Jonah George Mezger, a Dutchman, refined Dr. Ling's techniques and is credited with other popular techniques of massage such as effleurage, petrissage, tapotement, and friction—all techniques we still use today.

By the late 1800's, the full-body massage became part of the "rest cure" for the type of melancholy known as neurasthenia that was popular among society ladies who lived the wealthy life of the late 1800's. Even Sigmund Freud (1856-1939) experimented with massage in the treatment of hysteria, a form of mental illness that is characterized by hysteria, but has no physiological basis. In 1916, Dr James Mennell went on to use certain forms of tactile stimulation, such as stroking and light touch, mostly developed by him.

Massage is its own healing practice, and is the origin of many medical practices that later arose, such as physical therapy and chiropractic manipulation. It uses the most natural form of medicine (human touch) and transcends the particulars of human culture and history. While our scientific knowledge has changed over the centuries, massage as an applied healing practice has not changed dramatically, just as the human body has not changed significantly. We are still using most of the modalities learned through history; as our medical paradigms shifted in the West, however, we continued to learn about and to use more whole-system approaches with massage.

THE POWER OF TOUCH

I believe we all can attest to the importance of touch. Skin to skin contact has been encouraged as soon as babies emerge from the womb. Every mother touches, holds, kisses or caresses her child when they are in pain or in need of comfort. What is the first thing we do when we hurt ourselves? Usually we touch the hurt part of our body. This physical instinct sends signals to the part that was hurt to promote healing. Skin is the largest organ in the the body and is often referred to as one big sense organ. It has many sensory receptors that enable us to feel light touch, pressure, temperature, vibration, and pain. Skin contact is used to stimulate some of these receptors, leading to a particular reaction depending on which receptors are stimulated and what effect is achieved and determined by the nature of the skin contact.

Like our other senses, touch comes in gradations. An exquisite array of receptors can distinguish minute variations in the environment. Using fast, slow, deep, light, hot, cold will have different biological effects in the body. Pacinian corpuscles, one of the pressure receptors, send signals directly to a nerve bundle deep in the brain called the vagus nerve. The vagus is sometimes called "the wanderer" because it has branches that wander throughout the body to several internal organs, including the heart. It is the vagus nerve that slows heart rate down and decreases blood pressure. Some receptors react only to caress, while others send pain signals.

Each type activates a different part of the brain, making us feel soothed or hurt, comforted or distressed, angry or calm. David Linden, a Johns Hopkins neuroscientist, cites "the electric touch of romantic love, the unsettling feeling of being watched, the relief of pain from mindful practice, or the essential touch that newborns need to thrive" as diverse sensations that "flow from the evolved nature of our skin, nerves and brain" (Linden, D.).

In the mid-1970's , Tiffany Field (head of the Touch Research Institute at the University of Miami Miller School of Medicine), was a new mother. She massaged her infant daughter, who was born prematurely. The calming effects she witnessed inspired her to study prematurity and massage. The research showed that massage caused premature infants to gain more weight than their non-massaged premature infants (Field et al.). Even short bursts of touch—as little as 15 minutes in the evening—in one of her studies not only enhanced growth and weight gain in children, but also led to emotional, physical, and cognitive improvements in adults. Touch in general appears to stimulate our bodies in very specific ways (Field,T.).

Studies in Romania in the 1990s examined the sensory deprivation of children. The touch-deprived children, they found, had significantly higher cortisol levels (a stress hormone) and slower growth developments for their age group (Carlson, M.). Another study indicated that when pre-school aged kids and adolescents are touched less, they become more physically aggressive towards each other (Field,T.). Continuing to study touch, Dr. Field now is looking at the elderly.

One group of elderly participants received regular conversation-filled visits while another received social visits that also included massage; the second group saw emotional and cognitive benefits over and above those of the first. It is easy to see how an elderly person who is regularly visited by a massage therapist or who is engaging with touch in some way might be happier and healthier than one who is not. In studies with elderly people that had the elderly massage babies, versus receiving massage, interestingly enough they found the effects were greater when they were giving the massage rather than receiving. This goes to show touch is as beneficial both giving and receiving. Massage therapists are also getting some kind of benefit from stimulating the pressure receptors in the hands, elbow, or whatever body part they're massaging with.

One of the greatest losses during COVID and quarantine where people had to physically be distanced from one another definitely resulted in touch deprivation. As a massage therapist, I certainly felt it myself. In fact, a survey put together found that touch deprivation was highly correlated to anxiety symptoms to depression symptoms, to boredom and to loneliness. Every negative scale and rating on the survey was related to touch deprivation. What they also saw is that the immune system is being more compromised (Field, T.). So, as you can see, both touch and its lack affect our bodies in very specific ways.

MORE THAN JUST SKIN DEEP
I have always been enraptured by the physiological, biochemical, and emotional reactions massage promotes. The many benefits of massage include pain relief, relaxation, improved sleep quality, decreased stress and inflammation, decreased blood pressure as well as improved mental health and release of stored emotional and physical trauma. So how does all this work in the body? Let's go a little deeper

and discuss some of the mechanisms and benefits of massage.

Physiological, Biochemical, and Emotional Mechanisms of Massage

- Massage using light pressure releases oxytocin, a neurotransmitter that is produced in the hypothalamus. It is known as the "love hormone" or "feel good" hormone because its levels increase during hugging and orgasm as well as massage. It also regulates our emotional responses including trust, empathy, and positive memories. Oxytocin stimulates other "feel good" hormones such as serotonin and dopamine, which reduce the stress hormones in the body such as cortisol and nor-epinephrine.
- Massage produces a 'relaxation response". An involuntary response in which heart rate and breathing slow, stress hormones decrease, serotonin is released, and muscle relax. As discussed earlier, it is the vagus nerve that slows heart rate and decreases blood pressure.
- Massage decreases pain by disturbing signals to the brain and helping to "close the pain gate." It reduces Substance P, which acts as a neurotransmitter altering cellular signaling pathways and decreasing sensitivity to pain.
- Massage reduces inflammation in the body by improving circulation and removing fluid build-up. Massage releases cytokines known as Interleukin-4(IL4) and Interleukin 10(IL10), which have anti-inflammatory effects.
- Massage reduces stress by decreasing muscle tension and increasing body temperature, which promotes relaxation. It also reduces ACTH (adenocorticotropic hormone), which stimulates cortisol, a stress hormone.
- Massage increases available level of serotonin, which has positive effects on emotion and thought.
- Massage, using moderate pressure, increases theta brain waves, which accompany relaxation.
- Massage enhances sleep by releasing serotonin, which is derived from the amino acid tryptophan. Serotonin is converted to melatonin in the brain, which influences the sleep stage of an individual's circadian rhythm.
- Massage boosts our immune system by flushing out toxins and increasing circulation and lymphatic flow. It also works on the immune system by increasing natural killer cells (an immune cell), which are the front lines of our immune system and kill viral infected cells.
- Massage boosts the lymphatic system, stimulating circulation and the

159

removal of metabolic wastes generated in the body.

- Massage promotes release of histamine, a neurotransmitter, that increases the permeability of blood vessels, increasing vasodilation. Vasodilation, which causes blood vessels to widen and become closer to the skin, increases relaxation, decreases pain, and can help with preparing the body for exercise or competition.

These are just some of the many mechanisms and benefits massage brings.

THE BODY REMEMBERS AND SPEAKS ITS MIND

How Emotional Trauma Manifests in the Body

Albert Einstein has speculated that rational science reveals only the external experience of some deeper reality. Understanding how emotions and trauma get trapped in the body is extremely valuable. As a hands-on practitioner, I believe it is more critical than ever toUnderstand not only how these get trapped, but to be able to know how they can be released with bodywork. Emotions are mental stimuli, a complex reaction pattern involving experimental behavior and physiological elements (UWA, Psychology and Counseling News).

Often confused with feelings and mood, emotions are physiological states and should not be interchanged with feelings and mood. Feelings arise from an emotional experience, and mood is a shorter-lived emotional state of usually low intensity; both lack stimuli and have no clear starting point. For example, when we experience the emotion fear, our heart beats faster, and we may sweat, shake, or freeze up. This is a physiological response and is the result of the autonomic nervous system's reaction to the emotion that was experienced. There can also be a healthy counterpart to emotions. Fear may paralyze some, while for others it provides the stimulus and motivation to move to higher and deeper levels of awareness and achievement. All emotions are inevitable and normal when they arise in daily life. They only become problematic when they're excessive, prolonged, or both. When traumatic experiences aren't consciously dealt with they can result in chronic fear, stress, and even occurrences of PTSD.

Trauma is considered anything that keeps us locked in physical, emotional, behavioral, or mental habit. When trauma occurs, our bodies activate a protective mechanism. A stressor that is too much for a person to handle overloads the nervous system, stopping the trauma from processing. This overloads and halts the body in its instinctive fight/flight/freeze response, causing the traumatic energy to be stored in the surrounding muscles, organs, and connective tissue. Whenever we store trauma in our tissue, our brain disconnects from that part of the body to block the experience, preventing the recall of the traumatic memory. Any area of our body that our brain is disconnected from won't be able to stay healthy and heal (Barnes, JF). As Peter Levine so effectively states, "No animal, not even the human has conscious control over whether or not it freezes in response to threat."

This state of immobility is beyond conscious control and becomes a vicious cycle maintaining physiological high levels of activity of both the parasympathetic and sympathetic nervous systems (Barnes, JF). The body is a map of every experience we ever had. Any area of our body that our brain is disconnected from won't be able to stay healthy and heal unless we properly address it.

UNLOCKING THE CAGE USING EASTERN & WESTERN MODALITIES

Certain bodywork styles effectively reduce stress and tension, allowing release as well as function to reconnect the brain with the stored trauma. As I mentioned earlier, my first teachings of massage and understanding of the human body were of Eastern tradition. The first bodywork I ever learned was in Thailand, studying Traditional Thai Massage at Wat Pho (The Temple of the Reclining Buddha) in Bangkok, continuing on with advanced training in Medical Thai massage on the magical island of Kho Phan Ghan with my teacher Nipha Sankhawai. It is through these teachings that I first came to understand Eastern tradition of a whole-body approach through bodywork.

Thai Massage
The basic principles of Thai massage ensure the flow of energy through the energy channels (meridians)m improving blood circulation throughout the body. Thai massage can benefit almost every organ in the body. For example, a headache is not just in the head according to Eastern medicine, nor is it merely a pain or something to be stopped with regards to its origin, and never, ever treated on the basis of someone else's headache. Rather, it is an obstruction of qi (energy) that can be related to one's lifestyle. Treatment might include work on other areas like the legs and arms as well as or instead of the head, and may bring more lasting and positive changes that will attempt to block the superficial systems. Eastern philosophy regards everything as mutually conditioned rising together.

Shiatsu

Shiatsu is a holistic discipline developed in Japan. This comprehensive treatment system is based on the same concepts and roots with Chinese Acupuncture and Traditional Chinese Medicine (TCM). According to this theory, the human body and its internal organs function with the power and influence of Qi (energy). Shiatsu restores this balance of energy in our body, bringing harmony between these aspects of our life. It is a whole-body approach treatment. Although Shiatsu literally means "finger pressure," the essence of Shiatsu is communication through rhythmic touch. The treatment also uses stretching and is focused mainly along specific channels (meridians) from where the body Qi (energy) passes through. Using the bladder/kidney meridian as an example will give you a glimpse of how it works.

In Traditional Chinese medicine, the bladder is one of the six yang organs that are paired with the kidney, one of the six yin organs. Yin organs store vital substances (such as Qi, blood, yin and yang), whereas the yang organs are more active and have a function of constantly filling and emptying. The bladder is a yang organ whose main physiological function is storing and excreting the urinary waste fluids passed down from the kidneys. For this to happen, the bladder uses Qi (energy) and heat from its paired yin organ, the kidney. Therefore, the bladder system in Traditional Chinese Medicine has far more influence in the body than over just fluid transformation and excretion. And as an energy system, the bladder channel is initially related to the autonomic nervous system. This is because the bladder meridian (the longest meridian channel) runs along the back of the body from the eyes to the little toe, with two parallel branches flowing along each side of the spine. These 4 branches of the bladder meridian directly influence the sympathetic and parasympathetic trunks of the autonomous nervous system, which regulates our fight or flight response and in turn all the body's basic vital functions. I particularly pay attention to the two branches of the meridian that run along both sides of the spine. This is where the nerves emerge from the spine to enervate the body.

Massage to the bladder meridian has the palpable effect of relieving headaches and back pain, and can be helpful when one has eye pain, lack of bladder control, or a cold virus. Working this meridian not only has physiological effects; there also can be an emotional response. In Traditional Chinese medicine there is an emotion connected to the organs. The emotion associated with the kidneys and bladder is fear. So, if the bladder meridian is not regulating, you can be experiencing an emotional/psychological response as well. As mentioned earlier, massaging this channel directly stimulates the parasympathetic nervous system and encourages one to feel more relaxed and peaceful. As you can see, releasing tension in the back and stimulating the bladder meridian will automatically release the stored psychic tension, resolving many physical and psychological problems.

Mayan Abdominal Massage

Another of my favorite, profound techniques that I had the privilege of studying in Guatemala is Mayan Abdominal Massage, a technique using mostly external massage to the abdomen and pelvis. My trainings were taught by Doña Dominga, a Kakchiquel midwife from the San Marcos La Laguna region of Guatemala.

The Mayans believe that many human emotions are stored in the abdomen. They aren't alone in that belief, as many cultures focus on the abdomen as a source of healing and power. In addition to physically releasing deep tension and refreshing the blood flow to muscles and organs, Mayan abdominal massage also reopens blocked energy paths and can release blocked Qi, life force as they call it, that has accumulated due to pent-up emotions (Avrigo, R.). This massage can be done on men, children and women. In women it is used specifically to help the uterus contract back to its adequate place after birth. After performing Mayan abdominal massage, a long woven fabric (commonly called a faja) is tied around the abdomen to help support the work, keeping the heart down (Mayans believe the heart is in the stomach) while at the same time supporting the body to directly affect the lower back. This a deep work acting as an energetic surging on the body, emotionally and physically. Allowing and supporting the release is part of the healing process.

Myofascial Release & Unwinding

With regards to emotional and physical trauma, the most profound teachings I had were taught to me in the West through "The John F. Barnes Myofascial Release Approach," taught by Barnes himself. John Barnes is a trained physical therapist who studied manipulative procedures from Dr. James Mennell, one of the forefathers of massage, mentioned earlier in my section on the history of massage. Barnes then went on to conceptualize his own theory of treatment. It was in the John Barnes approach that I learned extensively about the connective tissue system as well as soft tissue mobilization as a means to relieve pain and restore function. It focuses primarily on the fascial system.

Fascia is an incredible tough connective tissue that spreads throughout the body like a spider web from head to foot without interruption. Fascia supports, protects, envelops, and becomes part of the muscles, nerves, organs, and blood vessels, from the largest structures right down to the cellular level. When all is well, the body functions in harmony. However, when injuries occur, the fascia has the ability to reorganize along the lines of tension imposed on the body. Physical trauma from direct injury or accidents can cause the fascia to tighten down in an involuntary attempt to protect the body from further harm. As an injury remains unresolved, the reorganization of the fascia becomes more pronounced. Fascial strains slowly tighten, causing the body to lose its normal ability to act and react to its environment. It has been estimated that myofascial restrictions can create a tensile strength of up to approximately 2,000 pounds per square inch (Katake, K.). This enormous and excessive pressure of the myofascial restrictions on pain-sensitive structures can produce many of the pains, headaches, and undesirable symptoms that many people suffer. Most of these go undiagnosed because our standard medical tests (X-rays, CAT scans, EMG) do not show fascial restrictions (Barnes, JF.).

Patients with fascial restrictions are usually told that nothing is wrong with them or that their condition is arthritis and in some cases psychosomatic. Sometimes the patient is never even touched. Touching patients with skilled hands can be one of the most potent ways of locating fascial restrictions and effecting positive change. Touching through massage, movement therapy, or refined touch of myofascial release helps to enhance function and movement of every structure in the body. Myofascial release helps remove the pressure caused by restricted fascia, easing symptoms of pain, headaches, spasm, and fibromyalgia, and restoring range of motion. Myofascial release is a whole-body approach designed to rectify the fascial restrictions that caused the effect or symptom. While having been trained in all of John Barnes' myofascial release courses, it wasn't until his myofascial unwinding course that I experienced the most profound experience connecting mind and body releasing both emotional and physical trauma on a much deeper level. Let me first state that before taking any of the myofascial courses, although having been trained in many Eastern whole-body approaches, I was working in a more traditional medical rehabilitation center in stroke and brain trauma, using more linear thinking and sometimes being skeptical of what might be known as esoteric or "energy" work.

The best way for me to describe myofascial unwinding is the spontaneous movement of the body via the mind in response to the therapist's touch. During fascial unwinding, the therapist stimulates mechanoreceptors in the fascia by applying gentle touch and stretching. The client responds with spontaneous bending, rotating, and twisting of the upper or lower limbs or of the whole body in either a rhythmic or a chaotic pattern. Despite how mystical this sounds, its results are effective and profound.

My first experience as a student in myofascial unwinding took place in a hotel's ballroom at one of Barnes' seminars. When he first demonstrated the technique on the stage, using one of the students as his model, I was stunned, shocked, and overwhelmed. This was exactly the type of "energy" work I steered clear of for many years. The emotional energy coming forth in the room was disturbing and at first disruptive. In the darkness of the room I became deeply fixated while working as the giver, then I was jolted by someone screaming, moaning, choking, or doing all three at once. I wondered to myself, "Am I experiencing an exorcism?," I was beginning to get scared and leery of this technique. After performing the unwinding on my partner, I was becoming more and more skeptical. Some of the people sitting around me were stressed to the point of wanting to escape. We looked at each other in disbelief, at the same time consoling and supporting each other.

It was now my turn to be the receiver. I was steadfast in my thinking that none of this emotional release would ever happen to me. As I lay on the table, my practitioner began with touch to my head and neck. Within moments, I suddenly felt my eyes start to flutter, my head began to roll from side to side, and heat rushed to my throat, at which point my practitioner placed her hands on my throat. I began to cough and choke. The throat has always been a spot I have weakness in. Growing up as a very shy girl, I often felt I didn't have a voice. There were master practitioners walking around and one approached my table and begin to assist my practitioner, repeating over and over, "let it go, scream, yell, let your voice be heard." In my head I kept thinking, "this can't be happening to ME." My left arm began to circle around receptively (I had a previous injury to my left shoulder).

Before I knew it I was thrashing about the table, proceeding to go into a complete headstand (one of my greatest fears in yoga) and here I was on a soft massage table actually doing one. I then continued to contour my body in all shapes and forms I never thought possible, continuing until I was slithering off the massage table to the floor, the entire time being guided by two practitioners. Oddly enough, I felt completely safe. When I completed my "unwinding" I could feel a sense of peace, as if 1000 pounds had been lifted off me. A few years earlier, I experienced an allergic reaction to an antibiotic resulting in severe neuropathy throughout my entire body. I had been dealing with the pain trauma for many years, explaining my intense response to the unwinding.

This may sound extremely esoteric to some. To better explain it, studies show that during long periods of trauma, people make indelible imprints of experience that have high levels of emotional content. The body can hold information below the conscious level, as a protective mechanism, so that memories become dissociated. The memories are state- or position-dependent and can therefore be retrieved when the person is in a particular state or position (Rossi, et al,16). It has been demonstrated consistently that when a myofascial release takes the tissue to a significant position, or when myofascial unwinding allows a body part to assume a significant position, the tissue not only changes and improves, but memories and associated emotional states also rise to the conscious level. The therapist acts as a facilitator, following the body's inherent motion (Barnes, JF).

In the days to come during the seminar, I looked around the room and I could see the difference in the faces and body language of all the students. I noticed the ones who did the most unwinding were walking taller, their faces glowed, shoulders were relaxed, and most important their hearts were open to everyone around them. This work is powerful. I continue to practice it today on clients and have seen incredible physical and emotional releases. I have seen patients relive car accidents, athletes go into the exact position they were injured in, and many suffering from fibromyalgia get an enormous sense of relief. The list goes on. It"s extremely gratifying to see clients relieved from pain and emotions they were holding for years, with most of them having tried numerous modalities that failed to address the pain or injury. My own testimonial as well as the experiences of my many clients speaks to this incredible healing through myofascial unwinding.

I am grateful to all to my clients and patients who have taught me in my path. And I am honored to have had the privilege of learning this wonderful technique from John Barnes. He has not only taught me but shown me that "the body keeps the score." These techniques I have described are just a few examples of whole-body system approaches.

KEEPING IN TOUCH WITH YOURSELF
It is of utmost importance to not only listen and get to know your body, but to take time to receive treatment. If treatment is not an option, teaching ourselves the tools to meet our needs can be as beneficial. To restore your body and dissolve stored

blocked emotions, first allow yourself to feel them. One of the best ways to get rid of muscle tension is to actively feel and let go of emotions as they come. Feeling the emotions might involve any form of catharsis like running, dancing, deep belly breathing, screaming or crying. This is called emotional regulation, which is our ability to cope with stress in a flexible, tolerant, and adaptive way.

Our attitude matters, and it is important we come from a place of non-judgment. When we consider our emotions as something bad or wrong, we actually deepen our suffering and solidify the tensions within our bodies. Instead, surrender to each emotion. Become aware of yourself. Our deepest challenge is to recognize the emotion and feel it in our body. This is where mindfulness is helpful. Notice what is happening, and accept and feel it fully without judging. Be gentle and kind with yourself. This might sound simple, but it's profound. Muscle tension tends to add to our inner voices, which cause us even more tension. Find a trained practitioner and receive bodywork. If this is not an option, self-massage, meditation, and breathing techniques are all extremely beneficial. While self-massage caters to our physical state, it can also unwittingly play a role in our mental state. Self-care helps us learn to identify and care for our physical and emotional needs.

Self-Massage Techniques

- Take time to do self-massage in a relaxing setting. Dimmig lights, lighting candles, or even going in nature can help promote more relaxation.
- Using aromatherapy is extremely beneficial. Your brain responds to smell and aromas. Essential oils added to a cream or a base oil like almond oil complement touch. Never apply essential oils directly to skin. Besides smelling, good essential oils also stimulate specific brain action.
- Grapefruit oil can promote release of endorphins, neurotransmitters that act as natural pain killers.
- Marjoram oil can boost your levels of serotonin, helping you feel calm.
- Sandalwood oil releases both dopamine and serotonin.
- Lavender, one of the more familiar oils, is known to promote relaxation and sleep.
- Ylang-ylang, a tropical plant native to India, Indonesia, and the Philippines, triggers the release of the "feel good" endorphins and serotonin.

When practicing self-massage techniques, it is more beneficial to use less physical pressure. When too much pressure is applied, our bodies naturally fight the pain by contracting our muscles, making the massage harder to enjoy. We have tightness in our body due to overuse, stress, and anxiety. Stress and anxiety are more mental responses, so keeping the pressure light is best for these. You can use a deeper pressure for soreness or injuries.

Shoulders & Neck

These always comprise an area of muscle tension and stress. Begin with one side of your shoulders at a time, hooking your fingers over the trapezius muscle (your bulky shoulder muscle that is easily palpated) and knead with your fingers, being sure to focus and keep pressure on areas of increased muscle tension. To create deeper depth, lower your ear to the opposite shoulder to stretch the trapezius muscles as you continue to massage the area.

Abdominal Massage

Abdominal massage can ease bloating and encourage waste to be dispersed. Use both hands to stroke the stomach, going in a circular motion including the sides of the waist. Lastly, stroke the abdomen up the right-hand side, across the top and down the left hand side. This is the pathway of the colon. Remember that the abdomen can be a place where emotions get stored. Massaging this area can release anything that is blocked.

Reflexology

Reflexology, a type of massage using pressure to the feet, is based on a theory that areas of the feet are related to certain organs and body systems throughout the body.

- **Diaphragm Reflex** - located along the entire mid foot. Using your thumb, work across the middle of the foot 3 times. Working this point helps to release tension held in the entire body.

- **Pituitary Reflex** - Using your thumb, press and circle the middle of the big toe for a few seconds. The pituitary gland is found at the base of the brain and is often referred to as "the master gland" of the body. This gland produces many hormones and is responsible for releasing hormones that stimulate the adrenal glands, the thyroid gland, the ovaries, and the testes. Repeat at least 3 times.

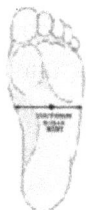

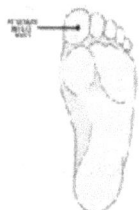

- **Spinal reflexes** - Using the thumb, press and circle down the side of the foot, starting from the big toe down towards the heel. Next, press and move across from the heel to the ankle to the big toes along the side of the foot. Repeat at least 3 times.

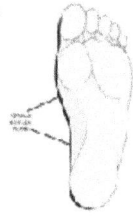

Shiatsu/Acupressure

The acupoint LI 20, English name Welcome Fragrance and Pinyin name Ying Xiang, is a very powerful point to treat all kinds of conditions related to the nose and sinuses. With so many suffering from allergies, this is a wonderful point to work. In Traditional Chinese Medicine the large intestine is paired with the lungs (yin and yang). Both of these organs represent our ability to be "open" or taking in, and "letting go" or releasing. In the body, their channel-pathways can be used to create space in congested areas.

This point can be located at the level with the midpoint of the lateral border alanasi (also known as the side of the nostril). It lies right above the largest sinus pocket in our head and is the last point on the large intestine meridian. You may wonder why a large intestine point is on the face. The concept of "letting go" on the face is analogous to that of our bowel function: both are a physiological process of releasing what no longer is needed to nourish our body. When we experience cold symptoms such as sinusitis, this is also a form of releasing accumulation, a clearing out of what does not serve the body. By pressing into this area we can improve fluid circulation and open the airway for better breathing, releasing any pressure you may have in this area. It is a good point to use when suffering from rhinitis, sinusitis, acne, abscesses of the mouth, and toothache, to name a few.

ACUPOINT: LI20

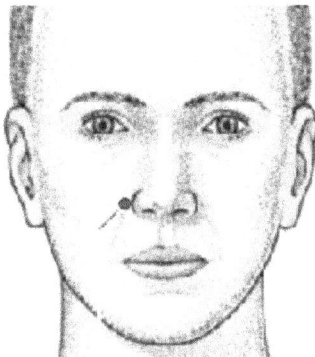

Thai Massage Stretch

A beneficial pose in Thai massage is Supine Spinal Twist. Start by lying flat on your back. The first thing to do is bring one leg across the body, slowly rotating your body in the opposite direction. Let your gaze follow, then take a moment to pause and breathe while holding the position.

The many benefits of Supine Spinal Twist include quieting the nervous system, and stretching the gluteals, external obliques, and abdominal muscles. Internal organs are toned during abdominal stretching. Supine Spinal Twist is also conducive to digestion and relieves constipation. Tension in the back is also relieved and fatigue is alleviated. In general, twists allow more nourishment to reach the roots of the spinal nerves, and this has a positive effect on the sympathetic nervous system. There are some contraindications that should be noted with Supine Spinal Twist. These include pregnancy, spinal operations, herniated discs, degenerative disc diseases, and sciatica.

~ ~ ~ ~ ~ ~ ~ ~ ~

Most important to understand is that your biology, experiences, environment, careers, and emotional states are your own and unique to you alone. These are all connected to who you are and what manifests within you. In listening to your mind, body, and spirit you can best determine what makes you feel nourished, what you need and how you can adapt and care for yourself. This is the first step to apply, which can be more profound than any application or technique.

It is then that you will be able to comprehend your structural relationships, which can assist you to seek a practitioner with these needs in mind. Find the right person or modality that fits your unique being. A qualified and experienced practitioner will guide you in your journey to heal from pain restrictions, injuries, trauma, anxiety, or whatever it is you may be experiencing, but remember it is your journey and you are your best guide. It may never be as simple as one modality or treatment, and it may be as simple or not so simple as learning to breathe, relax, or calm your mind and body. You and only you will be able to know what is right and how you can expand on it. Life is a process of multiple states we encounter. Embracing each one is part of the journey. It is when we remain in a state that restrictions and holding patterns are created.

Be present, expand, and dare to blossom!

WORKS CITED

Avrigo R., Epstein N. Rainforest Home Remedies: The Maya Way to Heal Your Body & Replenish Your Soul 2001)

Barnes , JF. Myofascial Release: The Search for Excellence. Philadelphia: Rehabilitation Sciences Inc. 1990)

Carlson, M. & Earles F. (1997) Psychological and neuroendocrinological sequel of our social deprivation in institutionalized children in Romania

Engel G. The Need for a new medical mode: a challenge for Biomedicine Science.1977; 196:129-136

Field, Tiffany M., et al (1986) "Tactile/Kinesthetic Stimulation Effects on Pre-term Neonatals Pediatics. 77(5): 654-658)

------- (1999), Pre schoolers in America are Touched less and more aggressive than pre-schoolers in France, Early Development and Care, 151:1, 11-17.
------- Massage Therapy Research (1st edi.) Edinburgh: Elsevier Churchill Livingston, 2006

Katake, K.1961: The strength for tension and bursting of human fascia.J. Kyoto Med. Univ. 69:484-488.

Kurtz R. Body centered psychotherapy: the Hakomi therapy, Ashland,OR: Author of the Hakomi Institute, 1988

Linden, D. (2015) The Power of Touch, The New Yorker

Ni, Maoshing, Ph. D., The Yellow Emperor's Classic of Medicine: A New Translation of the Neijing Suwen with Commentary. 1995.

Rossi, E.L.(1987) From mind to molecule. A state-dependent memory, learning and behavior theory of mind-body healing. Advances, 4(2). 46-60
"The Science of Emotion Exploring the Basics of Emotional Psychology," Psychology and Counseling News. UAW Online, June 27, 2019.
https://online.uwa.edu/news/emotional-psychology/

CHAPTER X

My Eastern Paths to Healing

We have heard the poets say it and the astrophysicists alike: we are nature. We are the universe. We are both creation and creators, one with the source of life. We are the sun and the stars and the earth we walk upon. Our luminous beings are made up of the same elements that make up the entire existence of the cosmos. We are governed by electromagnetism and the laws of nature. Yin and Yang. This is who we are as individual beings and collectively as a whole.

How connected we are to these truths directly affects the quality of our human experience. When we live in accordance to the laws of nature, we are in a state of balance. Balance is health, the alignment of body, mind and spirit. Our energy is fluid like a river. Perhaps you have had the experience of being in the flow. You have seen athletes in the zone, masterful artists who have taken your breath away. The confluence of body, mind, and spirit working in concert with each other is the balance of life itself. Balance also occurs as we are harmonious with nature. Like a tree in the spring, when buds form, soon to flower and bloom, such is replicating in our own bodies too. Our energy in the beginning of spring is beginning to expand. By summer, like the sun, our life energy is its most expansive. By the autumn, we enter the gathering phase, not unlike the harvest to prepare for winter, where we contain stored fuel. This is the cycle of the seasons as well as the cycle of our body. We are created to follow nature.

Sickness, on the other hand, happens when we break that natural cycle. When a patient comes into my office, chances are, their systems are off cycle, even compromised. Like those of many holistic professionals, my services are often sought after exhausting other more mainstream avenues. Perhaps patients have a sinking winter pulse in the middle of summer, indicating a cold or kidney/bladder issues. They might be suffering from symptoms like lethargy, frequent urination, thirst, or back pain. Together, we begin the process of restoring their system to harmonize once again with the laws of nature.

Balance—I wish it sounded sexier. If only we could choose the red pill or the blue pill. Beginning with formulating a diagnosis, I am confronted more often than not with what I describe as a knotted chain that needs to be unraveled. Piece by piece, we undo the blocks created by a myriad of causes, from poor diet, physical injury, emotional and psychological imbalances, trauma, insomnia, viruses, and pathogens, to genetic predispositions. While Western medicine focuses on treating illness, holistic medicine addresses health and wellness in a biopsychosocial approach. We treat the cause of the imbalance where mainstream medicine focuses on the treating the effects. Each treatment is a building block to remove old patterns and blockages in order to restore the system to its full potential.

Eastern medicine is a road map. In the body, there are points that form part of a meridian, which is a pathway of energy. We refer to this energy as Qi or Ki. Every meridian relates to the function of an organ in the body and its system. Every system correlates with the elements of nature. As we return to health, we are restoring all of nature. When we live in accordance to nature, we are repairing nature itself and protecting ourselves from pathogenic sickness. I can't properly articulate the wonder I experienced hearing this for the first time, that there is a harmony in the universe which expresses itself in the form of sound, frequency, energy, electromagnetism, light—and that our enlightened ancients, connected to the source of life, were able to preserve in detail an innate understanding of the laws of life and to preserve a detailed medicine that we still use today, a medicine that has more relevance as people seek to heal.

Life, as I knew it as a child, couldn't have been farther from the life the ancients described. My story is a common one you hear all the time, of a practitioner whose interest in healing was sparked by her own health challenges. When I was a child, I suffered from ongoing pain, doubled over from pain, and staying home from school kinds of digestive issues. This often led to my attraction to foods which only increased my discomfort. In a continuous spiral, I resorted to strong laxatives, on which I became dependent before I was 13. On my own, I would put myself on severe diets, hoping that would make me feel better. Even though I was athletic, I was dysmorphic, my body a source of struggle and pain. Not a single doctor could diagnose me, neither my pediatrician nor my parents' primary doctor—or the cadre of specialists whose tests and diets often made things worse. During one of those times, when I was eleven, I decided to eat only sugary fruit yogurt for breakfast, lunch, and dinner: mono-eating, what I now know is a sure sign that the system is off. There were the protein powders given to me by a specialist, a famous doctor who inaccurately diagnosed me with hypoglycemia, low blood sugar. His dietary guide of an all-protein diet made me even sicker and more sluggish. There was the summer I ate only mixed salad. I was intolerably hungry, but afraid to eat.

My teenage years were marked by cystic acne and an overactive, unbalanced hormonal system. I rarely felt good. My emotional state was so out of whack, I often medicated with recreational drugs. Doctors gave me ongoing antibiotic therapy to help my skin. My digestive system worsened. I no longer remembered what feeling good, or well, was like. I was anxious and couldn't sleep. Then came the muscle relaxers for a nervous stomach.

Nobody could correctly diagnose me. However, I had an inkling that something was missing. When I was around 12, I found a book on the street called The Herb Book, by John Lust, a book on herbs from the Northern Hemisphere called the most complete catalog of "miracle plants" ever published. I was riveted and dog-eared all the pages. The book contained recipes for concoctions and teas to heal various conditions, including infusions for my digestive woes, but I had no idea where to find the herbs. Where was Google when I needed it?

One day, I entered a store that sold hippie products like lava lamps, rock and roll posters, candles, and silver jewelry. I found packets of Belladonna and Damiana, which I excitedly bought having seen their names in the The Herb Book. I took them home, but when I read that Belladonna was poisonous if not dosed properly and Damiana was an aphrodisiac, I left them untouched. I was a little kid and I didn't want to accidentally poison myself, nor was I ready to have sex. Through the years, I accumulated books on metaphysics, herbs, tarot, hand analysis, crystals. I had a nagging sense that there was something more to life, but it was just not yet revealed to me.

On a trip to Chiapas, Mexico, when I was 17 years old, I picked up a book on medicine of the Ancient Maya at the library of Casa Na Bolom, an inn and sanctuary created by anthropologist Frans Blum and his wife Gertrude. I read through the healing methods of the local shamans, the extensive knowledge of ethnobotany, the connection to the divine life force and the cycles of nature, and even some dangerous remedies including putting feces on your head, as a last resort to ward off death (not to worry, I have never prescribed that in my practice!). The book described the animal spirits, the power of the Nahuatl (the jaguar), and all the different deities. For me it was a mix of plant wisdom and the spirit world, of which I had zero understanding. I was surprised how comprehensive the system was for something that was recorded so many hundreds of years ago.

Everything changed for me during my college years. In my freshman year, my faculty advisor, a professor of Eastern and Indian studies, took 15 of us to see Swami Jiddu Krishnamurti. He was seated on the floor on a large stage at an outdoor arena, talking about life to an enthusiastic crowd of devotees. I think I might've fallen asleep, lulled by the drone of his voice and my resistance. However, listening to him was also a catalyst for a journey that has never ended: the world of spirit and the search for the meaning of life. By my senior year of college, I was hoping to embark on a career as a Classical musician; I didn't know it then, but in the summer of 1984 I attended a weekend workshop that was going to change the course of my life.

His name was Sensei Masahilo M Nakazono, the founder of a school in Santa Fe, New Mexico called the Kototama Institute. There, he and his two sons were training students to be doctors of an esoteric form of Eastern Medicine called Inochi, based on the Kototama Principle, the sounds according to Shinto that make up our entire existence. We spent that weekend in August, 1984 learning about the governing laws of life, energy frequencies, sounds, nature, and health. He talked about universal truths as told by the ancestors. I cried for days, with an inner knowing, like coming home.

That week, I also met Dr. Neal, a naturopath who would start me on my personal journey to healing. It was determined that I had, among other things, an overgrowth of yeast in my system, the prime environment for pathogenic bacteria to thrive. The cause? Overuse of antibiotics. I had almost no healthy intestinal flora. Additionally, my diet was making it worse. He muscle-tested me, which led to dietary changes, such as the removal of yeast, wheat, sugar, meat, dairy, caffeine, alcohol, nightshades, vinegar, etc. He replaced them with whole grains, fruit and vegetables, chicken, fish, legumes, oils. I added therapeutic levels of probiotics, homeopathic remedies, exercise and other supplements to support holistic healing from within. I followed the regimen religiously and it paid off, finally knowing what it was like to feel good, and well. My mind was clear, my energy was vibrant, my digestive system became regular. I slept well, and my body both felt and looked fit. My outlook on life improved as I felt a sense of gratitude and well-being. I wanted everyone to feel this way, to know what it was like to be integrated.

In 1985, after a year in Italy amid a failing marriage, playing and teaching music, studying natural medicine from anyone who'd teach me, metaphysical workshops, and diminished health from stress, Italian food, and an abundance of despair, I returned to New York to pursue my Master's degree in music at NYU. Meanwhile,

I was invited to attend a two-week workshop on healing with Inochi Medicine by Nakazono's son Jei, exactly a year after I attended his dad's seminar. I dove in. Jei handed out his translation of The Yellow Emperor, The Lost Books Of The Su Wen. It further opened my eyes to a holistic world, where everything turned out to be part of the laws of nature. Its prologue says:

> The ancients thought that there were five indispensable qualities for living. These are Wood, Fire, Earth, Metal and Water, and they are otherwise known as the five phases. They each possess different characteristics, and all phenomena and substances within the universe belong to one of these five phases. The idea which has developed into the five-phase theory is that all phenomena and substances in the universe are the products of the movement and mutation of these five phases. The five-phase theory, as described in the Neijing, is a philosophical theory of medical practice in ancient China. This theory has served as the guiding ideology and methodology of physiology, pathology, clinical diagnosis and treatment. The characteristics of each phase in this theory have been derived from the observations of countless generations over the millennia, and they are reflected in clinical experiences (Ni).

In addition to The Yellow Emperor, Jei handed us each a five element chart. It blew my mind how everything in the universe could be synthesized into five categories. There were five sounds, five directions, five yin organs, five yang organs, five elements, five emotions, five senses, five tastes, five virtues, the list was endless, showing how our entire world belonged within the system like a whole, interconnected circle of life. Everything exists within the flow of life; from matter, like a wooden table, to something subjective like worry. I learned about Yin and Yang, the laws of dualism. As defined by The Yellow Emperor, "The law of yin and yang is the natural order of the universe, the foundation of all things, mother of all changes, the root of life and death." I was taught that existence falls within the variabilities of darkness and light, and how yin and yang are both opposites, yet complementary, an interconnected circle from concentration to expansion and back, just like the seasons, the years, the months, the days, the hours, etc. There is even an Eastern Zodiac which also follows the universal cycle of Yin and Yang through twelve animal spirits. Anything that exists, I was taught, lives within the Taoist concept of time, space, and dimension. I learned what constitutes health, the harmony of the elements, and the disharmony that creates sickness.

During the two-week seminar, we practiced a form of handwork called Do-In, where we treated ourselves, using self-massage, and each other. My interest in bodywork and acupressure surprised me, as I was never that comfortable connecting to people through touch, but found myself feeling immense satisfaction at being both the patient and even more as the practitioner. More importantly, I started to get treated by Jei twice a week. He asked me many questions, the same ones I ask my patients to this day, to formulate a diagnosis. He read my pulses on my wrist and neck simultaneously to determine the root cause of my sickness. He told me that he was reading the state of my organs' systems and that he was going to use acupuncture to tonify and sedate my body's systems depending on what he deemed necessary. I so badly wanted to read what he was reading. My passion was ignited.

Through The Yellow Emperor, I also learned that these pulses have additional unique qualities which also correlate with an organ's system. For example, the heart pulse is a rapid pulse which has the sensation of a hook coming up and around on the finger, whereas the kidney pulse is a slow, sinking pulse. Liver pulse has the sensation of a tense violin string, and so on. There were also secondary and tertiary pulse qualities. 70 percent of treatment is diagnosis. I learned that to be integrated with nature, it is expected that you would have the pulse quality that corresponded to the season we were in. If you didn't, it was indicative of imbalance or even sickness.

In Eastern medicine, there are twelve primary meridians and eight extraordinary meridians. There are 361 main points and 48 extra points, The twelve primary meridians are pathways of energy (ki or Qi) of specific organs and viscera. The twelve meridians represent the flow of energy of the Liver, Gall Bladder, Heart, Small Intestine, Heart Constrictor (Pericardium), Triple Heater (the body's thermostat), Spleen, Stomach, Lung, Large Intestine, Kidney, and Bladder.

You read the condition of these systems on the pulses along the radial artery of the wrist. The Liver/Gall Bladder System relates season of spring, the phase of birth and consciousness. The Heart/Small Intestine System relates to summer, the growth and awareness. The Spleen/Stomach system is late summer (or the middle of each season), the phase of transformation and love. The Lung/Large Intestine system relates to the season of Fall, the phase of gathering and discernment or clarity. The Kidney/Bladder System relates to the season of winter, the phase of storing and wisdom. Here is a short Five Element chart:

	Wood	Fire	Earth	Metal	Water
Orientation	East	South	Middle	West	North
Season	Spring	Summer	Late Summer	Autumn	Winter
Climate	Wind	Summer Heat	Dampness	Dryness	Cold
Cultivation	Germinate	Grow	Transform	Reap	Store
Yin Organ	Liver	Heart	Spleen	Lung	Kidney
Yang Organ	Gall Bladder	Small Intestine	Stomach	Large Intestine	Bladder
Orifice	Eye	Tongue	Mouth	Nose	Ear
Tissues	Tendons	Vessels	Muscles	Skin & Hair	Bones
Emotions	Anger	Joy	Pensiveness	Grief	Fear
Colour	Blue/ Green	Red	Yellow	White	Black
Taste	Sour	Bitter	Sweet	Pungent	Salty
Voice	Shout	Laugh	Sing	Cry	Groan

The Meridians and their points are said to work with the nervous system. Our bodies look a lot like trees with a root system and branches.

Human body meridians

ANTERIOR VIEW
LEFT - YIN SUPERFICIAL MERIDIANS
RIGHT - SUPERFICIAL MUSCULATURE
ARM YIN MERIDIANS & SHICHEN   LEG YIN MERIDIANS & SHICHEN
LU - LUNG MERIDIAN 3-5 AM   SP - SPLEEN MERIDIAN 9 - 11 AM
HT - HEART MERIDIAN 11 AM - 1 PM   KD - KIDNEY MERIDIAN 5-7 PM
LV - LIVER MERIDIAN 1 - 3 AM   PE - PERICARDIUM MERIDIAN 7 - 9 PM
GV - CONCEPTION VESSEL (CENTERLINE)

POSTERIOR VIEW
LEFT - SUPERFICIAL MUSCULATURE
RIGHT - YANG SUPERFICIAL MERIDIANS
ARM YANG MERIDIANS & SHICHEN   LEG YANG MERIDIANS & SHICHEN
LI - LARGE INTESTINE MERIDIAN 5-7 AM   ST - STOMACH MERIDIAN 7 - 9 AM
SI - SMALL INTESTINE 1 - 3 PM   BL - BLADDER MERIDIAN 3 - 5 PM
TW - TRIPLE WARMER 9 - 11 PM   GB - GALL BLADDER MERIDIAN 11 PM - 1 AM
GV - GOVERNING VESSEL (CENTERLINE)

LEGEND
WOOD PHASE MERIDIAN
1ST FIRE PHASE MERIDIAN
2ND FIRE PHASE MERIDIAN
EARTH PHASE MERIDIAN
METAL PHASE MERIDIAN
WATER PHASE MERIDIAN
PRIME VESSEL

● STIMULATION ACUPRESSURE POINT
● SEDATION ACUPRESSURE POINT
○ ELEMENTAL ACUPRESSURE POINT
●● ALARM ACUPRESSURE POINT
●● YU (ASSOCIATED) ACUPRESSURE POINT
● ● SUPERFICIAL ACUPRESSURE POINT
○ "SHICHEN MERIDIAN STRIKING POINT
◇ SHICHEN ZANFU 12 HOUR VITAL STRIKING POINT

WRIST PULSE
LEFT   RIGHT
DEEP / SUPERFICIAL   DEEP / SUPERFICIAL
HT / LI   LU / LI
LV / GB   SP / ST
KD / BL   KD / PE - TW

□ GENERAL USE STRIKING POINTS

178

By the end of the two-week intensive, I was at a crossroads. Do I return to my marriage in Italy and my job teaching music, do I get my Masters at NYU, do I enter into the family business, or do I embark on a journey I never imagined for myself, studying to become a Doctor of Eastern medicine? At the time, there were so few people with careers in natural medicine. Almost nobodheard of acupuncture, let alone herbology. Anyone and everyone tried to dissuade me. But, it was a friend of my parents' friend, an American doctor who spent time in China, who encouraged me to follow my heart. In January of 1986, my marriage and my music career were to become a distant memory. I showed up for my first class of Kototama Life Medicine and never looked back.

Eastern Medicine Explained

It is nearly impossible in a single chapter to explain Eastern Medicine, as vast as the universe itself. As I mentioned, everything that exists belongs to a circle of transformation. Life is change, so it follows that Eastern Medicine is a guide as to how to live by universal law, given perpetual change. According to The Yellow Emperor, the ancients had an innate intelligence for thousands of years, in which they naturally understood the flow of life. Chapter One of The Yellow Emperor is called "The Universal Truth," written within 2698-2598, BCE. Here is an excerpt that still resonates to me today as it did the first time I read it in September, 1985, nearly 37 years ago. The Yellow Emperor, Huang Di, is discussing medicine, lifestyle, and nutrition, along with Taoist cosmology with his ministers, Qi Bo and Lei Gong.

'I've heard that in the days of old everyone lived one hundred years without showing the usual signs of aging. In our time, however, people age prematurely, living only fifty years. Is this due to a change in the environment, or is it because people have lost the correct way of life?' Qi Bo replied, 'In the past, people practiced the Tao, the Way of Life. They understood the principle of balance, of yin and yang, as represented by the transformation of the energies of the universe. Thus, they formulated practices such as Dao-in, an exercise combining stretching, massaging, and breathing to promote energy flow, and meditation to help maintain and harmonize themselves with the universe. They ate a balanced diet at regular times, arose and retired at regular hours, avoided overstressing their bodies and minds, and refrained from overindulgence of all kinds. They maintained well-being of body and mind; thus, it is not surprising that they lived over one hundred years. These days, people have changed their way of life. They drink wine as though it were water, indulge excessively in destructive activities, drain their jing—the body's essence that is stored in the kidneys—and deplete their qi. They do not know the secret of conserving their energy and vitality. Seeking emotional excitement and momentary pleasures, people disregard the natural rhythm and order of the universe. They fail to regulate their lifestyle and diet, and sleep improperly. So it is not surprising that they look old at fifty and die soon after. The accomplished ones of ancient times advised people to guard themselves against zei feng (viruses and flus) disease-causing factors. On the mental level, one should remain calm and avoid excessive desires and fantasies, recognizing and maintaining the natural purity and clarity of the mind. When internal energies are able to circulate smoothly and endocand concentrated, illness and disease can be avoided. Previously, people led a calm and honest existence, detached from undue desire and ambition; they lived with an untainted conscience and without fear. They were active, but never depleted themselves. Because they lived simply, these individuals knew contentment, as reflected in their diet of basic but nourishing foods and attire that was appropriate to the season but never luxurious. Since they were happy with their position in life, they did not feel jealousy or greed. They had compassion for others and were helpful and honest, free from destructive habits. They remained unshakable and unswayed by temptations, and they were able to stay centered even when adversity arose. They treated others justly, regardless of their level of intelligence or social position.'

I was like, WOW! No two patients have the same pulses or diagnosis even if they both have the same illness. Nor are their treatment protocols the same. We are the sum of our parts, therefore unique. One patient's life experience will naturally differ from another's. One patient might drink alcohol every day, the other not. Lifestyle differences and genetic dispositions create different needs from the practitioner. Hence, while they could both have arthritis, one might be needled at the top edge of the small finger's fingernail, which begins the small intestine meridian, whereas another patient will receive moxibustion (burning hemp) along the large intestine meridian. This is radically different from allopathic medicine, which takes a one-size-fits-all approach to treating illness. It is the work of an Eastern doctor to peel away the layers, to undo the pathogenic flow of energy to one that is in tune with the cosmos.

In modern society, this has gotten rather complicated. We are pressured to follow life-depleting goals. Out of necessity, we follow the dollar bill, get swayed by illusory societal ideals. We spend countless moments away from the now, diving into our barrage of thoughts, feelings, and stressors. We waste energy trying to change others and expend priceless moments worrying about what other people think. This leaves us fragmented. Our bodies are often sedentary for hours at a time. It hurts me to see school-age kids sitting for their entire school day without an outlet for their life energy. No wonder we're sick. We are more polarized and divisive than ever, careening away from the natural order.

The ancients believed then that we need to find our way back to a simple, more authentic way of life, connected and interconnected. To regain or even retain health, we need to honor the seasons and our place within them. The Yellow Emperor writes, ""Health and well-being can be achieved only by remaining centered in spirit, guarding against the squandering of energy, promoting the constant flow of qi and blood, maintaining harmonious balance of yin and yang, adapting to the changing seasonal and yearly macrocosmic influences, and nourishing one's self preventively. This is the way to a long and happy life." There are plenty of examples of how we can weaken or strengthen the body. How well we follow the laws of nature in the spring can determine the state of our health in late summer. If we follow the guidelines as related to summer, we will be strong as we gather our energy in autumn to help in the winter months. That's how interdependent the cycles of the seasons are.

Humans have developed technologies to mitigate the effects of the seasons, with air conditioners in summer and heating in winter. Our bodies have acclimated to living less harshly in the elements. However, I do believe that in summer we need to be active and to sweat. It is how we remove toxins and avoid sickness later on. We have an inner thermostat that maintains the proper temperature within the body called the Triple Heater, that while it has adapted to modern ways, still benefits from the seasons that regulate us. As we are made up largely of fluids, we need to drink water throughout the year. However, we need to drink more water in the summertime when it's hot and there is danger of dehydration. Or even in autumn, the dry period. Constipation can be prevalent in winter due to the use of heating in our homes, which dehydrates the body. While we need to drink water to counteract the dry heat, if we drink water that is too cold in the winter months it will hurt our kidneys. This can harm our physical stamina and life force. In winter, hot or room temperature liquids help us stay healthy. We will stay well if we abide by the common-sense rules. This includes doing what you can to preserve your life energy and not drain your ki.

Following the seasons and abiding by their rhythm is another way to protect ourselves. In winter, as the days are shorter, going to bed earlier will preserve our life force. Doing strenuous physical activity in extremely cold weather can weaken our kidney energy. Even the excess of sexual intercourse in winter can weaken our system. Overexerting is easier in the spring and summer months, when the life energy is at the most expansive.

We are what we eat!
When someone enters into my practice, the first order of business is to regulate the digestive system. There are too many illnesses to count either caused by or worsened by digestive irregularities or impairment. Inflammation in the gut alone is the cause of a myriad of sicknesses including autoimmune problems.

I cannot overstate the importance of not only eating according to the season, but internalizing that food is fuel or energy that nourishes us and keeps us alive, even helps us thrive. Many adverse health conditions can be mitigated or healed by diet. In a patient who is out of balance, I often use food as medicine, as what they are eating could be toxic, exacerbating their sickness. Not unlike what happened to me.

In the last 35 years, I have seen more and more patients with food allergies and sensitivities. Between overly processed, chemically enhanced food that is stripped of its properties, bodies have been compromised by their inability to break down and metabolize the food as it works its way through the digestive process. For example, simple sugar can cause havoc. Excess sweet taste causes an internal loosening which is the equivalent of an internal mudslide in our bodies. This can lead to symptoms like brain fog, fatigue, anxiety, aching, and stiff muscles, stomach pain, heartburn, even gout. In fact, too much of any one taste eaten repetitively can potentially make you sick. As all things, it all comes down to balance.

As a rule, a diet rich in nutrient-dense foods includes organic fruit and vegetables, locally sourced meat and fish, beans, whole grains, and fats. Nakazono used to recommend the 60/20/20 rule; 60 percent vegetables and fruit, 20 percent protein, and 20 percent whole grains.

Eating within a twelve-hour period and no later than 8pm, when the digestive energy is strong, is optimal. Of course, each person thrives on different things in any given moment. Food is fluid. Other food recommendations you would hear if you entered in my practice is to eat the colors of the rainbow. To incorporate all the tastes and their colors in your meals will nourish your organs and their systems. We need to strive for a balance of sour, bitter, sweet, hot (spicy), and salt, and the colors green, red, yellow or orange, white and black or purple to feed the liver, heart, spleen, lung and kidney systems, respectively.

There are five phases pertaining to our cycles. Spring is the birthing stage, when we can eat early foods like berries, cucumbers, asparagus, and sprouts, to name a few. Summer is the most bountiful, when we can eat the largest variety of seasonal fruits and vegetables. Spicy food is tolerated better during summer as it helps us sweat and dispel heat. Late summer, still abundant, we have broccoli, string beans, corn, peaches, plums and nectarines. By fall, we enter into the gathering period, the time of the harvest; apples, pears, cabbage, squash, beets, and potatoes can be picked and stored for the long winter ahead. Winter, the storing periodm is a good time for root vegetables, hardy winter squash, warming foods, grains, soup, and stews. Along those lines, the Locavore movement recently took hold. The definition of locavore is "one who eats foods grown locally whenever possible." Coined on Earth Day in 2005, the movement was a way not only for people to eat healthfully and more nutritiously, but also for its positive impact on the environment as we move away from agribusiness to local individual farmers who tend to employ farming practices more sustainable for the planet, which includes avoiding harsh chemicals like pesticides and preservatives used to keep the produce alive during long trips. Lacavore is a natural way to align our diet to the seasons.

Oftentimes, a clinician will offer dietary guidelines depending on the patient's diagnosis. This includes what foods and fluids will contribute to balancing the patient and which foods will continue the cycle of illness. Food can be medicine or it can be poison. Water is what we need to sustain ourselves, yet as in nature, too much water, with no place to go can be destructive. All of this can be complicated as people don't just eat for nutrition. I have discovered from my own experience that people have a challenging relationship with food: we also eat to placate an emotional need, which could be considered a form of self-soothing or other pathologies. It is often a part of our brain circuitry: food as reward, part of the Behavior Loop discussed in Chapter III (p. 50). On the other side, there is fear of food and the need to control. We have complicated a simple process naturally intended to use food as fuel.

Nakazono Sensei once told me that there was a time when we had the innate intelligence to know unequivocally what our body needed to thrive, including which tastes would make our body stay whole. This intelligence belonged to the hundred year-olds mentioned in The Yellow Emperor. He said that acupuncture, which is the system of needling the patient, was considered drastic and extreme, not unlike Western surgery, by the people already in balance. In time, however, our ability to ascertain what would create or maintain balance waned. Today we are drawn by images in store windows, ads, cravings that override our healthy proclivities and our intuition of the steps we can take to regain balance. I remember when I was around five years old, there was a Twinkies commercial where every time a kid ate a Twinkie, he would grow tall. I believed it. In my house, growing up, you never found junk food. You have no idea how hard it was for me to convince my parents to buy me Twinkies so that I could grow as tall as the kids on the commercial. Twinkies came in a packet of two. Honestly, they were vile, way too sweet. But, look at the power of advertising! For immediate satisfaction, we can be swayed, which distances us from what we truly need to be well. In my practice, I have seen the effects of frozen coffee drinks as a direct cause of stomach issues. The mixture of caffeine as a stimulant, ice, dairy, and sugar is a quadruple whammy. How people drink these in winter is the pinnacle of disconnection from what the body needs. You might as well be drinking arsenic.

As far away as we have gone from living with the cycle of nature, I believe we can get it back through conscious retraining. For example, women who are pregnant get clear signals from the body as to what they need. When I was pregnant with my first child, I was eating my usual way back then, very cleanly, no refined sugar, no dairy, no red meat, no wheat or yeast. One day, on my way to work, having the urge to stop into a typical NY deli, I ordered an egg with cheese on a white seeded roll. I remember to this day how surprised I was by the clarity of this need, yet I knew decisively that it was what my body needed. Another evening, I made myself a huge a bowl of sautéed organic spinach with garlic. It was always my absolute favorite meal! I sat down to watch the Yankees game and put a bite of spinach in my mouth and I recoiled! The smell, the taste, I couldn't even put it in my mouth. I never heard from my body that clearly around food before. I ate a piece of organic steak instead. My body was happy. There was also a time when I was at a party seated next to a tray of dried fruit. Normally, I stayed away from dried fruit for two reasons: they are hard to digest and, more importantly, my mother never allowed junk food in the house, considering dried fruit as a treat. Needless to say, my association with dried fruit was that it was the ultimate booby prize. They were not Yodels! Anyway, that day, my eyes were drawn to a dried fig. Usually not a fig-fan, something told me I had to have it. I put one in my mouth and the flavor burst in such a way that reminded me of how I felt when I would guzzle water due to intense thirst after severe dehydration from strenuous activity. I ate five more. This went on for about a week, where I would eat about five dried organic figs and my body totally welcomed them. Then, one day, I went to eat one and the taste changed. My body no longer wanted them. Perhaps I needed the fiber, calcium or even potassium. When my system was satiated, I was done.

We can train our bodies to know what tastes we need in any given moment, bypassing the mind and our temporal desires and instead learning a process which requires intuition and sensitivity. Here is an exercise I recommend to patients, a quick mediation to sensitize them to the energy of the food as it relates to your system.

Food Awareness Meditation
Whatever food you are planning to eat, look at it, think of the taste of it, imagine the feeling in your mouth, your body. If it's something you can hold, feel its energy in your hand connect to your body. How does it make you feel? Do you have a feeling of opening or closing or nothing at all? Does it awaken your desire to eat it? Do you feel repelled? Maybe you feel nothing. That is okay too. This kind of awareness develops over time. Let's say that your body feels open to it when you sit down to eat it: can you connect to the tastes, experience the consistency, the temperature? Take the time to chew. How does it feel? Are you attuned to the moment when your body signals that it has had enough? This is also something we can cultivate through mindful practice. As a rule, it is good to stop eating when you are 80 percent full. As it happens, as your body starts the digestive process, you will feel a hundred percent full within 10-20 minutes after eating. This is a re-education on the road to holistic health.

Connecting to the food we eat is a powerful process. Some people say grace as a way to show gratitude for the bounty. The Japanese clasp their hands together, bow slightly and say, "Itadakimasu," which is a way to thank the spirit of the organism for taking the precious gift of their life. Using your senses is a helpful tool, like triage. Looking at the food with your eyes, tasting the food, feeling the consistency, hearing the chewing. We use our physical senses to both derive pleasure and receive its full nutritional value. For the food to have the most healing properties, it is best to chew until it's liquid before swallowing, thus getting all the nutrients out of the food and easing the digestive process.

Of course this is easier said than done. In my family, we scarfed our food, eating in a maniacal way—yet another factor in my years and years of digestive hell. One more thing I would like to emphasize where food is concerned is that food is also a form of divine pleasure. While I am not advocating for cheeseburgers or a slice of thin crust pizza, neither am I making any proclamations against them. In a perfect world, if you are in solid health, you should be able to enjoy whatever you want from time to time. As long as you eat slowly and with good spirit, no harm should come to you, and your body should inherently know how to restore itself. In fact, your conscious presence and state of being while eating is the last piece of the puzzle.

In 1992, when I was living, studying, and working in Santa Fe, New Mexico with Nakazono Sensei and his wife, I assisted him with an extensive guidebook for practitioners he was compiling on Kototama Life Therapy (no longer called Inochi Medicine). We tested hundreds of foods, products, and medicines to determine which systems they belonged to and, alternatively, which systems they could damage, so that we could use our knowledge of food and supplements to serve our patients. We were conducting our experiments using applied kinesiology, a form of muscle testing, to see how the body reacted. One day, we performed an interesting experiment with a piece of chocolate and organic string beans.

We muscle-tested the string bean and it came up healthful. Then, we muscle-tested the chocolate and it came up weak. Sensei put the string bean in my hand again and asked me to think angry thoughts; then, when he muscle-tested me, the string bean came up as weak for my system. Next, he put the chocolate in my hand and told me to think of joy and gratitude; the chocolate tested strong. So, the final thing I have to say on food is to eat with good spirit. If we eat with fear or strong emotions, the food will harm us. Consciousness matters.

While eating smartly leads to positive outcomes, rigidity and religiosity can be limiting to our health. The gist is to be free and in- =the-moment, to eat with connectivity. The trick to eating awareness is paying attention to how you are filling your tank, so that we have ample enough fuel to live well and enjoy what we eat. This is about developing common sense and critical reason.

Tools for health

Nature

Humans used to be forced into the elements in order to survive. It was taxing, but we were strong and hearty. We didn't have machines and computers. My grandfather had hands the size of baseball mitts and spent a lot of time working the land. He was tough as nails. Whether we exercise, walk, dance, play sports, or take a martial art, it is important to keep moving for our muscles and tendons (liver system), our blood circulation (heart system), digestion (spleen system), our immune system (lungs) and our bones and brain (kidney system). As you can see, we need to approach health as a whole organism.

Another way for us to heal is to commune with nature. As we are of nature, communing with nature is a reminder of our cycle of life. Looking at trees, standing at the shoreline of a beach or lake can revive us. As we do with food, take in the colors, letting the elements of nature and their vibration feed your body, mind, and spirit. Personally, I find hiking restorative and centering. It incorporates the elements and minerals which nurture our bodies, a tremendous activity boosting one's metabolism, washing the senses with trees, rocks, streaming water, and the sun.

The Japanese call this Shinrin-Yoku or Forest Bathing. They did a study to assess the benefits of being in nature. "The findings were as follows. In the forest area compared to the city area, 1) blood pressure and pulse rate were significantly lower, and 2) the power of the HF (High Frequency) component of the HRV (Heart Rate Variability) tended to be higher, and LF (Lower enterocepFrequency)/(LF+HF) tended to be lower. Also, 3) salivary cortisol concentration was significantly lower in the forest area. These physiological responses suggest that sympathetic nervous activity was suppressed and parasympathetic nervous activity was enhanced in the forest area, and that "Shinrin-yoku" reduced stress levels. In the subjective evaluation, 4) "comfortable," "calm," and "refreshed" feelings were significantly higher in the forest area. The present study has, by conducting physiological investigations with subjective evaluations as supporting evidence, demonstrated the relaxing and stress-relieving effects of "Shinrin-yoku" (Tsunetsugu).

Similarly, children allowed to play in nature have less anxiety, good study habits, higher grades, better health, and fewer psychological and developmental behaviors, says a study by Louise Chawla from University of Colorado. This applies even to urban kids who are exposed to parks or community gardens. When children are outside in nature, putting their hands in soil and climbing trees promotes an enhanced sense of connectivity and a willingness to protect the earth.

> Opportunities for children to connect with nature are important for the preservation of the biosphere. A large and steadily growing body of research shows that access to nature benefits young people in multiple areas of their lives. Reviews of this literature show that when children have nature around their homes, schools and neighborhoods, it promotes their physical and mental health and cognitive performance (Chawla, 2015; Kuo, 2019; McCormick, 2017; Norwood et al., 2019; Tillman et al., 2018; Vanaken, 2018).

Nothing will make us understand the cycle of nature more than composting and gardening. We take soil and leaves from the ground in autumn, add ash from the fireplace to the soil in winter, and consistently enlarge the compost with scraps of organic food including corn husks and egg shells. Once the big, fat worms do their thing, the compost has the most wonderful earthy smell, rich in minerals, which provides fertilizer for our vegetable and herb garden in spring. We are utilizing the energy of all four seasons to begin the cycle of birth and growth again. I love the connectivity to the elements and seasons.

Another tool of health is to do things that let us receive light, or enlightenment. For example, learning something new or doing something out of our comfort zone can go a long way to a rich life. I recently taught a class that was live-streamed around the world. It was so out of my realm, but a beginner's mind enables us to grow towards mastery as long as we stay pure and wondering, never stagnant or static. I love being a student. I also welcome challenges which raise my frequencies. The self-expression of our authentic self through our pursuits leads us to a fulfilled heart. Knowing the laws of nature is often about common sense. As the ancients say, as we are nature itself, we already have the wisdom within us. It is my hope that you approach your everyday life, as purely and organically as possible, to be the healthiest, clearest, most vibrant you can be.

I am saying this at a time in our history when things are very challenging. We have been stuck in a pandemic, our lives on hold. As grueling as it is in present day, I always say it is one thing to thrive when times are good, but the question now is how do we find health and well-being when times are hard. More than ever, we need to double down on the principles of health, wellness, and spiritual fortitude. I think this time of global pandemic has given us great clarity to prioritize the things where we derive value in our precious lives and to discard the rest. It also solidifies feelings of gratitude for the things that bring us satisfaction. One way to honor ourselves is to practice self-care.

Self treatment (do-in)
Here are some tools to implement into your daily routine for optimal health. Dress comfortably,

A. You can sit on the floor in seiza (kneeling), cross-legged, or on a chair. Rapidly rub your hands together until it creates friction and becomes warm. Place your hands on your heart. Do this three times. Start with some upward motions with your hands on your forehead, beginning at the 3rd eye until you feel the area tingling. Put your hands on each eyebrow and press as you move towards your temples. Finish by pressing lightly on your temples. Do this three times (more if you feel tight).

B. Rapidly rub your hands together as you did before. This time, press lightly onto your closed eyes and leave the fingers there until you see light. Do that three times. You can do the same thing with your ears. Put your forefinger in front of your ears and the rest behind. Do an up and down motion.

C. Pay special attention to loosen the jaw. Open your mouth slightly. Put your fingers along your cheekbone, gently press, and move toward the outside of your face. You can stop and hold wherever there is tension. Put your hands on either side of your nose, moving them up and down. Press along your jaw line, above and below. Hold where there is tension until it releases. Put one hand above your mouth, another below, and move laterally in opposite directions. Press your fingers on your chin. Hold if there is tension.

D. Do upward motions on your neck. Do circular motions on your left shoulder, up and down motions with your upper arm, circular motions on your elbow, up and down motions on your forearm, circular motions on your wrists.

E. Press on the base of each finger and use the pressure to pull your fingers, much like cracking your knuckles (but without trying to crack your knuckles). Massage the inside and outside of your hand. Do the same thing on your right side. Open and close your hands on your chest. On your abdomen, if you are born female, move your hands to the left and massage in a circular fashion. Men go in the opposite direction, to the right.

F. For a kidney rub, put your hands under the back ribs and open and close to awaken the kidneys. Do the same thing on your pelvis.

G. Do up and down motions on the front and back of your thighs, circular motions on your knees, up and down motions on you calves and shins, circular motions on your ankles, up and down motions on your feet as you did with your fingers; pull the toes one by one all the way to the tip. Put your foot on your leg, massage the bottom of your foot with both hands like kneading dough, continue to press on an area that is sensitive.

H. To finish, go to your head and tap all over, including the back of your neck, the base of your spine. You can tap your face, anywhere. Put your hands together at the end in gratitude.

I have treated everything from structural injuries to chronic and severe illness. I see the effects of poor diet, stressed out lifestyles, long work hours, and dietary and alcohol excess, anxiety, obsessive thinking, and depression on the system. Meditation goes a long way to reverse the imbalance by bringing the mind and emotions back into balance. We address lifestyle, behaviors, diet, and all the influences that contribute to ill health and step by step as we go on the path to wellness. But, like any process, there are slips built in. This is not meant to be a rigid, punishing pursuit. We can find grace in the process of change.

Balancing emotions

Nakazono always said that the source of our anger and upset arises when we want something that we are not necessarily meant to have in that moment in time. As the poet Rumi says, "When I run after the thing I want, my days are a furnace of stress and anxiety; if I sit down in my own place of patience, what I need flows to me and with not any pain. From this what I understand is that what I want also wants me, is looking for me and attracting me. There is a great secret in this for anyone who can grasp it" (Rumi). A daily practice in mindful meditation allows us to experience spaciousness with the added bonus of living beyond or transcending the limits of our emotions. It also helps us release all the unnecessary phenomena which tether us to the world of illusion. Whether you do sounds, sit quietly, do hara exercises, or any of the many modalities and visualizations we can draw from, we will feel more aligned with the universe. If we can remember to turn our switch on to mindfulness as much as we can throughout the day, then we will heal. Of course, there is an ugly side to this. Spiritual practices can sometimes bring out our ego, feeling smug and superior: "Look at me, being enlightened!" Only nothingness in the here/now can abate our ego's tendencies. Let's not take ourselves so seriously. Laugh it off! We are not bound by dogma. Perhaps music transforms us! Singing on the top of our lungs, dancing, crafts, art, a brisk walk with a friend, aikido, yoga, watching baseball, going to a concert, our path is our own to evolve and enrich.

When I lived in San Antonio De Las Minas, Mexico, I used to take my bokken and jo (wooden sword and staff) up a mountain with the local dogs from nearby ranches to do sword cuts and jo katas (forms). This became my cleansing ritual. I love climbing up mountains just to feel the power of nature and to sit in solitude, at one with the flow of life. Purification rituals are endemic to many cultures. Baptisms come to mind. The Kabbalists write about the importance of Mikvehs, ritual baths for the purpose of purification. In Shinto, people perform Misogi, a purification which involves standing under a waterfall in a state of mindfulness. I once heard a story that Nakazono went to teach an aikido seminar in Montreal and did snow misogi, where he and his students stripped down and rolled in the snow as a form of spiritual cleansing. He used to suggest that at the end of a normal shower, make the shower cold and stand under it. Not only is it purifying, but it also invigorates and strengthens the immune system while improving circulation.

Clearing the body
Here is another self-treatment which also feeds your body, mind, and spirit. You can do this standing, seated, in seiza (kneeling), sitting cross-legged, seated in a straight-back chair or even lying down. This is the treatment I do on myself every morning, the way for me to put myself in the right consciousness, balancing my body and releasing the illusions I get myself caught up in before the day even starts. Take it as a clearing.

If you are standing, have your feet shoulder width apart, knees slightly bent, so that your back is in alignment. Tongue at the roof of your mouth. Eyes can be opened or closed. If you are in a seated chair, don't lean back. Keep your spine straight, yet supple. The pathway of energy within your body is like a spiral that is going up and down at the same time with every breath. The energy converges in the center point of your body, the hara or tanden in Japanese, approximately 3 inches below the navel. Take your mind and put it in your hara. Your consciousness is now the center of our body. If you'd like, you can put your hands three inches below your bellybutton by cupping them against it. Breathe in through your nose very slowly, as slow as you can. You can feel your abdomen expand into your hands. When you reach the peak if your inhalation, hold, and then slowly exhale through your nose. Feel each microsecond pass within the breath. At the very end of the exhalation, hold, in order to empty your lungs and begin to inhale again. Clearing your mind, be in the nothingness. Once you feel ready, breathe into your hara and feel the energy or ki radiating out and up through your body. Let the ki permeate your body and cells. Your breath emanating from your hara is oxygenating your entire body. Pay attention to areas that hurt or feel tight. Breathe into the tight spots. Breathe into your bones, your muscles, tendons and tissue. Breathe into your eyes, ears, mouth, tongue, jaw. Breathe into your skin and feel the breath expanding out beyond your body, like a cylinder of ki. Then breathe, guiding your breath through your legs and feet towards the center of the earth. Form live roots out the bottom of your fee. Breathe as far as the center of the sky out of the top of your head. You can start with a few minutes a day, gradually increasing the time, so that you will do this throughout your day.

My aikido Sensei, Yamada Shihan always says as a matter of fact that you can be Zen anywhere, at any time, even or especially on a crowded subway train. I love practicing mindfulness on the subway, on the city street, everywhere at any time. Meditation is a way to drop into yourself, to go deep within. What can we do as humans to live a rich, fulfilling life? What can we do to live our time on this planet in optimum health? If we live according to the assumption that we are nature itself, we can rely on the elements of the universe to guide us to be our authentic selves.

 What does that look like? We have a physical form. We have five senses, which are the antennae that perceive the world around us. We have our mind, which is the control center, the headquarters as it were. Lastly, we have our spirit, the purpose which drives our existence. Without soul, we are merely robots. If we prescribe that we are of nature, it would also stand that we are all part of a whole. The idea that we are divided or separate from one another is an illusion that over time has come to feel real. Our egos, in particular, like to differentiate our needs from those of other people. Our egos like to compete and compare. We judge. We want. We want more. A healthy ego has a sense of self, whereas a weak ego needs validation and separates you from me. It doesn't concern itself with the collective. It likes to be fed because it is hungry. The ego can be a great motivator, often the loudest voice in the proverbial room. And it often can drown out the soft breeze that is our soul.

192

Feelings and thoughts are mutable and in no way define us. Only we as the overseers of our own existence can put ourselves in balance by being the conductor of our own orchestra. How do we do that? We can start by moving through our feelings rather than negating them or sweeping them under the rug, only to have them rear their heads in the form of unconscious behaviors. It's beneficial to ask questions to make ourselves accountable. The Heart system is about awareness. Knowing our humanity, we ask, "to what extent are we enslaved by our story or the events of our past?" How does our past limit our growth? Can we let go of what we can't control? How can we use, even embrace these feelings as tools to our existence, but not let them damage our systems? Can we infuse a sense of radical acceptance to all that is, so that we stay in the flow of life? These conscious actions are part of the process on the road to balance. Excess emotion harms the liver and threatens our equilibrium. Each emotion can either be a catalyst for change or can be destructive.

For example, fear has its usefulness. We learn to be afraid of putting our hands in fire, lest we burn ourselves. Sadness can awaken us to an unhealthy relationship, like a warning system, so we can take appropriate action. However, what happens to us when we let fear or sadness run amok in our system? We get anxiety and depression.

Clearing the day and preparing for sleep
To a practitioner of Eastern Medicine, sleep is also an important way to restore life energy and optimize the body's healing power. Ideally, if you can be fast asleep before midnight, earlier in winter, getting 6-8 hours of uninterrupted sleep gives you the best chance to revive. Unfortunately, insomnia and sleep irregularities have been a common complaint in my practice these days. Overactive brain activity from technology, worry, stress, alcohol, the news, rich food, sugar, all impair the quality of sleep. To improve sleep involves a multi-pronged approach.

For example, a study by Oxford University did a study that determined that insomnia is often caused by worries and anxieties that arise at night while we are at rest. They discovered that one is more likely to fall asleep and stay asleep if we write in a journal before bed to clear the mind and promote inner peace.
Patients with insomnia commonly complain that they are unable to get to sleep because of unwanted thoughts and worries. One account given of this excess cognitive activity is that it results from the incomplete processing of daytime stressors and hassles. Previous research has demonstrated the benefits of writing

about emotional experiences as a method to facilitate emotional processing. This pilot study tested the hypothesis that writing about worries and concerns, with an emphasis on the expression and processing of emotion, will reduce sleep onset latency among an analogue sample of poor sleepers (Harvey, 1).

Scientists at Baylor University and Emory University of Medicine performed a sleep study that determined, more specifically, that a person who wrote a to-do list rather than a recap of the completed tasks fell asleep faster and easier. Additionally, making an effort to not ingest any food and drink (especially alcohol) after 8 pm helps the body prepare for sleep.

Prompts for journaling:
   1. I am grateful for…
   2. I forgive….
   3. I'm feeling…
   4. To-do list…

One way to clear the effects of the day is to sit, quiet your mind of thoughts, and be in your mind at your hara, conscious center, three inches below your navel. Give your mind a space vacation from overthinking and just feel life. You can follow your breath going from the center of the earth in the inhalation up to infinity and exhale from infinity to the center of the earth. Let the energy awash you completely. Slow down time to the microsecond. Release your thoughts and feelings. Let your spirit come home to its vessel. Just be. This is good to do in the evening or before bed.

Treatment starts with diagnosis, reading pulses on the wrist, asking questions. I palpate the abdomen, looking at the tongue, listening to the patient and the tone of their voice. For example, do they have a lung voice? This is the start of a profound process, as no two people heal alike. We are all the same and yet so unique at the same time; healing chronic illness or injuries therefore can be revealing and illuminating. Oftentimes, a patient has firmly established patterns of imbalance and there is a certain familiarity the patient might have with their illness or injury over time. It's the devil you know! Once we start to restore the body back to balance, we enter into a path together, guiding the body back to health, giving the system new messaging. Inevitably, there can be various points along the way where the patient feels stuck, often even more symptomatic again after a period of relief—discouraged, oddly protective, if not defensive of their sickness. This is often the phase in treatment when they start to doubt themselves, the process, and me. It reminds me of the moment during labor before the birth of the child, when the mother just can't go on anymore. She is experiencing the most pain at this time, the contractions at their strongest. This is usually when the cervix is in the process of dilating from 8 to 10 centimeters, referred to as the period of transition, the stage before the contractions change and the mother feels compelled to push. The transitional period is just this, the difficult moments before transformation. The same thing happens in the healing process.

I recently went through this with a patient who had eczema over his entire body. I recognized that he was suffering from an autoimmune response brought on by stress, anxiety, and diet. Needless to say, his skin appeared dry with a fiery redness and scabs from scratching himself silly. There came a moment after his treatments when he would feel relief, but his condition would revert back after a few days. This went on for some time. In the meantime, I muscle-tested him and concluded that he needed to eliminate dairy, which was difficult due to the fact that he was vegetarian, and not vegan, and struggled to get enough protein intake. I also prescribed a mixture of Chinese and Western herbs to his regiment. At one point, he said to me snappily that those herbs were not helping. I got it!! It sucks!! I told him to be patient and persist. He would need to be on them long-term. I could tell he was getting frustrated. It was right around the time of COVID, before everything stopped. He was feeling sick, and his skin worsened. He took baths in the middle of the night, in agony from itching. It was further drying his skin. He had a persistent cough, chest congestion. His throat hurt. His jaw was tight. He was not a happy camper. Then, one day, I read his pulses as usual and noticed that his condition had changed. For the first time in months, I needed to address a different system. The chain was unraveling. At the same time, his skin was looking good. He was healing.

When Sensei Nakazono started treating me, my pulses and my symptoms indicated an imbalance of my heart/small intestine system. In addition to abdominal pain, I had circulation issues, cold hands and feet, muscle stiffness, and my intestines were inflamed. After a few months of treatment, dietary changes, probiotics and other herbs and supplements, meditation, sound practice, and inner work to forgive and clear the past, I got really sick. I had fever. I had pain all over. I couldn't leave my bed. After a couple of days, I was back to myself. When I went for treatment, my diagnosis changed. The healing crisis was the culmination of my commitment to biopsychosocial wellness. I felt better than I had since I was a little girl. I was evolving on the road to healing.

Healing requires work inside and out. Everyone is different. However, to live pain free, to bring your body into balance, to change a pattern of behavior, to heal, requires fortitude, patience, resilience, and self-love. Pain, in and of itself, is a guide, a teacher which sends us on a process to find the balance we seek. These days, in my practice, I see a lot of patients with varying degrees of anxiety, from crippling and self-sabotaging to a general malaise. It has become commonplace.

When we are in the flow of the universe, our consciousness offers us a balanced way to experience the same phenomena. Feelings limit us, plus they are steeped in illusion. I can feel one way about something and, with some space, feel the opposite way a day later. Critical thinking, which I call the overseer, is the mindfulness to see what is real. Letting the overseer, the totality of us in the moment, question our limited beliefs systems, emotions, and patterns, can go a long way towards truth. This is what this book is about, to put us on the side of life, to make us whole. To unify our parts is to overcome their pathology to do us harm.

Joy and Compassion

To develop our emotional intelligence means to understand the fluidness and fleetingness of feelings, They don't create our identity nor even what's real. But they can be self-induced. For example, the emotion related to the heart system is joy, something we can generate from within. We need not wait for the world to make us happy. I mean, yeah, Kettle potato chips make me pretty darned happy, albeit temporarily. Because internal joy, like the warmth of summer, is expansive, putting ourself in that frame of mind attracts light from everywhere. One exercise that I recommend to access joy is to think of something or someone that makes you smile. Put the smile in your heart and the center point in the middle of your chest, between your breasts. It is the energy center of your spirit, your shen (Chinese) or shin (Japanese). Breathe into the point and back in the smile until it fills your body. Another way to attract light in our life is through compassion and sharing.

In Eastern medicine, the cycle of human life is such that from conception to birth, children are connected to their parents' life energy, specifically their mother's. Females are on a 6-year cycle and males are on a 7-year cycle. When a child enters into my practice, if the girl is 6 or the boy is 7, there is a chance that I would have to treat the mother as well. When a girl turns 12, or a boy turns 14, their energy converts from one of receiving into one of sharing as contributing members of their community. Their life energy is expanding out as they begin to relate to and interact with the world around them. By the time kids reach adolescence, they are oftentimes more invested in interactions with their peer group, forming their lifelong identity. Sharing is medicine for our heart, the language of love.

If you were to meditate on the word "compassion," how does it feel in your body? Where do you feel it? Can you feel it in your heart area? A nice guided mediation you can do to strengthen your spirit is to breathe into the "shin" point and heart. Feel the center of your chest open like the sun shining in the noon sky. Next, feel the same sun shining from the point in your back. Then, have the sun radiate down towards the body and up through your head. How can you share? Can you conduct yourself with grace? Can you inject space into a situation before you blow up? Can you breathe?

Are we enlightened yet? Healing ourselves changes the life energy of the universe. Nakazono Sensei talked about that often. As we subsist off the land, made up of the same elements, if we truly know in our cells that the earth is us, would we be less inclined to threaten it? Would we protect her? We can start by being present and practicing self-care. It is up to us to create our reality, to be in the silence where our true selves can emerge, our soul integrating inside our bodies as its rightful owner.

What I experienced back in 1985, when I dropped everything I'd thought made me who I was and instead immersed myself in this "new" path of life, as old as life itself, still fuels me to this day: the mind-body-spirit connection, that we are nature, the essence of creation, the infinite that is and our finite expression of it. Most of life to its source is both mysterious and unknowable. It even eludes the poets, the scientists, and the philosophers. Yet, the Ancients preserved wisdom for us which tells us we have the intelligent capacity to heal ourselves. As the universe seeks balance, so do we. Pain tells us when we veer off course, giving us the opportunity for change. I can never properly express my gratitude for being on my ongoing path to biopsychosocial wellness and the drive to guide others to do the same. In the midst of this are the place keepers of the ancient ways, the information for a transcendent life path. Just the coming together of this book, with the fusion of different perspectives of a single imperative towards holistic health, shows the push forward to a new paradigm, a way of unifying healing, interconnected, as one. Perhaps this is just the collective we need to tackle life's ills while making life meaningful and transcendent. Journey on!

WORKS CITED

Chawla, Louise, "Benefits of Nature Contact for Children." Journal of Planning Literature, 7/22/2015
https://doi.org/10.1177/0885412215595441

Harvey, Allison G. and Clare Farrell, "The Efficacy of a Pennebaker-Like Writing Intervention for Poor Sleepers." Behavioral Sleep Medicine, 1:2, 7 June 2010, 115-124,

Kuo, Ming, Michael Barnes and Catherine Jordan, "Do Experiences with Nature Promote Learning? Converging Evidence of a Cause-and-Effect Relationship." Frontiers in Psychology, 19 February, 2019.

McCormick, Rachel, "Does Access to Green Space Impact the Mental Well-eing of Children: A Systematic Review." National Library of Medicine, Sep 4, 2017.

Nakazono, Masahilo M., The Source of Present Civilization, Kototama Books. Dec. 1994.

Ni, Maoshing. The Yellow Emperor's Classic of Medicine: A New Translation of the Neijing Suwen with Commentary. 1995

Norwood, Michael et al., "A Narrative and Systematic Review of the Behavioural, Cognitive and Emotional Effects of Passive Nature Exposure on Young People: Evidence for Prescribing Change." University of Bath, 2019

Rumi. Rumi Poetry: 100 Bedtime Verses. Createspace Independent Publishing Platform, 2017.

Scullin, Michael K. et al., "The effects of bedtime writing on difficulty falling asleep: A polysomnographic study comparing to-do lists and completed activity lists." Journal of Experimental Psychology: General, Vol 147(1), Jan 2018, 139-146.

Tillman, Suzanne et al., "Mental Health Benefits of Interactions with Nature in Children and Teenagers: A Systematic Review." Journal of Epidemiology and Community Health, Vol 72, Issue 10, 2018.

Tsunetsugu Yuko, et al., "Physiological Effects of Shinrin-yoku (Taking in the Atmosphere of the Forest) in an Old-Growth Broadleaf Forest in Yamagata Prefecture, Japan." Journal of Physiological Anthropology, Vol 26 (2007) Issue 2: 135-42.

Vanaken, Gert-Jan and Marina Danckaerts, "Impact of Green Space Exposure on Children's and Adolescents' Mental Health: A Systematic Review." International Journal of Environmental Research and Public Health, Vol 15, Issue 12, 27 November, 2018.

van Leer, Bernard, The Beginning of Life (Documentary).

***** For a comprehensive list of Five Element Theory, Sound practice, or Do-In videos, please visit **www.kototamalifetherapy.com**

CHAPTER XI

YOGA:
EMPOWERING YOUR HEALTH THROUGH YOUR INNER EVOLUTION

Welcome to my Chapter! I am honored and grateful that you are here!

Since I was a little girl it's been my deepest desire to support and empower people's physical health and their overall well-being. So much so that I declared as a 9 year-old that I'd some day make a pill that would cure cancer and thus would help millions of people worldwide to be happier. However, in my own winding evolutionary journey I've come to the humble realization that the source and power to healing and to sustainable health and well-being does not lie outside the body but rather, it exists within.

My intention for you is that this Chapter will effectively support you in bringing forth a new, radical relationship with your health and well-being, and one that you can sustain for the rest of your life. How I am going to support you in achieving that is through a twofold model:

1. **Enlightenment:** Specific coaching distinctions that help you reveal your inner truth.
2. **Embodiment:** Specific practices with breath work at their core to help you embody your revelations and to directly support and empower your innate wholeness.

Enlightenment:	Coaching distinctions
Embodiment:	Energy Codes Breath work practices and BodyAwake Yoga

This is what transformation is: a revelation of truth—in an 'A-Ha' moment—that naturally brings the release of illusionary beliefs that have kept at bay the abundance, the wholeness, and well-being that we truly are and have. Rest assured that wherever you are in your own healing and empowerment journey is absolutely perfect. In whatever ways you are ready, open, and willing to listen to and integrate the teachings I bring you here, you will. As such, I am starting this Chapter sharing key aspects of my own personal journey, with the intention that they bring light to you and your own unique journey.

Section 1: My Own Personal Journey

Ever since I was a child, my heart saddened as I saw people suffer, and it's been my heart's desire to become someone who can effectively help millions of people to be happy. I've also been forever fascinated about how life works: Isn't it amazing that planet Earth gives us everything we need to live and thrive? Isn't it amazing that we can move around without being plugged into an outlet? How do the ~30 trillion cells in our bodies work, both individually and together to keep the entire body functioning properly?

So it may not be a surprise to you that at the age of 9 I declared to myself –and to my dad—that I'd find a cure for cancer. Achieving this goal would allow me to relieve suffering for millions of people on Earth, and restore them to their well-being and happiness. At that time I believed it would take a lot of effort, but it was definitively possible. And my dad believed it too! He would encourage me on Sunday mornings at the kitchen table—where I'd sit right after waking up to study science—telling me that I'd get the Nobel Prize some day. Seeing him be so convinced that I could accomplish that was so empowering to me!

I spent my days and nights studying and learning, walking my path towards college. A strong knowledge of chemistry would be necessary to develop a successful drug against cancer, so I went on to major in Chemistry. Being involved in research led me naturally to do a Ph.D. I joined an internationally recognized research group at the University of Granada (Spain), where after 4 years I obtained a Ph.D. on Biophysical Chemistry of Proteins. A couple of months later at 26 years-old I became a professor there and started teaching one semester a year to senior students. I loved teaching my students! During the rest of the year I performed research on folding and assembly of viral capsids as a Visiting Scientist at the Department of Biology at MIT (Cambridge, MA). This would end up being my 'bridge project' between my Ph.D. and finally doing research on cancer specifically.

I was accepted to work at a highly competitive laboratory at NYU Medical Center, with Prof Joseph Schlessinger, one of the most successful scientists in the field. They were already making great progress on the elucidation of some of the molecular and cellular mechanisms that are deregulated in cancer. Joining this lab was a dream come true, even though it meant leaving my position as a professor back in Spain. At NYU I spent 7 years learning and using the most highly specialized molecular biology techniques. The work required many skills, from the intellectual understanding of my projects to the fine work with my hands.

I loved working in the lab, designing experiments and doing all they required. Very good at this highly creative and intellectually stimulating activity, I published 7 articles in peer reviewed journals during that time and have published a total of 15 in my scientific career. It brings me great joy to see that some of my publications continue to be cited to this day, 20 years later.

My boss moved his lab to Yale University in July 2001. One side of me was thrilled that now I'd be able to spend much more time with my daughter, who was 18 months old at the time. However, I was also heartbroken, having fully dedicated the previous four years to a highly sophisticated project that did not produce the kind of striking results that would have granted its publication in the kournals Cell, Nature, or Science. And it was quite clear that my chances of ever going back to the lab were slim.

I fell into a depression with an identity crisis, not knowing who I was. I did not realize at the time that I was suffering because I had attached 'being a scientist' to my identity and that if I had known that, and had released that attachment, I would have given myself freedom. This is a perfect example of what healing and empowerment can look like and what this Chapter is about!

My son was born 10 months later. As I continued to unconsciously expect happiness to be delivered to me from the outside, my marriage started to tremble. During that time of my life I hid from the world: did not tell my family, and did not reach out to any of the few friends I had; I was too embarrassed of who I was and about what my world was, self-perceptions that I did not want anyone to know. I felt completely alone with my misery, and hired a therapist just to have someone to talk to. She put me on anti-depressants, which deepened my feeling of being a loser, all of which I kept as a secret from my family and the few friends I had. During this very painful period of my life I did not know that a different, empowered, joyful and creative life was possible. At least not for me. I was being a complete victim of my circumstances, which, as I now know, corresponds to the lower part of the spectrum of consciousness that I've depicted in Figure 1.

In early 2004 I had a key realization (enlightenment!) that took me out of the void I had been in for almost 3 years: "Intellectual stimulation is what I've been missing!" This led me to NYU Career Services and to start taking classes on management and all kinds of topics (including 'English Writing' with Bob Davis!) at NYU SCPS (School for Continuing and Professional Studies). What struck a chord big time for me was my class on Foundations of Coaching. I learned there that coaching is about helping others fulfill their potential, to facilitate the positive change that is required to achieve goals that are truly worth going for. Sitting in that class and hearing coaching's purpose caused me to experience a powerful 'A-Ha' moment: Being someone who gives people access to fulfill their potential felt completely true for me! I could not believe my ears! My heart was finally singing after 3 years of dark silence, and I was thrilled to start training to be a coach!

A few months later and as my divorce process began, I came across Yoga. I really did not know anything about Yoga, other than it could possibly help me with stress and posture, but felt I needed to experience it. Little did I know then the degree to which it was going to change my life!

So there I was at my first Yoga class: going to the back of the studio to hide, I sat on the mat crosslegged as everyone else but... I started to feel very uncomfortable right away, and I looked in the studio mirror and saw that my back was rounded, when everyone else's was straight. I didn't know what was going on, but plenty of self- criticisms such as "I am different," "I am broken," and "I don't belong" voiced themselves all at once. The class started and I was having great difficulty following instructions; I couldn't breathe and barely could do any of the poses. Half-way through the session I found myself hyperventilating, and had to stop. It seemed as if yoga was 'impossible' to do. However, somewhere in my being I sensed that there's "medicine" here for me. I immediately hired a private Yoga teacher and started working with him right away. The first thing he taught me is how to breathe. How come I did not know how to breathe?!

I started to have countless 'A-Ha' moments both on the Yoga mat and off the Yoga mat because of my regular practice on the mat. Looking back, I can now say that I had just started my journey of self-forgiveness, self-love, and compassion. At the time, I did not have the distinctions of Enlightenment and Embodiment, but now I know that that is what I was experiencing then: I was slowly but surely discovering more and more of my inner truth, and my life started to become more aligned with my truth.

Practicing Yoga and deepening my coaching studies became priorities for me, and in the next few months I established a collaboration with David Rock, one of my Coaching teachers at NYU SCPS, and I began to do research on the relationship between how the brain/mind works and coaching. This exciting research was used in the book Quiet Leadership that David was writing.

By the time my divorce process was complete, I had clearly experienced in my being that Yoga practice is a powerful practice not only to help with posture and flexibility, but for raising consciousness and for catalyzing personal transformation and becoming a more loving human being, so I naturally wanted to share it with others. I registered for a Vinyasa Yoga teachers' training program at my local studio, at the same time that I was learning NLP (Neuro Linguistic Programming) to further my coach training.

I came across Kundalini Yoga just a few days after I graduated as a Vinyasa Yoga teacher, fell in love with it, and also registered to do the Kundalini Aquarian Teacher's Training. During this time I also was traveling to attend Yoga retreats with world-renowned teacher Shiva Rea and others, and also meditation retreats in the US and France with Thich Nhat Hanh. What a privilege to get to learn directly from these Masters of Consciousness!

I started teaching to small groups of friends in my home in 2008. I also started teaching at Yoga studios but found it not as fulfilling; I discovered that it's important to me to personally connect with my students and follow their personal evolution. Teaching Yoga and coaching came together in a beautiful way as an integrated effective path that was healing and empowering me, as well as my students and clients.

In 2010 I participated in a transformational coaching program that allowed me to experience multiple 'A-Ha' moments and shifts in consciousness that allowed me to access and release illusionary beliefs, resulting in extensive forgiveness of self and others and access to more self-confidence and self- love than ever before, all in just three days. And just as with everything I find powerfully transformational in my own experience, and inside of my calling to give people access to their own empowerment, I immediately started to train to lead the program. This training typically takes several years, and with the intention to speed up the process in 2016 I took on a job as a full-time staff member, which I felt as an honor and a privilege. This job was the perfect training ground to learn and develop effective management and leadership practices as well as to cultivate my ability to making an even larger difference in people's lives. And little did I know that taking on this job was going to catalyze a major spiritual awakening!

Eighteen months into this position I started to develop a frozen shoulder. As months passed the pain intensified and the mobility of my left shoulder decreased so much that I had to stop doing my favorite physical exercises: Yoga and swimming.

Getting dressed in the morning was an excruciating experience. For many months I did not connect this pain with being in the job. Gradually it started to became a hint that grew louder and louder. At some point it became quite clear that this pain was a message telling me that remaining in this job was no longer aligned with my truth and that it was time for me to leave. However, I kept convincing myself that I needed to stay, with the main reasons being 'not wanting to look defeated,', fear of losing the appreciation of a like-minded community, and not wanting to disappoint the many people that were counting on me to stay in the job. Now, looking back, I can see that all of my reasons had to do with fear of being judged and, specifically, fear of losing others' love and appreciation. It's a very natural human reaction that is sourced by the ego or protective personality fighting fiercely for its survival.

The longer I went against my truth by staying in this position, the more my suffering intensified and the harder it became to do the job. Now looking back, it makes total sense! As I now know, the Soulful Self tirelessly waits for the mind to catch up, and sooner or later the light of its truth will shine on and melt the workings of the ego/false self. So, I finally surrendered and resigned, and the surrendering itself was the transformational action that tookme into the Void.

Three months later the Universe presented me with the work of Dr. Sue Morter; her first book, The Energy Codes, had just been published. I started listening to the audible version and, as I listened to her words, I was moved to tears with one A-ha after another! My heart felt so 'at home'! Dr. Sue, as she likes to be called, is all about empowering people to master their health and their lives, from the inside out, through embodiment practices. She has developed the Energy Codes (EC) principles and practices to give us effective access to a radical and sustainable transformation. This transformation is accomplished by activating dormant circuits in our electromagnetic energy and nervous systems (more on this later). Said in another way, this transformation is accomplished through embodiment practices that integrate mind, body, and breath together.

This powerful quantum technology was my new path in front of me, and I felt so joyful and grateful! Not only that, a couple of weeks later I found out that she'd developed her own Yoga style that integrates the EC practices into Yoga: BodyAwake Yoga. I went "OMG" and immediately registered for the Teachers' Training. And then, after over a year without being able to do any Yoga because of the pain and lack of mobility in my shoulder, I gathered enough courage to go on my Yoga mat and attempt to come into downward facing dog. My pose was highly asymmetrical due to my shoulder's condition, and tears of sadness and joy were running down my forehead. I continued to practice a little bit every day, incorporating the specific breath work from the EC while on the pose. That together with gentle swimming and receiving a specialized form of physical therapy helped me heal faster, regaining mobility and strength in my left arm again. By the time the BodyAwake Yoga Teacher's Training Program started in Oct '19, I had only about 5% left to have my shoulder back to normal.

In March '20 the Covid-19 pandemic hit and I realized I had with me a technology that could tremendously help the people who were in their homes frightened and not exercising. I found myself 'jumping in the pool,' nudged by my soul, and started reaching out to people and live- streaming four Yoga classes a week. Since then to this day I've live-streamed over 200 BodyAwake Yoga classes to students in 11 countries.

The summer of 2020 I 'threw myself into the pool' again, when I started teaching BodyAwake Yoga in Spanish. The idea of teaching Yoga in Spanish had crossed my mind in the past,; however, every time I dismissed it, mainly out of fear that I might freeze often during teaching, whenever I would not know how to translate a word or guide my students throughout the class effectively. I've now taught over 60 classes in Spanish. In this last year I've also become a certified Facilitator and a certified Coach of the Energy Codes, and I've been working with individuals and groups in those capacities in English as well as in Spanish. What a joy and what an honor to contribute to the lives of these amazing human beings!

I invite you now to take a moment and be in this inquiry:
What aspects of your life's journey are you finding that are mirrored by my journey? Can you see that moments of suffering in your life have also been catalysts for spiritual awakening and expansion and have supported you in finding what's next for you?

I have great news for you! There is no need to suffer anymore to catalyze this process! Embodiment practices that help us cultivate our innate wholeness are the answer. This will be covered in detail later in the Chapter.

First, let's explore how we can connect with our inner truth:

Section 2: Coaching distinctions that help you reveal what's true for you: Enlightenment

As I shared in my own journey above, we human beings have developed a protective personality or ego since childhood, giving rise to a false self that wants to please others to avoid judgment and to be loved. The limiting beliefs of unworthiness that define the false self are stored in our body, our energy field, and our subconscious mind. Our life's choices are driven by these protective patterns at least 95% of the time, and "Until you make the unconscious conscious," as Carl G. Jung noted appropriately, "it will direct your life and will call it fate." For you to live a more consciously created, freer and happier life, you will want to unveil what's really true for you, behind the mask of the protective personality. As this updated version of reality emerges in your awareness, your choices will be more congruent with what's true for you.

An effective way to shed light on what's really true for you is using coaching distinctions, linguistic constructs that allow for revelations of your inner truth as 'A-Ha' moments of insight. In effect, they help us bring what's subconscious ('from the dark') to conscious awareness ('to the light'). We all have experienced those moments: it's as if a light bulb went off inside your head! Therefore, coaching distinctions support the raising of your consciousness by inducing clarity, revealing to your awareness a new piece of what's true for you.

Different transformational programs offer their own specific coaching distinctions, even though many of them are basically the same, just named differently. In this section I've gathered some of my favorite coaching distinctions that are very effective in helping you reveal more of what's true for you. There are also coaching questions intermingled in the text. Thus I recommend that you have your lap top or a notebook and pen nearby, so that you can capture your revelations. I really hope you find it highly user-friendly and get back to it often!

In this section and in the chapter overall I'll use interchangeably Soulful Self, Higher Self, and True Self to refer to our divine aspects vs. our human aspects. The first distinction that I want to bring to you is:

1. VICTIM vs CREATOR

We are VICTIMS when we believe we can't do anything about the situation we are in (powerless). At the other end of the spectrum of consciousness, we can be CREATORS and create our own experience and outcome independent of the external world (empowered). A bit more conscious version of victim is when we are hopeful that our life can get better; we may seek therapy or self-help courses during this stage. It's the beginning of your awakening!

I invite you to take a look in your own life: you probably can identify some specific areas or situations you are dealing with right now where you're currently feeling like a victim (e.g., being inside of the Covid-19 pandemic at the time of my writing this chapter), and other situations/areas of life where you are trying to fix something and maybe resolve something with others when you are being the creator of your life experience.

Higher Consciousness Personal Power

Creator stage: I am a pro-active steward of my health and wellbeing

Self-help stage: looking for actions I can take to improve my health and wellbeing

Victim stage: I am at the effect of my circumstances (genetics, environment)

Notice, in your own experience, that as you move from victim to creator in more and more areas of your life, you're elevating your consciousness and experiencing more and more moments of freedom, self-love, peace, and joy, together with a life where there's more flow. When it comes to the area of your Health and Well-being, where are you at in that scale?

Here are some examples to help you look:

- dealing maybe with a chronic condition that does not heal and being hopeless about it, continuing to take drugs that don't really help? (Victim)
- dealing with a condition or physical symptoms and looking for what's out there that may help? (Self-help)
- doing daily practices that keep your vitality and immunity strong? (Creator)

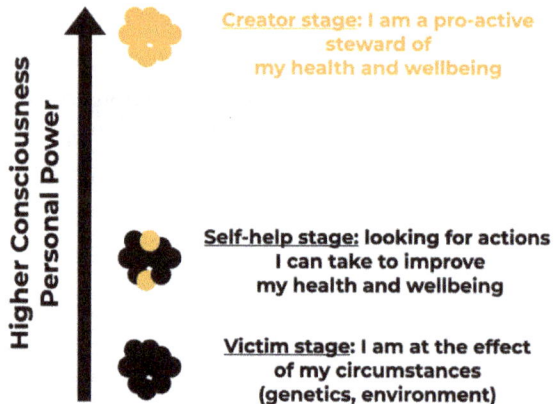

- I invite you to pause reading now and inquire where you are at.

A possible statement describing what may look to be a Creator in the area of Health and Well-being is:

> *"I am responsible for (and the creator of) my health and well-being. I am responsible for creating the environment inside of myself and around me that will support my staying healthy throughout my life."*

That may sound like a big leap for most people at this time. And that is what I am interested in bringing to you: A radical empowering of your wholeness.

This leads us to the next distinction:

2. CONTEXT = your "come from"

I define Context here as a belief or set of beliefs that give you a particular lens or filter to look from and look through whatever is at the forefront of your awareness. The contexts we operate inside of are mostly subconscious. They originated at very early ages when we faced moments of 'failure' and decided things such as "I am not good enough," "I'll never be X, Y, or Z," etc. These limiting beliefs create a false version of who we are. They shape and color what's actually happening in front of you, and automatically generate a particular meaning in your awareness which comes with particular feelings in the body, and will lead to specific actions/choices resulting in a particular outcome. So, every outcome in your life is correlated to and comes from a particular Context.

I also invite you to notice when you look at your own experience how there was a complete absence of love and trust in the moments in which limiting beliefs were generated.

Take a moment to look for yourself. Limiting beliefs are therefore coming from the reality of the FALSE SELF. This distorted view of reality takes the shape of wrong assumptions about ourselves, others, land ife, and often will lead to a great deal of suffering for ourselves and others. These false beliefs affect the electromagnetic energy field of the body, distorting its flow and causing energy to get stuck in the body. And the energy associated to the feelings that we don't embrace is pocketed away in the body's tissues (defense physiology). Energy stuck in the body will sooner or later produce physical symptoms and ultimately disease of the body

(Morter, 136).

Here are a few common examples of limiting beliefs and the impact of believing them:

1. While you believe that you don't deserve to be loved, you won't perceive love when people around you are loving you and you'll likely feel lonely and suffer.
2. While you believe you are not capable of becoming the leader that you know you are, you'll experience yourself as small and you'll suffer.
3. While you have a dream that you don't believe is possible for you, you won't manifest it and you'll suffer.

Maybe after reading these examples there's a limiting belief of yours that has brrm revealed to your awareness?

If of course you are operating from beliefs that are TRUE (natural laws, universal laws, cosmic laws), then your context is going to be one that empowers you, and the correlated actions will produce miraculous results in your life.

Here are a few examples:

1. I am a sovereign Creator of my life.
2. Everything that happens in my life is in support of my highest good.
3. My life's purpose is to bring more love to the Planet.

You may want to take the opportunity at this moment to bring to your awareness something that's currently challenging in your life, and I invite you to look at it through any of these 3 lenses. You'll gain a new perspective on it that empowers you and you'll find yourself taking new creative actions towards solving it. As you can see, different contexts result in very different life experiences. That is why it's key to examine both the context and the beliefs that are running your life, making them conscious. This is what the process of 'awakening' is.

The statement I wrote above, coming from being a Creator, "I am responsible for (and the creator of) my health and wellbeing. I am responsible for creating the environment inside of myself and around me that will support my staying healthy throughout my life," is a consciously created 'come from' or context that provides a new way of relating to one's health and well-being. If I choose to believe that statement because it empowers me, my actions will be correlated with it. So, if someone offers me a can of soda, the action that's aligned with this consciously created context is for me to say, "No, thank you." And I won't have to think about it. No effort. My reply will arise within me organically. That is the power of context. Therefore, the context, the 'come from,' what we believe, determines our choices, including our choices regarding our health and well-being. If we don't create our contexts consciously, they'll be created for us by our subconscious, which is filled with limiting beliefs from past experiences and other people's beliefs that we unconsciously took on as 'ours.'

What's your current context for your health and well-being? Have you created it consciously? Most of us have not. We did not even know about context! We may not even know that my choices regarding my health and well-being may be coming from what I learned watching movies and TV shows!

How you find out about your context in the area of health and well-being is by looking at your daily choices of food, drink, air your breathe, exercise, sleep, and thoughts. I invite you to pause here and start to make a list. Then brainstorm some possible contexts that empower you (feel free to use any of the three I offered you above) so that you consciously choose/create your own choices. Always create contexts as statements/declarations in the present tense, and make sure that you feel empowered by them. And if my statement above resonates strongly with you, feel free to make it your own!

When you are ready, move on to Distinction #3:

3. EXTERNAL vs INTERNAL OR INNER ORIENTATION

"Where attention goes, energy flows. Where intention goes, energy flows." -James Redfield

External: We human beings don't realize how much we are externally oriented. It may be obvious that we are using our 5 senses to receive information from the outside world; after all, that's what they are for. However, having an externally oriented focus has us look outside of ourselves for the things/people we believe we need in order to experience the freedom, love, joy, and peace we all seek (as I shared in My Own Journey section above).

How much time in the day DO you spend with your attention focused on your cell phone? And your lap top? TV? There's an App that counts how many hours and minutes a day you are on your screen, if you are curious to accurately know. But for now, just estimate. How many hours? Besides the hours, what are you watching? What are you feeding your conscious and subconscious minds with? What 'juice' are you getting out of this overloading of your senses? Notice if you already are feeling 'wrong' about it. There is nothing wrong. But by taking inventory of the reality of what you are doing, you get to observe your patterns and therefore to elevate your consciousness. This new, updated reality—which is much closer to reality than your previous perception—may lead you to take a new action or even a new habit (see Chapter III) that supports your health and well-being.

This external orientation also supports a victim disposition, since if the outside world does not deliver what we want, we feel bad, sad, anxious, depressed. And as our energy is projected outward, by the end of the day we are so exhausted and wonder why. Inside of this external focus we also tend to notice and point out what's not working, what is wrong or missing that needs fixing. If all we do is live life with this external orientation, what are we not experiencing? Foremost, the wholeness that we are! The vitality and joy that our cells are made to radiate! And this vitality and joy is precisely what we've been seeking, looking for in all the wrong places, outside of ourselves!

Internal: The importance of re-directing the mind's attention to the inner world is already described in ancient yogic texts and termed Pratyahara. Pratyahara is usually translated as

"withdrawal of the senses" and more literally means "gaining mastery over external influences," which frees the mind to attend to the inner world. Swami Sivananda tells us that

"Pratyahara itself is termed as yoga, as it is the most important limb in yoga sadhana."

There are a number of simple practices which we can do to practice Pratyahara and which create positive impressions in the mind:
- Turn off your electronics or put them in silence mode and close your eyes and focus on feeling your breath.
- Go out in nature and practice gazing at the horizon, a forest, a lake, an ocean, the blue sky… or practice being present with trees, rocks, flowers, etc.
- Visit temples, use altars, candles, incense, etc. to alert your mind that it's

time to go inward.
- Yoga, and particularly BodyAwake Yoga (see below).

Another key distinction that's related to this External vs Internal orientation is:

LIVING IN THE HEAD vs LIVING IN THE BODY

When you wake up in the morning, where are 'you'? You likely experience yourself somewhere in or around your head, don't you? I mean, you don't wake up and find yourself inhabiting your knee, or your hand, or your foot. You are in your head and that's where you live.

Therefore we make feeding our mind with knowledge and information a priority. And of course we feed the body when we are hungry, but other than that we largely ignore the body. And ignoring the body results in a diminution of life force or Prana, twhich will eventually cause symptoms and even diseases.

Even if you are exercising the body you may not be doing it consciously, as when watching a TV show while running on the treadmill. Nothing wrong with that—however, you are not in the body and therefore are unable to enjoy all the benefits you could get for your health if you were to bring consciousness to walking or running on the treadmill.

What does it look like, then, to be in the body, you may wonder? "Being in the body" is directing your mind's attention to the body, to any specific areas/tissues where any sensations are felt, no matter how subtle, and recognizing that what you are feeling is the energy that you are. This is a beautiful mind-body partnership that when coupled with conscious breathing through the area where you are experiencing the sensations, results in integration of mind-body-breath, which is the formula that allows for experiencing the wholeness that we are; this, therefore, is what needs to become our priority. The integration of mind-body-breath is also one of the definitions of Yoga, and it is what you will accomplish through the Energy Codes embodiment practices: a new health and wellness paradigm that focuses on cultivating the wholeness that we are.

Regarding 'being in the body,' there is an invisible and magical part of you, your central channel: a column of energy running across your body from the top of your head to the tip of your spine, also called Sushumna in Sanskrit. This central channel is home for the 7 chakra system, the place in your body where your life force resides in its highest concentration. Isn't this something that you really wanted to know about but didn't even know anything about? We want to master tapping into this infinite source of wholeness, which will result in healings in all areas of our life. That is what we do with the Energy Codes embodiment practices, directing our attention inward to the central channel and cultivating its presence.

This brings us to Distinction #4, whose subtle differentiation helps us better understand the invisible power of the Sushumna:

3. INVISIBLE ANATOMY VS PHYSICAL ANATOMY

This segment will act as a bridge between the Enlightenment and Embodiment sections.

It is a belief for most of humanity that who we are is the body (physical anatomy) that has a mind and a soul, because it is what we can see with our eyes. And therefore all will be over when breathing stops. In other words, we identify ourselves as the body/mind. However, besides our obvious physical anatomy, there is a subtle—and very exciting—realm not visible to the eye: the etheric body, the chakra system. There are 7 chakras within the body, from the tip of the spine (chakra 1/root chakra) to the crown (chakra 7/crown chakra). They are vortexes of energy or energy centers in the body, each of them corresponding to a different level of consciousness. These are the chakras that are familiar to most people, but I'll mention in passing that we also have less-known chakras—8, 9, 10, 11, and 12—outside of the body, corresponding to even higher levels of consciousness and vibrational frequency. We activate, balance, and integrate all of these chakras (1-12) when we practice BodyAwake Yoga, which I'll expand upon later in the chapter.

The chakras are also connected with the ~72,000 nadis (Johari, 2010) and the meridians —super-fine pathways through which energy travels within the body. The chakras may be invisible to us, but when they are partially or totally blocked, this imbalance has a profound impact on the body: sooner or later we'll experience pain, inflammation, and even diseases in the body.

I personally have known about chakras since I began my first Yoga Teachers' Training back in 2007, and have visited them in many trainings since then, but I never knew how to make that knowledge useful in my own life in any way, shape, or form. Through my studies with Dr. Sue Morter and the Morter Institute for

BioEnergetics I now know how to work with the chakras to support my health and well-being and I am sharing it here with you. In the following Table I've gathered information about the chakras that's relevant for our discussion.

CHAKRA	Symptoms	Consciousness	Breathwork and other practices	Yoga poses
1st (Root) chakra, base of the spine	Mental lethargy and spaciness, osteoarthritis, poor general health	"This is my life, and I get to choose my experience moment by moment." "I belong." Vibrant health	Mula Bandha Central Channel Breathing	Chair pose, Warrior I, Pyramid pose, Tree pose, Standing forward fold
2nd (Sacral) chakra, just below the navel	Feelings of isolation, impotence, low back pain, prostate and bladder issues	"I create joyful relationships and my communication flows with ease." Development of intuition.	Take it to the Body	Boat Pose, Pigeon Pose, Yogic Bicycle, Seated Spinal Twist, Breath of Fire
3rd (Solar Plexus) chakra, base of the sternum	Digestive issues, stomach ulcers, allergies, diabetes, chronic fatigue	"I allow my own way and I allow yours." Confidence, self-esteem, power.	B.E.S.T. Morter March	Camel Pose, Bow Pose, Reverse Table Top, Crescent Warrior, Breath of Fire
4th (Heart) chakra, center of the chest	Codependency, shallow breathing, high blood pressure, heart disease, cancer	Love and compassion, vulnerability "Everything is in my favor." Abundance.	Heart Coherence Breath Generating Loving Presence exercise	Triangle Pose, Thread the Needle, Fish Pose, Reclined Spinal Twist

5th (Throat) chakra, base of the neck	Perfectionsim, inability to express emotions, sore throat, thyroid issues, neck aches, asthma	"I hear and speak the truth with grace and ease." "I manifest easily."	Breath patterns for Healing	Cobra Pose, Plow Pose, Bridge Pose, Toning with Sound (Om, Ma, Ha)
6th (Third Eye) chakra, middle of the brain	Nightmares, glaucoma, headaches, learning difficulties	High intuition. Perceives beyond the 5 senses, creative genius	Saliva pH to gauge alkalinity in the body Conscious Exercise and Body Awake Yoga	Downward Dog, Shoulder Stand, Child's Pose, Peaceful (Exalted) Warrior, Balancing Poses
7th (Crown) chakra, to of head	Depression, confusion, epilepsy, Alzheimers' disease	"I am a divine being."	Central Channel Breath Meditation	Corpse Pose, Headstand, Rabbit Pose, Wide Angle Forward Fold

*Information for this table has been mostly extracted and curated from Morter, 76-77.

In the first column we find the name of each chakra and location in the body. The text has been highlighted with the corresponding chakra color. In the "Symptoms" column we find common symptoms and types of illnesses. In the "Consciousness" column there are some examples of statements that we'd say when the corresponding chakra is operating at its highest power. In the "Breath work and Practices" column I've listed one breath work and one other practice for each chakra. There are more practices in The Energy Codes book for each chakra. I've selected two per chakra here to keep it simple. In the "Yoga Poses" column we find some poses that focus on the activation of the corresponding chakra.

HOW TO USE THIS TABLE TO SUPPORT YOUR HEALTH AND WELL-BEING:

For example, if you have a heart condition, you'll find that it is a symptom of the heart chakra not functioning properly.

So, you'd go to the "Breath work and other Practices" column corresponding to the heart chakra and find that the recommended practice is the Heart Coherence Breath and the Generating Loving Presence exercise. In addition, it's important to realize that the heart condition is a symptom and the cause of the symptom may reside in a different chakra. So you will also want to ask your body: "Is there any other chakra related to this symptom that I need to work on?" Sense and feel your body for the answer and go to work there!

Section 3: Embodiment Practices that Activate your Innate Ability to Heal And Empower your Wholeness

When we have an 'A-Ha' moment, we are in the presence of so much clarity that we believe we are never going to forget it. But I bet you've had the same 'A-Ha' more than once. Why? The light that was present in the first moment of insight was not embodied; it remained at the level of the mind, only. In order for transformation to be sustainable, we must embody our revelations.

What follows is a selection of specific practices for embodiment, which help integrate mind, body, and breath together as one. They allow for empowerment at all levels of your being, beyond your physical health. I've made a selection of some of the embodiment practices described in The Energy Codes book, focusing on 1-2 practices per corresponding chakra (as in the Table above). It's been challenging to choose, since each practice is so meaningful and empowering! For more detailed information on these practices and for learning about all the others that Dr. Sue has developed, go to Dr. Sue's book The Energy Codes.

Rather than starting with Chakra 1 and going one by one to Chakra 7, I'm going to place my analytical mind to the side, allowing my true self to present this information 'out of order' and to start with Chakra 4, heart chakra. Why? Because your loving presence resting in and moving through your body is the healer within: "To heal the body, we have to be in the body. To heal most powerfully and quickly, we have to be in the body in love" (Morter, 185). It's important that we are in the vibration of love and joy while we do the practices.

At some point, with enough practice, being in this vibration of love will be your 'come from' rather than your 'go to.'

Chakra 4:

Love is the healer within. For most of us, the love that we are used to experiencing is conditional. This is a natural result of wanting to protect our heart from getting hurt. Loving this way is also an experience of attachment: when I love you, and you love me, you must stay. It's as if you belong to me. However, "When we land in the core of our being, love is easy to experience because it's what we're made of" (Morter, 186). Further, and in fact, "The magnetic field produced by the heart is more than 100 times greater in strength than the field generated by the brain and can be detected up to 3 feet away from the body, in all directions" **(HeartMath Institute). (To access fascinating research on the heart-brain-emotions connection, visit: https://www.heartmath.org)**

Generating Loving Presence Exercise (Self-Love):

Things or people external to us can and do activate the vibration of love within us. This is why we tend to think that the love we feel is coming from them, when the truth is that their presence happens to activate and reveal the vibration of love within ourselves. This exercise will give you the experience that the love you feel is generated by you and received by you and, therefore, unconditional. This is how to do it:

1. Start breathing in your belly, and allow high frequency energy from the cosmos to pour through

2. your crown down the center of your body. Allow yourself to receive this energy, cosmic intelligence. You realize you can choose how to use this energy.

3. Now think of something that you love. Something that brings love and joy every time you think of it. Perhaps it's your beloved and the gratitude that you feel for having this kind of connection in your life. Or it could be your pet, or your best friend. Or the magnificent view of a sunrise or a sunset over the ocean. Feel this love and appreciation. Imagine you are eye-to-eye with this. Let yourself be loved back as you are loving it.

4. Notice how you feel in the body and turn up the volume of these sensations: keep loving it, let yourself be loved back, and notice how it melts you in the inside. Continue to amplify this feeling, letting it emanate off of you, even bigger than the room you are in. Notice how it feels in your body, and memorize it.

5. Now place your hand on your heart and claim it all for you. Whisper to yourself, "this is for me"; all of this energy is rushing in and you are now

receiving it. Feel it. It's unconditional love, since you've generated it and you're receiving it. Feel this love that you have generated.

This is the love that now you know is possible. This is your self-loving presence. You can memorize it and return to this vibrational state as often as possible. Practice all the time, even while doing the dishes or driving down the road. Allow it to be your 'go to' until it becomes your 'come from.'

Heart Coherence Breath: The breath of the Cosmos

This breathing pattern has become one of my favorites to practice daily. I also love to bring it to my BodyAwake Yoga classes, particularly when we are holding downward facing dog. This is how to do it:

1. Visualize a sphere of golden light all around you (at least 4 feet radius).
2. Begin to inhale, drawing the high frequency light from the sphere, from all directions, into your belly (in front, behind, right and left, above and below).
3. As it enters your belly, start to move it up the central channel, passing through and stretching the solar plexus, and opening the heart. Keep inhaling as the light (it's you) continues to be drawn upward towards the upper lobes of the lungs. Keep inhaling even bigger than the body. Now exhale long in all directions.
4. Repeat as many times as you want. I do at least 3 cycles. This is, by the way, the most simple and effective breath to relieve anxiety and stress.

Chakra 1

This is our anchoring chakra. Its activation helps us come down from the head into the body and anchor on the Earth. It helps us feel safe, complete, and at home, as we integrate mind, body, and spirit.

Mula Bandha or Root Lock:

The activation of Mula Bandha is similar to Kegel exercises, requiring a contraction of the muscles of the pelvic floor. It's a lifting up of the pelvic floor muscles towards the navel, as if we're drawing energy from the Earth up into the body through this section of our body. At first, if you are new to this, you may need to contract all the muscles in the pelvis. It's totally OK. Practice makes perfect. Try it now and notice how you feel in the body. With this practice we easily anchor our consciousness into a single point and we feel grounded and stable instantly. We are awakening those tissues with life force and establishing a new—higher—vibration in that area of the body. This will become a simple, instantaneous practice that will change your life! Practice as often as you can during the day!

There are 3 additional anchor points, at the heart, throat, and third eye chakra levels. Engaging the 4 anchor points at once is a key practice of the EC that effectively helps us embody our consciousness.

Central Channel Breath (CCB):
This is the foundational breath of the Energy Codes. Imagine a funnel that opens up to the cosmos on the top of your head and becomes a channel through the center of your body, to the tip of the spine. Now, get yourself seated in your heart, activating the vibration of love within you, maybe visualizing an image of a person or something that brings you lots of joy. As you are feeling that way, now inhale as you let high frequency light (your Higher Self) pour down through this funnel and enter through the top of your head down the center of your brain, center of your throat, center of the chest, to your belly; let your belly expand with this breath, then begin to exhale drawing the navel to the spine down the tip of the spine and into the Earth.

Now start the breath from within the Earth, inhaling to the belly, letting it fill with high frequency light (Soulful Self) and exhale rising up through the channel and out the top of the head. As you consciously follow the breath, inch by inch, you are activating all the circuits along the path. This is a whole cycle of CCB. Repeat as many times as you want.

In summary: you breathe in from beyond the body to the belly, and exhale out to beyond the body, in one direction first, then the other. As you do this breath, you are activating the presence of your Higher Self in your body, rejuvenating yourself and drawing cosmic intelligence onto you. As you become more and more familiar with this breath, you'll find yourself doing it anytime anywhere. You'll no longer 'kill' time: any open time can be used to give yourself the gift of the benefits of practicing CCB.

Chakra 2
This is our wisdom center and also our feeling body. This feeling body refers to the physical feelings, or sensations we experience in the body, which correspond to movements of energy. When we label our sensations as good or bad, pleasant or unpleasant, we are in duality and being conditional about them: We like the

good ones and we don't like the bad ones. However, they are all energies. So, this resistance or rejection to feeling certain energies that arise in our body is what causes the short-circuits in our energy field that will likely end up leading to physical symptoms and disease. Only when we get to embrace ALL OUR ENERGIES will we be able to heal and experience the wholeness of our being.

It's paramount that we learn to work with ALL THE ENERGIES that arise in our system, particularly those that we have labeled as 'bad.' Dr. Sue discovered that the sensations that arise in our body when we are experiencing a charge, like a knot in the stomach, or tightness in the chest, are pointing us to where in the body we have a short-circuit, a gap in the energy flow. It's our Higher Self talking to the mind through the body. Knowing this allows us to work with these energies in a very effective fashion towards healing our system. We accomplish this with the practice of "Take it to the body," which is why I consider this practice foundational to the Energy Codes and foundational to anybody's health and wellbeing! This is how to do it:

Take It To the Body (TITTB):
Whenever you feel emotionally triggered by a person or circumstance, rather than going to your head, come into the body: There will be a place in the body where you'll feel a charge.

First, note:
1. where in the body the sensation is,
2. what the sensation feels like (hot, cold, pressure, buzzing…) and
3. what chakra may be the one affected.

Then,
1. go there with your consciousness and love, and
2. squeeze the area from the inside, as if you were hugging it, intimately, as if taking care of a frightened child.
3. Then begin to breathe up and down the central channel with as much love as you can generate, integrating this area into the channel flow until you feel a shift in the energy. It will probably take at least 4 complete cycles of CCB.

For those of us who have been living in our heads all our life, it may be hard to feel where the charge is, simply because we have not been living in that area of the body and the circuits responsible for letting us feel that area are asleep. If that's the case, you can ask your mind (with as much love as you can), "Where do I need to activate circuits in my body so that I can be with this situation without getting triggered?" Whatever the first place where your mind lands, trust that that is the place.

I suggest that you start to get familiar with this practice when you are calm, and consciously with your imagination bring in front of you a person or situation that typically triggers you in some way. Practicing in the 'in between moments' is how it will eventually come naturally to you when the challenging moment shows up. And fewer challenging moments will show up!

This practice can also be used to work towards healing any painful area that already exists in the body. Consider that the area is painful because, as a result of a gap in the circuitry, the stuck energy is overstimulating the surrounding tissues, which may be causing inflammation and/or may have already manifested as a chronic condition. So, give this painful area a loving squeeze from the inside, tell it that you are 'moving back in' as you breathe up and down the channel, activating the circuitry for health and wholeness in the area. And don't forget to ask: "where else can I build circuits in my body to relieve this pain?"

Chakra 3

When something happens that is really upsetting to us and we reject it, resist it, and are unable to embrace it, a short-circuit is created in the energy field, and the energy flow stops there. And then that area of the body starts to show a disfunction: "What starts as an energy issue eventually becomes a tissue issue" (Morter, 158).
To manifest a vibrant life, we need to start to accept life as it comes. You may say, "I may be able to do that moving forward, even though it does sound challenging enough!" "And ... what about all of the short-circuits that already exist in my energy field from all the times I've resisted life? What can I do about those?" To answer the latter question, that is precisely what all the Energy Codes practices do: All of them reconnect this disconnected circuitry. This is the path towards self-healing and self-empowerment.

B.E.S.T.: BioEnergetic Synchronization Technique

In this section I want to bring your awareness to the existence of this healing technique, developed by Dr. Sue's father in the '70s. A pioneer in energy medicine, he developed B.E.S.T., which is a very powerful hands-on, self-healing technique. During a B.E.S.T. session, a number of circuits that were short-circuited due to the rejection of stressful events get reconnected again, and the moment the energy starts to flow again as designed in the body, self-healing occurs. "We are rarely stuck for the reasons we think we are," Dr. Sue reminds us. "There is almost always something deeper that is really the cause" (Morter, 159). I also want to mention that there is a self-administered version of B.E.S.T. called B.E.S.T. release. It was developed jointly by Dr. Sue and her father and you can find it in Morter, 168-174.

Morter March:

The Morter March is a powerful practice that helps us heal from traumas. It activates and unifies multiple areas in the brain and systems of the body at the same time, thereby creating a reset of the nervous system that allows us to release emotional unresolvedness from our subconscious and to replace it by a new message to the subconscious with the sense of well-being and love that we want to feel. This is how to do it:

1. Stand with your feet hip-width apart and your spine straight and tall.
2. Step forward with your right leg, bending it into a lunge, with the knee over the ankle. Back leg remains straight.
3. Place both hands together in front of you and lift up your arms to about a 45-degree angle. Now, lower your right arm until it's back and behind you at a ~45 degree angle, pointing to where the wall meets the floor. Notice that your right thumb is pointing down. Extend all the fingers awake.
4. Tilt your head slightly to the left shoulder and look directly up to your left thumb. Close your right eye.
5. Standing in this position, allow yourself to feel a deep sense of wellbeing, and then take a deep belly breath and hold it for as long as you can. Then exhale and step back with your right leg.
6. Repeat on the left side. And then once more on each side.

This life-changing healing practice is recommended twice a day, first thing after getting out of bed and last thing before going to sleep, since those are the times in the day when the communication between the subconscious and the conscious mind is most enhanced.

Chakra 5:

The throat chakra governs our breathing, our ability to manifest, to speak our truth, and to listen to others. We are going to bring mind, body, and breath together, as we place our attention in a particular area of the body and we breathe through it. This is how we activate self-healing.

There are specific breath works that allow for activation of each of the chakras (see Chapter 8 of the Energy Codes), but in this section I will focus on teaching this one powerful healing practice called:

Breath Patterns for Healing:

"Pain exists in the body because of a lack of energy flow through the affected area" (Morter, 226).

With this powerful and elegant breath work we'll be able to start to move energy through any area requiring restoration of proper energy flow and the integrity of that area. Let me give you a quick overview of the practice first, to make it easier: With the affected area squeezed, you'll inhale from beyond the area to the heart, being the light that's moving through the body, as if 'stripping the area through with healing light,' followed by an exhale out the other end of the central channel. This is how to do
it:

1. To begin, let yourself get into the vibration of your loving presence, as best you can.
2. Now, choose the area you are going to work on. Come inside that area with your consciousness, with your loving presence, with intimacy, tenderness, and care, as if hugging a frightened child.
3. The first inhale is from beyond the area to the heart. Squeeze the muscles along the route and stretch them at the same time. This may take some practicing, it's all good! For example, if it's your left shoulder, extend your arm out to a position where you can feel enough intensity, then inhale through your fingertips, up the arm (being inside the tissues and as if you're the energy that's being drawn with the breath—you actually are) through the painful shoulder, to the heart, then exhale down the central channel and into the Earth.
4. Next, inhale from within the Earth to the heart, and exhale through the painful shoulder (continue to squeeze and stretch the muscles along the route) down the arm and out the fingertips.
5. Now, you could take a regular central channel breath as described under 'chakra 1.'
6. Repeat steps 3, 4, 5 several times as needed.

This breath work can be used for any part of the body that hurts or does not feel totally healthy.

Thousands of people have had remarkable healings doing this practice. And you can, too!

Chakra 6:
The third eye chakra is associated with the pineal and pituitary glands, which are in the center of the brain precisely where the cerebro-spinal fluid is made and from where the chemistry of the body is managed. I'll now summarize a couple of very important practices   that contribute to a healthy third eye chakra:

Nutrition and Saliva pH:
The cells in the body need an alkaline environment to thrive. When the pH is too acidic, they begin to die. "Ninety-five percent of all diseases occur when the body is in an acid state. Cancers are the extreme result of a highly acidic state" (Morter, 238). So, we want to keep the body in an alkaline state, which is the state needed for healing and rejuvenation. No wonder the 40 years of research on nutrition that Dr. M.T. Morter Jr. did showed that, to facilitate healing when inflammation or disease is present in the body, our diet needs to contain ~75% of fruits and vegetables. Measuring our saliva pH regularly allows us to monitor the alkaline or acidic state of our body in a very simple and quick way. Additional recommendations are presented in Morter 244-250.

Conscious Exercise and BodyAwake Yoga:
As I mentioned earlier in the chapter, most people while exercising are either watching TV on the treadmill, or listening to music. Nothing wrong with that, but those activities distract our mind from focusing on the body. Dr. Sue has trained professional athletes and champions to break their own records by the simple practice of doing CCB (as described under Chakra 1) while they work out. As you do CCB, you're drawing high frequency light into your core, therefore tapping into a larger quantity and quality of energy than when not breathing this way. This allows you to do more in less time and without fatiguing.

When Yoga is practiced with this conscious awareness in the central channel, we have the most robust combination of healing and wholeness practices all in one: That is BodyAwake Yoga. See below the last segment of the Chapter for a detailed description.

Chakra 7
Chakra 7 is about our connection with God Source, Spirit, or Higher Self. Energy

medicine techniques work with moving the energy in the body. Something that's unique about the Energy Codes practices is that we identify ourselves with this energy that moves up and down and through the body. This energy is our true, essential self, and its presence in the body—its embodiment—is what we are cultivating with the energy codes practices. We want to learn to still the mind so that the true self can rise through the very noisy mind and we can perceive it with the mind. There are several practices that activate this chakra and help us still the mind. One is the CCB that I taught in 'Chakra 1.' Another is:

Meditation:
There are many kinds of meditation. I am going to focus on a type of meditation that's very easy and even fun to do, where you chant along a Sanskrit mantra. Chanting mantras may be easy and is incredibly powerful, because not only do these mantras still the mind, but they are also vehicles or pathways for commanding transformation, as we focus our dispersed consciousness into the sound waves of the Higher Self. There are many amazing artists who specialize in chanting mantras. My favorite ones to listen to and chant with are:

Deva Primal & Miten

Snatam Kaur

The two mantras that I feel the most joy chanting are:

1. The Gayatri Mantra

Mantra for enlightenment. Roger Gabriel tells us that "All of wisdom, knowledge, and the entire Vedas are concealed in the 24 seed syllables of the Gayatri Mantra." For detailed information about this mantra, go to: https://chopra.com/articles/the-gayatri-mantra-for-enlightenment

2. OM Tare Tuttare Ture Swa-Ha

This is the Green Tara Mantra and has the power to liberate us from our attachment to suffering.

For an in-depth description and understanding of the power of this mantra, visit "The Sophia Code" by Kaia Ra, 132-138

BODYAWAKE YOGA/SUMMARY/CONCLUSION

In this chapter you have become aware of and learned of the importance of being in the body and of cultivating the integration of mind-body-spirit to support your healing and sustain vitality and optimal health. You've become aware of and learned simple and powerful practices that can be done anywhere, anytime, and that allow you to activate the circuitry responsible for your healing and wholeness—a pioneer technology for self-healing and self-empowerment that does not require anything from the external world. The fact that most of these practices can be done seated, standing, or even lying down makes it even easier. That is pretty amazing! Whether you are already a yogi or not (yet), you don't want to miss the fact that when we move the body while doing the EC practices, we get to activate more circuits, faster. And if the movement involves putting the body in sacred geometries—Yoga asanas—even more so! Yoga asanas are specific shapes we can put our bodies in that allow our energy to rush through the body in specific ways and directions that support our wholeness. In BodyAwake Yoga we make this process conscious, using visualization to direct our awareness to the flow of energy up and down the central channel and consciously rushing high frequency light— unconditional love—to and through the specific areas in the body that feel tight, begging for love and healing. Pocketed emotions that were stored in the tissues as a result of traumatic experiences causing emotional and maybe even physical pain for many years can now be released, and energy can flow freely through that area, again resulting in healing right there on the mat. You are healing your inner child while on the mat! You are letting go of illusionary beliefs and re-writing your past while on the mat!

Consequently, with BodyAwake Yoga we not only become more flexible, stronger, and faster, but catalyze our own healing process exponentially. It is the most robust combination of healing and wholeness practices all in one. Because of all these benefits, practicing at least a few minutes of BodyAwake Yoga daily is my #1 recommendation towards cultivating your healing and well-being. If you are not a yogi, or if your body feels tight and your poses don't look like those in books, it's totally OK. You can still do BodyAwake Yoga. What matters is your desire to support and sustain your healing and vitality throughout your entire life.

~ ~ ~ ~ ~ ~ ~ ~ ~

To learn about my online and in-person coaching and Yoga offerings for individuals and groups as well as to explore co-creating a personalized wellness program for you or your organization, you can reach me at marisa@marisagalisteo.com

ACKNOWLEDGMENTS
I want to dedicate this Chapter to my parents: To my father, who recently transitioned (1932-2021), for his never-ending joy, for always believing in my potential, and for his loving support not only for me but for everyone who crossed his path during his time on Earth. Te quiero, papá. And to my mother, for her passion for learning that was passed down to me, for her dedication to her children,

her love and support, and for being my mom. Te quiero, mamá.

I want to express my heartfelt gratitude to each of the multitude of outstanding teachers and students that have come across my path so far and have contributed to my awakening, my healing and empowerment, and to my becoming a more loving—and happier—human being.

A special gratitude note for Robert Davis for his continual support and encouragement all these years since we met at NYU back in 2005, and for trusting that I could be a qualified contributor to this book.

WORKS CITED

Gabriel, Roger, and Deepak Chopra, "The Gayatri Mantra for Enlightenment" **https://chopra.com/articles/the-gayatri-mantra-for-enlightenment**

HeartMath Institute, "Science of the Heart: Exploring the Role of the Heart in Human Performance" **https://www.heartmath.org/research/science-of-the-heart/energetic-communication/**

Johari, Harish, Chakras: Energy Centers of Transformation. Rochester, VT, Destiny Books, 2000

Morter, Dr. Sue, The Energy Codes: The 7-Step System to Awaken Your Spirit, Heal Your Body, and Live Your Best Life, Simon & Schuster, Atria Books, 2019

Ra, Kaia, The Sophia Code: A Living Transmission from The Sophia Dragon Tribe. Mount Shasta, CA: Kaia Ra & Ra-El Publishing, 2016

Rock, David, Quiet Leadership: Help People Think Better- Don't Tell Them What to Do: Six Steps to Transforming Performance at Work. New York, NY: Collins, 2006

CHAPTER XII

Practical Pilates for Every Body

Pilates is a comprehensive exercise system with an extensive history. It has the potential to positively impact every area of the body that benefits from actualized and visualized physical movement. If you have never tried Pilates as such, chances are you have done some semblance of it or sampled some pieces borrowed from the vast array of exercises that harkens back to the 1930s. In that respect, it is time-tested and continued to be informed by the broad expansion and appreciation that physical exercise now has in contemporary life. What was once novel and experimental is now commonsense and backed up by research.

It is widely claimed that in Pilates there are more than 500 exercises and innumerable variations. Since every body is uniquely proportioned and idiosyncratically developed, the movements are tailored, often in real time, to those individual needs. One universal truth I hold as a teacher is that the better you seem to get at Pilates, the more challenging the work becomes on multiple levels. Going right to the edge of one's physical point of control is instrumental to building strength in Pilates. Muscles that start to shake and tremble, for example, indicate that the body has the potential to create a stronger neuromuscular connection to underutilized muscles that have already been developed. Imagine tapping into strength that usually remains dormant. Myogenic development, on the other hand—the generation of new muscle fibers—is durational, taking three months or longer. Pilates can help integrate these two important modes of strength building.

Another tenet is that basic movement fundamentals are present, utilized, and reinforced throughout the system. As these movement principles are drilled and attempted with varying degrees of success, a thoroughly embodied logic begins to permeate the practice: it becomes systematic. We know it is true that progressions and regressions complement each other to develop strength, stability, mobility, agility, balance, and all our other goals. Regression is the simplest form of a complex dynamic movement. If doing a push-up is difficult, then regress to just the plank position or place your knees on the floor; if walking is difficult, work on simply pointing and flexing through your feet. At root, Pilates helps us feel and look better as we advance though our lives. Like yoga, it is certainly a lifetime practice and can be successfully utilized at every stage of one's physical and psychological development.

Resting, Assessing, and Making Headway

One of the best ways to start a Pilates session is simple and effective: "Lie down on your back, knees bent, feet flat on your back, arms at your side." Then, a few specifics: heels lined up with the sitting bones, and the center of the knees lined up with the hip sockets. If you find satisfaction in this level of detail, that's good news: there's much more to come. Thankfully, our nervous systems respond to novel experiences and feedback, which helps us tune-in and make positive changes more readily. If you are already a seasoned practitioner, and this is familiar ground, then the intimacy you have attained can be comforting and you can infuse it with self-generated cues and imagery. Pulling in positive material from other practitioners with whom you've learned or from information you've read can yield powerful results. For example, you might couple the bio-mechanical imagery with information learned about how to break your negative neurolinguistic conditioning about a "frozen" shoulder or those damaging self-perceptions about your weight and age. Merging source material helps us create something unique to address the true idiosyncrasies of each individual.

The other benefit of starting simply is that pupils have an immediate sense that they have already done something well. We don't want to give empty praise, but positive reinforcement tends to have a greater impact than its opposite. By resting on the ground, we've already accomplished something impactful and have started reaping the benefits of dedicating time to this endeavor. The floor specifically provides ample support for the spine and the limbs. The back of the head and back of the pelvis are automatically aligned, which is something we can then aim to find when we're standing or sitting. Surplus weight and pressure are taken off the supporting structures between our joints, including our intervertebral discs. Overworked muscles have a chance to reset so that we can start finding support from muscles that might be underworking or are inhibited. Before any intentional movement begins, the pupil and the teacher can fill this container, what is commonly called the Constructive Rest Positions (CRP), with a range of imagery, information, questions, and suggestions that can prime us to move better. Here's a partial list of nine of those cues to practice.

1. Visualize a very clear centerline: nose, sternum, navel, public bone, space between the knees and the ankles aligned. Couple the idea of the midline with the idea of a central axis, thevery middle of the body, our true cores. In other words, the body has a right side and left side. It also has a front and a back. It may sound obvious, but exploring the body in this way

through movement can yield some profound results: anytime we veer off or away from center we are like a structure whose parts don't stack up. This means, ultimately, that we'll have to apply an excessive amount of effort over time to maintain what's already less than optimal positionally, which can lead to overly contracted muscles, strain, and heightened tension—all things we want to lessen in the body.

2. Imagine the downward slope of the thighbones (femurs) pouring down and resting into the hip sockets. Visualize the hips as being deep sockets, and the head of the femur fitting and floating in the acetabulum, the socket of the hipbone. Refining our sense of the shape and size of our own joints can help us clarify our movements and untangle less helpful embodiments.

3. Feel the 26 bones in each foot spread into the floor. Do the same things with the hands —note the extra bone in the wrist—and remember that our fingertips and toes are dense with nerves, which is why they are so sensitive to touch. The hands and feet have varying degrees of dexterity, but in general there's a fair amount of brain space allocated to what happens in distal points. Later, initiating and reaching fully through our extremities can help us activate entire muscle-chains more fully: reaching away from our centers pulls us back together.

4. Widen the back of the pelvis and the sacrum, the triangular bone just below the lumbar vertebrae. Visualize the front of the pelvis narrowing— especially on the exhale. Finding a neutral pelvis can be thought of as a three-step process—pubic bone level with the floor and ceiling, hip bones parallel to one another, two sides of the pelvis evenly weighted like scales.

5. Commit to the inhalation. A five-count breath functions nicely with work that comes later. Try breathing into the abdomen and the chest simultaneously. Breathe front-to-back, side-to-side, and top to bottom. Sense how the air entering the body is cooler than the air leaving the body. Notice the gentle stretch of skin and fascia as the body expands—how the spine elongates, how it calms the nervous system, how it lengthens the spine. For an added layer, visualize the heart beating slightly faster on the inhale and slowing down slightly on the exhale.

6. Find equal weight across the right and left side of the body. Check in with the back of the head, back of the rib cage, and back of the pelvis specifically. Balance the two sides like you would balance a set of scales.

7. Reach through the fingers' tips gently and press the palms of the hands

into the ground to check in with the back of the arms and upper back. Widen across the collar bones and roll the shoulders gently back. Instead of pulling the shoulders down, allow the shoulders to elevate subtly on the inhale to allow more room for the lungs and ribcage to expand. Let the shoulders rest down and spread out on the exhale. There's no need to pull or jam your shoulders into position.

8. Proprioception is our awareness of where are bodies are in space—many of the cues above rely on fine tuning how the body is oriented in space. On the other hand, enteroception is an awareness of what's happening internally. The awareness of our heart's beating, or bringing our attention to the organs and glands including where they are located inside the body can be especially useful: the ascending colon on the right, the descending colon on the left. The liver underneath the lower ribs on the right, the spleen on the opposite side. Focusing on the internal organs can also precipitate a shift to a parasympathetic state, where we are able to rest, digest, regenerate. The body really is a vast and remarkable universe that we should be learning about on an ongoing basis, not just when something goes awry.

9. In addition, orient your body in time and space very specifically. Notice the room you are in, its dimensions and features. Bring your focus to the mat or the equipment you are lying on. Know that we function and express ourselves in an environment, never in a vacuum. It's how we interact and connect with things that matters. This might be termed exteroception, how we interpolate external stimulation into our internal landscape. Combining all this sensory information gives us better stretch, helps us increase strength, move with more grace and fluidity. We want our whole being involved in the movement, giving ourselves permission to take up more space; to move like animals or elite athletes is part of this integrating process. Even though there are many times where we look piecemeal at the body, be certain to take some time to live, breathe, and feel the organic oneness and wholeness of your own body.

In addition to these generalized cues, the first five or ten minutes of a session can yield a vast amount of information, and additional cues can emerge on the spot to address the particular imbalances in the body. Funny head tilts, scoliotic deviations of the spine, muscles gripping extraneously are some common dysfunctional patterns that can be addressed here. This is also an opportunity to converse freely. We certainly do not need to be stoic about our aches and pains.

We don't want to reify or reinforce pain structures through an internal or external dialog. Self-fulfilling prophecies notwithstanding, one of our main goals is to have the experience of something having been improved in a short period of time. By acknowledging and affirming that something's been ameliorated, that something just feels a little better, we can potentially work our way out of the labyrinth of chronic pain.

The Impetus to Move

The question of where to begin is always paramount. One unique feature of the Pilates method is that there are always multiple entry points. There are a number of what could be called closed-systems that intersect with more open-ended approaches to the work. These approaches, not mutually exclusive, ensure that we don't get bored or run out of challenges. For example, the original mat work developed by Joseph Pilates himself is comprised of roughly 34 exercises that are completed consecutive to one another. His book Return to Life is still the definitive text for what truly constitutes Pilates as such, which was originally called Contrology. The set sequences can easily be modified, exercises can be omitted as needed, and contemporary approaches have created a layered or tiered approach so that there are beginner, intermediate, and advanced levels within the larger scope. The same holds true on the piece of equipment known as the Universal Reformer or on the Cadillac.

Another truth is that Joseph Pilates was a consummate inventor. A fully-equipped Pilates studio has a vast array of equipment, props and tools, which indicates that even the progenitor of the method was aware that for many people a one-size fits all approach would not bring about the desired results of a uniformly developed body. The use of springs or straps to help people accomplish things that they are not able to on their own exemplifies this. Assistance, sometimes called spotting, helps make us stronger as much as actual resistance does.

Still, the best place to start is always with the basics, the fundamentals, which are a container that we can fill with the vast storehouse of human movement potential. Sometimes this is called pre-Pilates. Here listed are ten useful basic or fundamental exercises from the repertoire:

1. Position the head on the floor so that the crown of the head extends to the wall directly behind you, nodding the head gently to create a gentle stretch and release in the back of the neck. The heads sits on top of the spine somewhere between the ears and behind the nose, and we attempt

234

to move the skull on the very first cervical vertebra. Above all, this should feel good. Turning the head slowly side-to-side and circling the nose on the ceiling can be very beneficial in restoring balance around the neck muscles.

2. Reaching the arms up to the ceiling, imagine the back of the shoulders resting onto the floor. Visualize the top of the arm (the humerus) as a little ball resting on the floor; some people call this plugging, but let gravity and the weight of the arms help make this more sustainable. Notice the movement potential in this position: little circles, turning the upper arm in and out, we can also try reaching the arms back overhead, taking the arms into a big T-shape, and reaching the shoulder blades around the sides of the ribcage to protract the scapula intentionally. All of these movements can become further refined as you make additional progress.

3. If spinal flexion hasn't been contraindicated as in osteoporosis or cervical herniations, then curling the head, shoulders, and chest off the mat is a cornerstone of the Pilates work. This does not mean that Pilates is out of the question for people who need to keep their heads down. However, if you can lift up, try taking the hands behind the head and peeling off the mat one bone at a time. If you come up for 2 counts, hold for 2 counts, and lower down for a slow 4- counts, you'll tap into all three kinds of muscle strength—concentric, isometric, and eccentric. The upper back muscles release nicely when this movement is well executed, and it is a great way to start strengthening the abdominals.

4. From the head, let's move to the tail and think about the ways we can move the bones of the pelvis. Visualize the pelvis as a sphere and roll it back and forth, toward your chest and then to your toes. We call this action tilting the pelvis. Of course, the nomenclature (posterior and anterior tilt) is less important that feeling and sensing the movement. Common language like tuck and untuck works just as well as any technical terms for some people. I encourage people to do this exercise if as many ways as possible. Try it with some gluteal activation—squeeze the butt a bit, then try it another way, by curling the tailbone and lifting up through the pubic bone. Play with the feet pressing down, the heels pulling back. Come up a little higher and lift the pelvis and a few of the low-back (lumbar) vertebra off the mat. Improvising subtly within the form is often the best way to ignite new strength.

5. Picking the legs up is one of the first things infants do before they find the strength to turn themselves over and push themselves up. In fact,

many of these fundamental exercises tap into that developmental process. Start with picking up one leg at a time; placing hands on the side you are working can help the abdominals contract to create stability through the torso so that limbs can move with ease around the strong central column of trunk. There are so many ways to refine this movement. Imagine picking the leg up from the back of the leg just below the buttocks. As the knee comes towards the chest, imagine the top of the leg moving subtly in the opposite direction. Keep some weight on the opposite hip: often the weight of the lifted leg creates some unnecessary torque of the pelvis. Stay curious and, when you are ready for a challenge, lift and lower both legs at the same time but be mindful of the lower back, which you can protect by revisiting earlier work. As the legs lower, the pelvis counterbalances by rolling, zipping up, in the opposite direction.

6. The foot is pivotal for walking and standing and deserves special treatment. Extend one leg out to 45 degrees, draw the legs together, and begin by simply pointing and flexing the foot and ankle. Again, the technical names of these movement (dorsiflex and plantarflex) are less important than feeling and sensing the complex movement of the foot. The simple ideas that the big toes have their own muscle and the little toes have their own muscles and that there's a third that connects to the top of the foot helps really flex the ankle fully, which in turn widens the ankle bones. We need strong ankle flexors when we walk—imagine the heel striking softly and then rolling through the foot. Full ankle circles are also a great way to strengthen the muscles all around the circumference of those joints.

7. Lying on the stomach is a crucial part of this fundamental work. To start, lie prone with hands stacked and forward, your forehead resting on the hands. Let the upper chest spread into the mat, because this will help to lengthen the upper back, which tends to round forward slightly. Spend time visualizing the front of the body elongating: stretch the sternum forward, lengthen everything underneath the sternum forward, lungs and heart forward, and keep spreading the chest into the mat. This is also a great place to focus on breathing. Remember there's no one right way to breathe, but try sending the breath into the back of the lowest set of ribs where the kidneys and adrenal glands are located. When ready, try lifting the head, hands and elbows just barely off the mat, extending the upper back. Bend back between the shoulder blades, behind the lungs and the heart. A couple of degrees of movement will train those spinal extensors

to support us better when we're sitting and standing. Before moving on, try lifting one leg at a time followed by bending one knee at a time

8. Quadruped position is commonly referred to as "all fours" and is a great strength building position. If knees are sensitive, padding helps. If wrists are sensitive, try making a fist and placing the knuckles on the ground, which stacks the wrist nicely. Start with a simple cat/ cow—flexing and extending the spine. Then find a neutral pelvis: back of the pelvis level with the floor and ceiling. There are so many movement possibilities to explore here. Try shifting the spine forward and backward in space. Simple stability exercises are all challenging progressions, as for example lifting up one limb up at a time, taking opposite arm and leg off at the same time and reaching in opposite directions, adding a small tricep push-up, and eventually floating both knees off the ground together. Making this part of your exercise routine will yield benefits over many years.

9. To finish standing after all the work above is really to recapitulate one's developmental process. Standing well is an art in and of itself that's worth studying and practicing. Start by thinking about the width of your stance. Try standing with the heels lined up with the sitting bones and the knees lined up with your hip joints. Distribute the weight across the sole of the foot, half the weight in the heel and half the weight in the front of the foot. Make sure you have weight balanced from left to right. Now that the front of the pelvis is level with the wall in front of you, lift the pubic bone up in the front and lengthen the tailbone down to a spot just behind your heels in the back. Elongate your spine by reaching up through the crown of the head and continue to breathe deeply. Adding some additional spinal mobility here can be a way to ensure that the spine has been moved in all directions. Place hands behind the head, look up towards the ceiling with the center of the chest for some spinal extension, and bend sideways for some lateral flexion, rotating right-to-left. Keep the movement controlled and work safely in the mid-range.

Now that you have some fundamentals, including moving the spine in all three planes if safe, you may be ready to start doing some of the beginning Pilates exercises. But remember that these restorative movements are also key to the most challenging exercises. For each of the exercises listed above, there are deeper, more nuanced ways of understanding the exercises, which is why working one-on-one with a trained practitioner is so vital whenever possible. Pair some of the pre-Pilates exercises with some of the cues from the rest position. For example, allow the shoulder girdle (collarbone, upper arm, and shoulder blade) to float up and elevate on the inhale while standing: fill up the lungs more efficiently by expanding the ribcage.

Basics of Breathing

Before we dive any deeper into the Pilates mat repertoire, let's circle back to the breathing since Joseph Pilates said, "Above all, focus on the breath." Remember, there is certainly no one right way to breathe—but there are many ways to play with and explore the breath that can be beneficial. This can be done pragmatically and doesn't require any metaphysical overlay. For example, practice drawing air in through the nostrils and visualize the air swirling or spiraling in. The nasal passageway is ridged and curved so the air doesn't travel in a straight line. Rather, it is filtered and warmed as it travels through the bronchial passageways. Simply noticing that the air entering the body is cooler than the air leaving the body can be a powerful tool.

Remembering that the oxygen enters the bloodstream on that particular breath is another simple way to deepen the breathing. Just as the ribcage expands on the inhale, imagine all your branches (bronchial and arterial) expanding and dilating on the inhale to allow for more flow. Perhaps the image of the heart beating slightly faster on the inhale and slowing down gently on the exhale, what's called vagal tone, will enhance our experience of breath here too.

Ultimately, the focus on the breath becomes centered on the diaphragm— our primary breathing apparatus and arguably the most important muscle in the body. The dome-shaped muscle located within the lower portion of the ribcage— underneath the lungs and the heart—contracts and shortens on the inhale; it literally works to create a vacuum pump to help suction air down into the lungs. The feeling of breath moving into the abdomen and the upper chest simultaneously is a powerful indicator of how effectively we are breathing.

In traditional Pilates, a vast majority of the movements are initiated on the inhale. Because Pilates uses body-weight and spring resistance there's generally less compressive load on the supporting structures of the body. We are rarely lifting static weight overhead or in a manner in which that weight would bear down on the body. In those cases, initiating movement on the exhale makes better sense because the abdominal muscles create a better brace on the exhale so that you can "power-lift" the weight up. Pilates is not weight-lifting in the traditional sense but can reinforce and help clarify certain instruction when looked at closely. In other words, don't adhere to rules alone, but look deeper for the underlying reasons.

Here are three simple ways to reinforce moving on the inhale—as a way to strengthen the diaphragm in coordination with a variety of movement.

1. In the supine position, press the palms of the hands into the ground on the inhale and slowly decrease the pressure on the exhale. Remind yourself that the arms (triceps and lats) are working in the same way at the same time as the diaphragm: they are working and contracting analogously. Then, take the arms up to the ceiling and pull them down to the floor on the inhale. Now the arms are also moving in the same direction as your diaphragm, modeling or mirroring the movement of the diaphragm inside the body. Furthermore, imagine how the space between the fingertips and the shoulders externally demonstrates how the lungs also expand and contract inside of the chest internally.

2. Revisit hands behind the head to lift the head, shoulders, and chest. This time curl up on the inhale so that the abdominals and the diaphragm, again, start working synchronously; they're contracting together, reinforcing the action of the other. However, it can also be useful to reverse this so that the abdominals and the diaphragm work inversely to each other. Remember the abdominals can contract and help send the diaphragm back up and under the lower ribs. In this respect, the abdominals are secondary breathing muscles; they help facilitate a deeper or more rapid exhale but they are not fundamental to it. You can certainly breathe functionally without the abdominals' assistance, especially when you are resting and simply breathing diaphragmatically. There are times where it is vital to recruit the abdominals' help, as when lifting weights or in fight-or-flight stress response, but then other times where you may want to reduce their presence from the ever-changing equation. Given that fact, try one more pattern here: curl up and hold the position and take a number of deep breaths. Pay close attention to all the changes, some subtle, and some very apparent as you alternate between the inhale and the exhale with the head lifted.

3. If you were able to lift the head comfortably and would like an additional challenge, try maintaining the position while bringing the knees into the chest, heels together, toes apart, knees lined up with the shoulders. Press the legs straight out to a 45-degree angle on the inhale and pull them back in on the exhale. Now you can put some of the pieces together more fully:

imagine the diaphragm contracting and pressing down towards the pelvis on the inhale as you send the legs out. You can even imagine sending the breath down into the toes. As the knees come back in, pull the abdominals in and up, then visualize reeling the knees back in from the abdominals, sending the diaphragm back to its starting place.

Matwork— Approaching the 100

In the traditional Pilates group class, this is often a first exercise, which assumes a great deal of bodily awareness and facility. If an individual has a strong movement background and exercises regularly, this can be a great place to start. Otherwise, private instruction and a methodical exploration of some of the fundamentals listed earlier lead up to this. For anyone who's had trouble lifting the head with the hands behind it, slow down: if you've already found your edge with some of the pre-Pilates exercise, spend more time with them.

Additionally, keep seeking the advice from a trained movement professional and give them time to share their wealth of information. If you continue to experience difficulty, try using a prop or piece of equipment. For example, place a folded towel underneath the upper back— press down into the towel to lift the head up and see if shifting how you create leverage changes anything. You can use something larger (yoga block, Pilates barrel) as a wedge to keep your back elevated, then adjust with the amount of weight you have resting on the supporting structure. There are so many different tricks, slight adjustments, shifts in perspective that keep us from getting stuck, complacent, or satisfied with the status quo.

Before we look at this quintessential Pilates exercise, assuming you are ready for the challenge, let's try something that may help explain the rationale for having this exercise come so early in the system.

1. Lying with your head on the ground and legs long on the mat, reach the arms back overhead—reach for the wall with fingertips, stretch the heels in the opposite direction—and pull the abdomen taut. As the arms return to the ceiling, allow the weight of the arms to sink down through the back of the ribcage, connecting lower ribs more deeply to the top of the pelvis.

2. Try the same movement (shoulder flexion and extension) with the head raised. If this strains the neck, stop immediately. Otherwise, see how far back the arms can go without the head and shoulders coming down at all. Generate a commensurate amount of force with the abdominals equal to the weight of the arms going back. It's a cantilever and you want

the supporting structure to maintain its integrity, resisting gravity's pull down. Don't let your own arms—or anything for that matter—pull you back or down.

3. Now contrast the arms reaching back to bringing the arms just above the pelvis. Notice how reaching the arms forward past the toes with the fingertips helps hold the position.

4. Set up the position with the arms reaching forward. Start pumping the arms straight up and down with a degree of vigor within a controlled range of six to eight inches. Keep it strong and contained. Emphasize the downward action of the arms at first, connecting to the back of the arms and the upper back and using the strong thrust of the arms forward and down to keep the part of your back on the floor firmly grounded. Inhale for five pumps and exhale for five pumps, keeping an even inhale to exhale ratio. Take 10 breaths, which equals 100 pumps of the arms. It's a sprint and will get the heart beating faster when completed correctly. Pilates has an element of interval training: the heart rate rises and falls moderately over the duration of a session.

5. For an added challenge, when ready, practice lifting one leg at a time or lift both legs a few inches off the ground so that the toes are at eye level.

The Roll-Up

The Roll-Up is a benchmark exercise and is performed exactly as it is aptly named, building on the skills already performed in the previous exercise. The idea here is not to foist the weight of the spine and ribcage off the floor with the neck muscles, which are primarily designed to lift the head and cervical spine up solely when lying supine. In order to get the abdominal muscles engaged, effectively remember the important of leverage. We press something down in order to lift something else up, allowing us to lift up more weight than force we are applying to lift that weight up, a hallmark of bio-mechanical efficiency. There's also a subtler aspect to this: leverage allows us to move where we want to move, bend where we want to bend, extend where we want to extend. For a joint to be healthy it needs to be moved in its full range of motion. With roughly 360 joints in the body, there's so much movement potential that can be actualized to keep all those joints rolling, sliding and gliding. Here are some basic ways to start building a more functional and effective roll-up.

1. Bring the legs all the way together to create a nice boundary or bolt for the pelvis. Make sure the heels are together to help level the pelvis. Lift the head up and check out the position of the legs to see if they appear

241

aligned. If they are veering off to one side, move them center. Placing your own eyes on your body is an important tool. Don't always take someone else's word for it. We want to learn to trust our own perceptions and pair that with information relayed by the outside observer.

2. Remember how important the weight of the arms was in the 100. Start by reaching the arms back overhead again, enjoying the flexion of the shoulders: the collarbones rolling back, the top of the shoulder blades tilting down towards the floor, the side-body lengthening, the low back spreading long and wide. As we bring the arms up to the ceiling, connect the lower ribs to the top of the pelvis and let the upper back get heavier on the mat; use that leverage to bring the chest up and the head will lift up in response. Try reaching the arms forward and down and keep peeling away from the mat. Come up one vertebra at a time by pressing one vertebra at a time down into the mat, by pressing one set of ribs down into the mat at a time. The ribs roll forward as the vertebrae flex forward. Elongate the back muscles as you come all the way up to sitting, reaching forward for the toes with the fingers and the crown of the head. If you find yourself getting stuck on the way up, resist for now the temptation to toss the head or arms down. Truly be patient and teach yourself to appreciate the hurdles you can't quite get over. The body will thank you in the long run because that's where the additional strength is required. It's also the way to build that strength which won't happen if you cheat it. In other words, we get stronger when we don't bypass the places where our weaknesses are revealed. Coming up part-way with good form is often better than coming up all way with a toss or a jerk. In the traditional Pilates mat work, we roll up half-way on the inhale and the rest of the way on the exhale: one full breath cycle on the way up and one full breath cycle on the way down.

3. If rolling up from the lying down position left you stranded slightly, give yourself permission to rock or lift yourself up so we can practice rolling down. If you rolled up all the way with good form, congratulations: now it's time to keep working and to find new ways to stay challenged. One of the best ways to better and master rolling up is by rolling down with precision, quality, support, and control. Rolling down is initiated in a reversed manner. If the legs are still glued together, reach through the heels without lifting them off the floor, which would indicate knee hyperextension. Without moving the upper body, send the tailbone toward the heels and start rolling the pelvis back, rolling it under. If you

keep moving from the pelvis, the upper body will respond by rolling back slowly. See if you can roll back to the base of the sacrum or the waistband of your apparel, pull the abdominals in, and exhale to come back up. Next time, roll down through the five lumbar and see if you can contact the two lowest sets of ribs in the back to the mat, pull the abdominals in, and exhale to come back up. The lower tips of the shoulder blades are the next landmark we encounter before we attempt to roll all the way down to the back of the head again.

4. Pulling the abdominals in when we lift up the weight of the trunk in these exercises is truly paramount. If we neglect pulling the abdominals in, we tend to overwork the hip flexors. Pulling the abdominals in on the exhale in those key moments means you are fulfilling two good fully functional objectives at once. Sometimes we start tuning out details or language that starts sounding rote. Needing constant reinforcement and real concentration is the knowledge that pulling the abdominals as you lift up the trunk is imperative, that it inhibits the psoas and protects the guts and lower back, which has less skeletal support and more weight to bear than the vertebra above. Imagining the abdominals as scooped out, hollowed out, concave like a valley, like a crescent, is integral to these exercises. If we are not pulling the abdominals in when we lift up the weight of our trunks, we are simply using the wrong muscles—just because it feels like we are using the abdominals doesn't mean we are truly activating them.

5. If you are having trouble with the roll-up, there's one more helpful trick. Give yourself more support by placing a small pillow between the pelvis and the ribcage. Pressing down into the pillow on the way up reminds you to create leverage at the right moment and gives you a little extra lift, a little bit of a head start or boost. These moments can also be refined on the Pilates equipment. Using the spring-loaded bar on the Cadillac can help people who can't do the exercise on their own and can challenge people with added resistance for those who feel they can roll-up with ease.

Bridging

In my teaching practice, we do the Bridge after the Roll-up to build on the skills and concepts that have already been introduced. Traditionally, one would roll the hips all the way over the head and shoulders, and then roll back down. I think the two are closely related and the one can be substituted for the other to help refine and clarify the movement principles. We'll look at the way to start rolling-over, which is suitable to beginners at the end of the section.

1. The Bridge begins with a clear posterior pelvic tilt from the pre-Pilates work. Start with knees bent, feet firm to the mat, heels lined up with sitting bones and the center of the knees aligned with the hip joints. Notice how if the knees open too wide it forces the weight onto the outside of the foot (supination), and if the knees narrow together it rolls the foot onto the inside (pronation). We keep the knees tracking over the second and third toes in general to keep the angle of the knees from getting too acute or obtuse. This prevents strain on the knees and distributes the weight more evenly across the surface of the joint. We can even project way ahead and start thinking about how these principles can help in our everyday activities and other kinds of training. This kind of focus can help us refine how we go up and down steps, how we sit and stand, how we do our squats.

2. Just as in the Roll-Up, we bridge sequentially through the spine by creating leverage. To lift the pelvis up, we press our low backs softly down. The low back rolls up as we press our lower ribs down in the middle back. The upper back between the shoulder blades becomes thefoundation as we lift the middle back up. Of course, we are trying to integrate the strength in our arms and legs with our torso. Pressing the arms through the extension of the shoulders all the way down to the palm of the hands and fingertips is satisfying and strengthening. Feet can press down and heels can pull back to engage the hamstrings and lengthen the spine past the feet. Feet can also press down and away from the body to engage differently. It's all fair game in the world of movement if done mindfully, with curiosity. Dogma and rigidity do not help us become more integrated. There's no one right way to do any exercise, but we do aim to adhere to the principles of physics and bio-mechanical efficiency such as we understand them in the moment.

3. Rolling down from the bridge is another reversal. Instead of dropping the hips back down, try keeping the hips lifted as you internally curl the ribs and spine back down. We come down one vertebra at a time by lowering one vertebra at a time back to the mat. Imagine the keys of a piano, playing one note at a time. Make sure you do come all the way down and give the pelvis a chance to release fully into the floor before you come up again. Every aspect of the movement is valuable—no moment is more important than any other. This means we are trying to stay connected through the transitions.

4. The breathing in the Bridge is truly fascinating. Inhaling on the way up

244

is a way to strengthen the diaphragm because it places the resistance on a downhill slope. The simplest way to visualize this is to imagine the muscle pushing something up a hill on the inhale, where there's more weight to lift. Rolling down of the exhale helps us contract the abdominals as we try to keep our hips lifted and curl the chest forward internally without lifting the head up.

5. Once you are ready to progress, try rolling your hips off the mat with your feet off the ground, knees bent into the chest. It requires a tremendous amount of effort in the arms. Eventually, we come all the way up to the spread of upper back between the shoulder blades— always being careful not to place too much weight on the back of the head and neck.

Single Leg Circles

Like many Pilates exercises, the single leg circle is a variation on a theme and is linked to the pre-Pilates movement fundamentals. After doing some version of the roll-up and some version of rolling over (bridging), the spine is stabilized again after being mobilized, and we begin to explore the movement in the hip joint again, moving the lower limbs around a strong and steady spinal column.

1. Before circling an extended leg, start in the constructive rest position and place one hand on the hip, reminding it to stay in place, to stay evenly weighted with the opposite hip. Then practice lowering and lifting the knee laterally, foot grounded without any attendant movement in the pelvis. At times, we want to ensure that the movement of our limbs does not destabilize other parts of the body. Later, we will explore integrating fuller movements consciously with sufficient underlying muscular support.

2. Limbering up can always be helpful before doing larger motor movements. Draw one leg in and place the hands behind the hamstrings. Extend and bend the knee with a real sense of ease. Enjoy how the two conjoined sockets of the tibia can glide and slide around the two conjoined balls at the bottom of the femur. Try this with the head and chest lifted. If you find it easier to stretch the back of the leg with the abdominals engaged, we start to become aware of how the body's reflexes, here reciprocal inhibition, help us move more freely. Remember, if you spend a significant amount of time on one side, it is always helpful to pause and feel the consequences of our actions; taking a moment to appreciate the effects of what we've done is a way to maintain those benefits. In other words, we want our sessions to have a lasting impact on our biomechanics and our

biochemistry.

3. Single leg circles sometimes seems like a bit of a misnomer: sometimes the movement is more elliptical, D-shaped. We can circumduct our legs through fuller ranges of motion as we get more agile, or reign it in and find the strength in the mid-range. Circling with the leg at a 45- degree angle can be beneficial for people who are tighter. The farther away from center, the heavier the leg becomes relatively, like carrying your grocery bags with the arms out in front compared to letting the arms hang at one's side. Factoring in how gravity is at play in each exercise can yield powerful results. Exploring a range of movement in a safe and balanced way within the relative constraints of a certain exercise is another way of building strength and body awareness.

4. Eventually the movement of the limbs, pelvis, and trunk becomes more integrated. Returning to the CRP, try rotating the pelvis subtly side-to-side, alternating where the weight is placed on the back of the pelvis, moving the pelvis side-to-side like a see-saw, and allowing the knees to move like windshield wipers. For added challenge, try the same movement with the knees up in a tabletop position; add a circular motion of the pelvis and imagine you are moving through all the numbers of a clock face or all the points of a compass. Eventually, one leg extends out long on the mat, and with the knee bent or extended the entire spine rotates over into a supine twist.

Rolling Like a Ball Preparation

1. Transitions to come up to sitting by rolling up, rocking up, or turning to the side all work well. The next exercises capitalize on a number of our fundamentals, including pelvic tilts and breathing. From a seated position, knees bent, feet on the floor, hands behind hamstrings, practice rolling back a quarter of the way, perhaps to the base of the sacrum and coming back up. Initiate from the pelvis on the way down by tilting the hips back intentionally from the lower aspect of the abdominals. Return by hugging the abdominals together and exhaling fully. It's worth my repeating that pulling the abdominals drawn together, in and up as you lift the weight of the trunk back up, is functional on two-levels: it inhibits the hip flexors from doing the work that the abdominals are better suited for, and it is aligned with proper breathing mechanics. We don't trust our feelings on this. Rather, we trust our intellect, interrogating ourselves and the movement for maximum gain: are we really drawing the abdominals

in when we lift up the weight of our trunks? This is imperative: it protects the spine, the organs, and helps us breathe more efficiently.

2. Try the same exercise with the feet lifted just off the mat. Start with the hands behind the hamstrings and eventually place the hands on the front of the shins. Visualize the spine growing taller over and around the knees. See the armpits rising over the knees or be extravagant and see the lower ribs in the front rising over the knees. Sometimes we imagine the impossible to find out what is possible. Pelvic tilts with the feet lifted will start to rock the body back. How far back can you rock without tipping all the way over and rolling all the way back? Hone in on the moment of initiation. Keep pulling the abdominals in when needed and pairing that engagement with the breathing.

3. One other way to feel the power of this suggestively embryonic shape is to return to the back and practice lifting the head and tail off the mat simultaneously, especially if the spine is known to be healthy. Try placing the hands behind the head and lifting the head and feet at the same time, bringing the knees to the elbows at the same time that you bring the elbows to the knees. This position engages the abdominals fully, from top-to-bottom and bottom-to-top. If there are concerns about spinal health, this movement can be performed lying on the side with a much smaller range of motion.

Series of Five

Pilates exercises tend to get more challenging. They follow a pattern of moving up a ladder. Generally, the exercises get progressively more difficult through the workout. Regressions—doing easier or modified versions—can also be seen as helping us work harder. Giving oneself a spot or assistant, for example, should deepen the work rather than allowing a way to skip over or bypass a tough spot.

1. One example of giving ourselves a helping hand also teaches us how to use our own body as a better training partner. Draw one leg into the chest and place the hands on top of the shin. Then, press the shin up into the hands, pull the hands down into the shin, pull the knee into your chest with your arms, and press the leg away from the chest just as strongly. Find just the right amalgam of push and pull here, and then feel the body working together. Try lifting the head up and notice how the arms, the abdominals, and the leg all conspire to help you stay up— we're stronger when we use the body in a unified way, finding the gestalt, the totality greater than the sum of its parts.

2. When ready, lift the opposite leg off the ground and slowly switch from side-to-side. Playing with the tempo, sometimes slower and sometimes at a quicker pace, is another way to keep building dynamic strength. We never want the movement to become pat or routine.

3. Eventually, we progress to taking both legs out for a double-leg stretch; move to straight leg scissors with the hands placed behind the leg or ankle. Practice double-leg lower lift with the hands behind the head, and criss-cross right elbow to left knee with right leg outstretched to the other side, then left elbow to right knee with left leg outstretched to the other side.

4. Variations of the exercises above include doing the entire series with the hands behind the head, or with hands or even a pillow placed underneath the back of the pelvis. The sky's the limit when it comes to doing the Pilates exercises, and this is just an introduction to the breadth of movement possibilities we aim to consider, the wide-range of movement patterns we hope to explore. For the more advanced practitioner, weights and other forms of resistance, including industrial-grade springs, add increasing levels of complexity and challenge. Pilates should not overextend or overexert the body but instead should take it right to the edge of what can be done with good form.

5. 5Before the end of the workout, coming back to a standing posture is generally a good idea. Additional ways of ending might include a set of calf-raises, further exploration of spinal mobility (flexion, extension, side-bending and rotation), and perhaps some standing roll-downs.

Pilates is a time-tested method that continues to evolve. It serves to help us become stronger and more aware in our bodies and can be a container for exploring all manner of biomechanics. It is motivational—it teaches us to hold our ground, stay calm, and work through myriad challenges. It also pairs well with all other activities we aim to achieve: it supplements rather than supplants. Pilates has a rich history with a host of colorful and diverse characters. It truly is a vast system. Individual teachers are the lifeblood or Pilates; much of what is learned and taught is done orally and in-person. At best it isn't scripted or formulaic but discursive and responsive, intuitive and analytic. In short, it must be lived, felt, and experienced.

CONCLUSION, with Summary Review
& Motion & Exercise + Workout Plans

When I meet people and introduce myself as a personal trainer, quite often I'm met with innocuous questions like "How should I work out?" or "What should I eat?" I'm sure I annoy people when I reply with the classic, go-to response: "It depends." Admittedly "It depends" is, on its own, a pretty useless answer. We need more context. Some people are interested in the discussion that follows, as I hope you are. For better or worse, there is no one-size-fits-all approach.

This chapter will focus on two primary objectives. First, we will explore the process of setting clear and measurable goals that align with your values and direct you to action. We will also start to examine how your goals should guide your approach to training, nutrition, and other lifestyle decisions. As nutrition, sleep, stress management, and other essential aspects of healthy living have been examined at length earlier in this book, we then will pivot to a more focused discussion of human movement and exercise. While we cannot pretend to provide a detailed understanding of these topics here, you should nonetheless conclude this chapter empowered; armed with a practical understanding of exercise fundamentals, you should feel confident to assess and revise your existing training routine as needed, or begin a holistic training routine that serves your needs as well as your goals. At the very least, you should feel well equipped to know what to look for if you choose to seek professional guidance and coaching.

PART 1: CLARITY IN THE GOAL SETTING PROCESS

OUTCOME GOALS
After you've asked "How should I work out" or something to that effect, and I've told you "It depends" (and you either visibly roll your eyes or just do so in your mind), the first thing we need to explore is your goal. What do you want? I'm going to have a hard time providing a map and directions if you don't know where you'd like to go.

When most people set health and fitness goals, they think about a desired outcome, a result they'd like to achieve. Often, these results are objective and easily quantified: get stronger, lower blood pressure, lose weight. Other times, the outcome is a bit more fuzzy or subjective: feel more confident, feel more comfortable playing golf, have more energy. Either way is fine—not all things that matter are easily measured.

Most important is that we have a guiding compass so that you're not spending your effort inefficiently, working hard while moving in the wrong direction. That said, even if your goal is more qualitative in nature, it is useful to establish clarity and specificity. After you decide what you want in broad terms, we can translate your goal in such a way that we can more easily assess progress over time. One such method is to develop a SMART goal. SMART is simply an acronym that stands for Specific, Measurable, Attainable, Relevant, and Time Bound.

Specific: This is the overarching umbrella—think who, what, when, where, why, and how. If your goal is to lose weight—how much? By when would you like to lose it? Are there any other parameters or conditions that you'd like to meet while losing the weight? You want to be muscular…so, like Arnold Schwarzenegger? Or are we just talking about filling out a medium size T-shirt instead of a small? Even though we probably share some thoughts on what it means to be healthy, fit, or lean, I want to know what exactly that means in your head. If your goal is to have more energy or feel more confident, think of concrete examples of what that would look like in your life. Tell me what your goal means to you.

Measurable: Again, how do you know if you've achieved your goal, or at the very least are making progress? "Get in better shape" is hard to measure, and doesn't tell me nearly as much about what you want as "lose body fat" or "improve cardiovascular endurance." Certain goals, of course, are harder to quantify—an example earlier referenced, "feel more comfortable playing golf," can be very difficult to judge objectively, since you're probably evaluating highly subjective feelings like muscular tension, energy levels, or pain. In cases like these, you can still come up with proxy measurements that help you understand if you're making progress. Maybe this is your score at the end of a round of 18 holes, or just feeling like you don't need to pop an Advil while you play.

Attainable: Wouldn't it be wonderful if Amazon Prime two-day shipping applied to our health and fitness goals? For many of us, there's a Goldilocks effect at play when we set goals; something that feels too easily achieved may not be sufficiently motivating, while too much ambition increases the risk of failure (or compels you to adopt strategies that may not be in your best interest). Are you hoping in two weeks to swim the English Channel, but don't currently know how to swim? Maybe your goal for the next two weeks is just to buy a swimsuit, find a nearby pool, and sign up for lessons! When in doubt, start small, especially if you've struggled with your goal in the past. Sometimes the most important part of this whole game is to continually experience the feeling of success and develop a sense of self-efficacy. With long-term goals, by all means you can and should have ambitious goals, but in plotting out your map to victory it's essential to create reasonable expectations. Dream big, but make your way there one step at a time.

Relevant: At surface level, you can simply judge whether your goal connects with something broader that you're working toward. Perhaps you tell me your specific training goal is to increase your one rep max (the most weight you can lift one time) in the bench press. That's great if you're a powerlifter! If your broader goal is to lose fat, a higher one-rep-max in the bench press might not be particularly relevant, since you can get a lot stronger without much change to how much muscle or body fat you have. Something like a 10-rep-max in the bench press or the time it takes you to row 2,000 meters would likely be more relevant, from a training perspective.

At a deeper level, it's important to consider whether or not your goal fundamentally connects and resonates with your values and priorities in life. Perhaps you associate gaining muscle with increased confidence, and in turn you associate higher confidence with performing well at your job. Ask yourself whether or not your health and fitness goals really connect with what you want in your life. We all know people who have a six-pack and are still insecure about their appearance. Take the time to consider what really matters to you. The more deeply your health and fitness pursuits connect to your most important values and priorities in life, the easier it will be to do the work necessary to accomplish your goal.

Time-Bound: Simply put, we're putting a deadline on your goal. It's not always critical to achieve our goals by a specific moment in time, and we rarely (probably never) have full control over whether or not we succeed. If you're looking to decrease your blood pressure from 150/95 to 110/70 in 6 months' time, but in actuality "only" lower it to 126/82, I sincerely hope you'll still be proud of the work you put in and happy with what that suggests about your improved health status! It may feel like cognitive dissonance to insist on deadlines without always taking them too seriously. The importance of deadlines is that they promote action and dictate the intensity. You might not have ever taken the steps to lower your blood pressure if it was just something you wanted to achieve "someday."

It's okay to occasionally create your own arbitrary deadlines (many of us do this naturally, anyway—birthdays, trips to the beach, competitions and races, etc.). It's easier to procrastinate and "start next week" when there's no pressure to do the work now, and there's a massive difference in how you'll approach your training, nutrition, and other lifestyle elements if your deadline sits one month away as opposed to one year.

DIFFERENTIATING HEALTH, FITNESS, AND BODY COMPOSITION

Let's revisit the idea of creating relevant outcome goals. Exactly what is it you'd like to improve—health, fitness (aka performance), or body composition, or some combination of the three? Let's explore some definitions.

Health deals with both the quality and duration of your life. In truth, thanks to the blessings of modern medicine, plenty of people live long lives without being particularly healthy. Heck, you can meet most of life's basic needs at the tips of your thumbs on a smartphone. Humans are one of few (possibly the only) creatures for whom physical activity is more or less optional. You don't see cheetahs ordering their meals on Seamless. Realistically, the types of things we can do to promote a state of good health—staying physically fit, maintaining a healthy bodyweight, getting adequate sleep, etc.—will probably help you live longer, all things being equal; however, with respect to longevity, these elements are necessary but insufficient.

To live a long life, go to your doctor's appointments, get your bloodwork done, and be on the lookout for major red flags. Running marathons and drinking kale smoothies can't do much for you if you're living with undetected tumors. Learn your family history and control what you can. Other than that, wear your seatbelt, look both ways before you cross the street, don't smoke, and try to avoid deliberately engaging in stupid or dangerous activities (basically, don't act like a college-aged undergrad). Be careful not to slip and fall in the shower or when walking on an icy sidewalk. Try not to get stuck by lightning. Yes, luck matters. When it comes to longevity, good genetics go a long way, too. Choose your parents wisely.

To achieve a high degree of health and prolong your healthspan, we might start to branch out and think of things like eating enough vegetables, getting plenty of sleep, and training an appropriate amount (we'll speak more on exercise from a health perspective later in the chapter). That said, please consider health beyond the purely physical. Paying attention to your nutrition, sleep, and movement can do amazing things for your cognitive and psychological health as well as your physical well-being; just be careful of extremes. Spending more time at the gym than you do with your family? Forgoing a dinner invitation with friends so you can adhere to a diet best suited to a professional bodybuilder? From the standpoint of your mental and emotional health, you might be better off reading Harry Potter with your kids or grabbing a beer with an old friend (or water, whatever floats your boat). By all means, eat well, sleep, and exercise, but also go take a long walk in nature, from time to time. Mindfully spend time with loved ones and in contemplation. Strive to be a lifelong learner. Dedicate time and energy to work that fulfills you and allows you to wake up each day with a sense of purpose. Practice compassion and forgiveness toward yourself and others. Give back. Be grateful. Find opportunities to laugh and to play. As they say, it's not the years in your life but the life in your years.

Fitness—aka performance—deals with your ability to perform a given task. Achievement at the highest levels of sport isn't always healthy (true for some activities more than others). Becoming a professional football player likely means multiple joint surgeries, chronic pain, and some amount of brain trauma. Even disregarding the injury potential, becoming a champion wrestler or gymnast often involves manipulations of bodyweight that risk acute dehydration and, over time, may result in eating disorders and metabolic disregulation.

Fitness is relative to the task at hand. Being fit as a powerlifter means being able to squat, bench press, and deadlift heavy weights for 1 repetition at a time; who cares if a tortoise beats a powerlifter in a foot race? An elite distance runner may not be your best bet if you're looking for someone with tremendous upper body strength. The next time you crack open a fitness magazine and get tempted to follow a training program meant for Navy SEALS, ask whether or not you really need to perform at their level in your daily life.

Most of us don't. Most of us can approach fitness as you would an undergraduate college education. Pick a major! Find something you like and get…decent at it. In the meantime, take courses in other subjects to create a broad base of knowledge, thereby avoiding major gaps as well as providing personal enrichment. Major in swimming, but take some classes in Pilates and kettlebell-based strength training. Major in powerlifting, but take some classes in yoga and modern dance. Major in running, but take some classes in rock climbing and Brazilian jiujitsu. The world is your oyster. Amateur athletics, should you choose to get more serious, resemble a master's program; professional athletics, a Ph.D. The deeper you go, the narrower your focus becomes. Specificity and specialization come at a cost. When your personal definition of fitness relates to navigating daily life with ease, variability is generally preferable. More breadth, less depth.

Another aspect of fitness, body composition deals with relative amounts of body fat and lean body mass. Aesthetic goals, focused on changing physical appearance by reducing body fat and/or adding muscle, certainly fall under this umbrella. Many measures of physical health (and, depending on the context, fitness) also improve when relatively lower levels of body fat and adequate lean body mass are maintained (approximately 8-20% body fat for men, 16-30% for women). However, changing body composition certainly does not always overlap with health. Elite bodybuilders, particularly near competition, achieve incredibly low levels of body fat while maximizing muscularity… and, by the time they're onstage to compete, often feel terrible. Women who reduce body fat past a certain level can lose their period. A lineman in American football might deliberately add substantial weight (both muscle and body fat) to become a more effective human wall on the field of play, but nobody said that this will benefit their long- term physical well-being.

Where do you fall in the Venn diagram? There isn't a right answer, truly. What you value and prioritize is for you to choose, and you alone. What's most important is that you have clarity with where you land and that your behaviors (e.g. training, nutrition, etc.) align with your goals. Nobody said you're permanently stuck in one spot on the Venn diagram for all time. When I was younger, I, like many young men, cared mainly about the circumference of my biceps and how much I could bench press. Meeting and marrying the woman I love did a lot to dissociate my confidence from what I saw in the mirror or how much weight I could lift. As I write this, I'm training to run a marathon. Cardiovascular training carries myriad benefits for physical well-being, but if long-term health were my sole concern, I'm sure I could get away with far less. When I was a kid, I reliably got bronchitis and generally detested cardiovascular exercise; when I heard about people running a marathon, I was quite certain it was something I was incapable of. I'm training to overcome a perceived limit I once imposed on myself. I imagine that, after I've finished that last mile, I'll scale back the running substantially. Most of us, as we get older and wiser, think more about the consequences of our actions, both immediate and enduring (hopefully!). We think about training, eating, and living in a way that is sustainable and supports long-term well-being. Nonetheless, it's nice to take on challenges every now and then.

When it's all said and done, almost all the clients I've worked with—almost all people I know—land somewhere in that middle area of the Venn diagram where the three circles overlap. Common sense suggests that health, fitness, and body composition usually overlap, especially for the general public. Maintaining a certain degree of fitness improves your quality of life and can potentially increase your longevity. Eating a "healthy" diet, based mostly on fiber-rich fruits and vegetables, lean proteins, whole grains, and beneficial fats, will likely make it easier to achieve a relatively lean physique. It's true that you can lose weight eating nothing but candy and fast food, but I'll bet that process is a lot easier eating the "healthy" foods previously mentioned ... and, over time, your bloodwork will likely look a lot better, too. Thankfully, that Venn middle region is also pretty darned big. Below is a list of basic behaviors I believe fall in that middle realm and serve as a good foundation for most people, most of the time:

- Consume an adequate amount of protein (0.5-1.0g/lb bodyweight)
- Eat a wide variety of colorful fruits, fibrous vegetables, starches, grains, and healthy fats, in appropriate quantities for your goals
- Walk 10,000+ steps daily
- Spend time outdoors, in nature if possible
- Sleep 7 hours nightly, more if needed
- Find a form of exercise you enjoy and do it 3-5 days weekly for 30+ minutes, with 2-3 sessions breaking a sweat. Try to include some form of resistance training at least 2x weekly
- Manage physical and psychological stresses

PROCESS & BEHAVIOR GOALS

Once you've established a clear sense of what you'd like to achieve, we dig into the real work of determining how you'll achieve it. In many cases, people actually know enough about what to do. Where most people need help is in figuring out how to consistently perform the basic behaviors, habits, and routines that will help them get there. Want to get more flexible? Stretch. Want to improve your cardiovascular fitness? Go run. Don't like running? Pick a cardio machine at the gym—no, I don't care which one. Want to lose weight? Be more physically active and try eating more lean protein and vegetables. Want to have more energy? Turn off Netflix and go to bed; I'm guessing you've watched that episode of "The Office" at least 5 times already anyway.

I didn't say anything too revelatory there, right? Obviously there's a lot more nuance to nutrition, sleep, exercise, and most other elements of health and wellness (presumably that's why you're reading this book), but the basics will get you pretty far most of the time. We all know it's good to drink water…so, how much have you had so far today? If you're like most people I know, not that much! Your outcome goal isn't a verb. Losing weight isn't a behavior, it's a result. You don't just magically build muscles by showing up at a gym; you lift weights, eat sufficient calories, and get enough sleep. What we need is to bridge the gap between knowledge and action.

Take your outcome goal—the thing you really want to achieve. From there, make a list of basic behaviors that you believe will help you achieve it. Some of these might be one-time actions, but most of them will likely be ongoing habits. Author and kettlebell specialist Pat Flynn ingeniously refers to such lists as "Pirate Maps"—follow the steps to get to the buried treasure. To offer a slight alternative, I'd like you to think of your list as a "behavior menu." Here's an example behavior menu I might use with a client whose primary goal is to lose fat (note the deliberate overlap from the list shown earlier):

- Consume adequate protein (~1.0g/lb bodyweight)
- Consume lots of water and vegetables throughout the day
- Focus on eating slowly and thoroughly chewing your food
- Walk 10,000+ steps daily
- 2 or more days weekly resistance training, additional cardiovascular training if needed
- Sleep 7+ hours nightly
- Manage physical & psychological stresses
- Create an environment conducive to fat loss behaviors
- Seek support from your community (family, friends, coworkers, etc)

Though I'd guess you know enough to get started (and our good friend Google is right there at your fingertips), seek expert guidance if you're unsure what basic behaviors will help you make progress!

Once you've created your list, begin by identifying areas you're executing at a high level and on a consistent basis. There's nothing wrong with making further improvements in these areas, but you'll probably see a greater return by investing your efforts elsewhere. From there, we can examine those other areas where you have more of an opportunity to improve. Among this latter group, pick 1-2 areas where you are both interested in making a change and feel capable of doing so.

Maybe you understand sleep is important for recovery, but have a newborn child and feel that improving sleep would be really difficult right now. That's okay! You can still facilitate recovery by working on other habits such as incorporating meditation or doing five minutes of stretching every day. Interested in working on your diet, but really hate the idea of adding more vegetables? If adding more protein sounds more appealing, let's do that right now and worry about the vegetables later!

Rome wasn't built in a day and you don't need to overhaul your whole life right away to make progress. In fact, I'd discourage it. People often underestimate the positive cascade of benefits that can come from small changes (e.g. even if you only explicitly focus on getting more sleep, you might find you have more energy in your workouts, have more mental bandwidth to eat healthier foods, or feel less stressed because you're more productive at work).

Once you've made your menu selection, it's up to you to think about the specific actions you'll take to get it done. There aren't any right answers here; this is where you have to find options that make sense for your unique life circumstances. You want to add more protein? Awesome! What type of protein will you consume? During which meal? How much will you add? Adding more protein might include adding a protein shake post-workout, snacking on hard-boiled eggs instead of potato chips, or ordering extra chicken in the salad you get every day for lunch.

Now, let's scale your new habit. Determine how much and how often. Let's say you currently drink an average of 32 ounces of water each day and would like, over time, to increase to 96 ounces. You don't need to immediately adopt a goal of drinking 96 ounces of water seven days a week. You might, for example, set a goal of drinking 48 ounces of water Monday through Friday. How will you accomplish this? By two glasses of water each day, one at breakfast, one at lunch.

Part of the scaling process is also considering potential obstacles and developing contingency plans. Returning to the water example, let's say your tactic to drink more water is to bring a water bottle in to work and keep it at your desk. What do you do if you forget to bring the water bottle one day? What will you do in order to stay on track? Other possible obstacles might simply involve specific actions you need to take to execute your habit. Maybe this is as simple as buying a water bottle if you don't have one yet or setting recurring calendar reminders to drink your water if you're not confident you'll remember.

Give yourself a high chance of success! When scaling your habit, give yourself a target that feels substantial enough to make an impact while remaining conservative and realistic. You should be at least 9/10 confident that you can execute your habit of choice—I guarantee things will come up that you don't expect. Many people get derailed by setting unreasonably high expectations for themselves and then, feeling as if they failed, quit when they are unable to live up to them. The all-or-nothing approach too often results in nothing.

Let's imagine you haven't worked out in years and now set a goal to suddenly begin working out seven days a week (sound like a familiar New Year's resolution?). If, over the next month, you exercise four days a week, you score a 57%. That's a failing grade. If, on the other hand, you give yourself a far more reasonable goal of working out twice a week and consistently go four times, you doubled your goal. Same outcome, very different emotional response. Go celebrate being a rockstar! It may sound cheesy, but understand this crucial point: you are not celebrating working out four times a week; plenty of people do that already. You're celebrating honoring a commitment that you made to yourself in service of a goal you really care about. That is big. Setting small goals doesn't mean you're not allowed to do more, it just means you give yourself a legitimate chance at feeling success.

After a couple weeks (or some other pre-determined amount of time) of working on your new habit, reassess. You should evaluate your progress with both quantitative metrics (like your weight, body fat percentage, or strength) as well as qualitative metrics like your mood, energy, quality of sleep, etc. While it's next to impossible to single out the impact of any given change (assuming your daily life is not so tightly controlled as that of a lab rat), we want to know if the behavior you're working on is making a positive impact in helping you achieve your goal.

The first question to ask yourself is whether or not you were consistent—think 80% or greater execution on your chosen behavior. If you were not consistent, how can we fairly determine if your chosen behavior is moving you closer to achieving your goal? If you were not able to consistently execute your habit, you may consider if it's not the right thing for you to work on right now, or if perhaps you just need to scale it differently for the time being (i.e. lower your target). If you consistently executed the habit, we can then gauge if this is something worth preserving or even expanding. If you enjoyed this new behavior (or at least it didn't make your life miserable) and it seemed to make a positive difference toward your goal, you might keep doing it. On the other hand, if it made no measurable difference (or even if it did but you hated doing it), you might direct your efforts elsewhere.

Ultimately, the whole journey of working toward your goal is simply a process of conducting experiments. Whether you're looking to add a new behavior or reduce/stop an existing behavior, there's no need to be afraid. You're not making lifelong commitments, you're experimenting to see what feels sustainable, what you like, and what helps you achieve your goals…and what doesn't.

PART 2
HUMAN MOVEMENT AND EXERCISE CONSIDERATIONS
Having explored the process of creating meaningful and specific goals and creating a path of action, we will spend the latter half of this chapter discussing human movement. The aim is to help you identify any critical gaps in your current training routine or to provide an initial direction if you have not exercised consistently for a long period of time. We will consider common types of movements that most people should incorporate into their training as well as different physical qualities that can be developed through the training process. We will finish with some simple but effective examples of how to thoughtfully organize training as well as training considerations to promote successful aging.

FUNDAMENTAL MOVEMENTS
reductiLet's start with fundamental movements, that is, broad types of movement that your body performs on a routine basis, both in the context of structured exercise as well as in daily life. It should be emphasized that we are focusing now on movements, not exercises. When we speak about squatting, for instance, we are talking broadly about a movement in which the hips, knees, and ankles all bend and extend against resistance (generally gravity) while a relatively upright posture is maintained. From the root movement of squatting, we can create countless exercises by manipulating variables such as the equipment used (barbells, kettlebells, bodyweight, machines), how we position the body or external load, and the direction of movement. People who have dealt with injuries and pain in their lower back are sometimes told by doctors or physical therapists to avoid deadlifting (an exercise involving lifting weight from the ground), yet often perform a similar movement when pulling up their pants in the morning or bending over to pick something up off the floor. Deadlifting is an exercise; the "hip hinge" is the movement. A powerlifter performs barbell squats, bench presses, and deadlifts; a yoga practitioner may perform Chair Pose, a Chaturanga Pose, and the Downward Dog Pose. We give these exercises different names, but they are,

259

respectively, the same fundamental movements.

Specific exercise selection may be most directly impacted by the style in which you train (e.g. Pilates vs. CrossFit vs. ice skating) and the equipment you have at your disposal. Exercise selection can also be an important variable to consider if you are dealing with physical constraints related to coordination, strength, mobility, or injuries/pain. A machine bench press might be far more appropriate than a pushup for somebody who has wrist pain. Kettlebell swings involve a motion almost identical to kettlebell deadlifts, but involve a quick and explosive motion; a trainee who cannot perform the kettlebell deadlift proficiently will likely struggle with the coordination and strength required to perform the relatively more advanced swing.

Psychological factors such as confidence and preference are tremendously relevant as well! A lat pulldown may be better than a pull-up for someone who is afraid of falling from the pull-up bar; people who sees themselves as inflexible and clumsy may be highly reluctant to go into a yoga or gymnastics class. It's okay! Don't like running as a way to improve your cardiovascular health? Try the elliptical, rowing machine, or a bicycle instead. Exercises, ultimately, are just tools - a means to an end. You can't always avoid doing things that are difficult or that you don't enjoy, but you are far more likely to adhere to a training routine that is at least somewhat enjoyable! Unless you participate in a sport that demands you perform specific exercises, make selections that give you the best benefit toward your goal with the least risk and cost.

To speak in greater depth about how to select specific exercises is outside the scope of this book. Rest assured, beginning with relatively simple tools and exercise variations can be a wonderful introduction to improve your movement literacy and physical capability. Any personal trainer or coach worth their salt will perform assessments to help in selecting specific exercises that are most appropriate to you given your training history, preferences, and goals.

Many trainers approach exercise (strength training in particular, perhaps) through the lens of training individual muscles—at times in combination, sometimes in isolation. We ask, "what muscle does this work?" when introduced to a new exercise, and seek to create balance in our training by incorporating sufficient exercise variety to address the entire body. There is nothing wrong with focusing on specific muscles or performing exercises that isolate muscles individually; this is likely the preferred approach for aesthetically focused training (bodybuilding, at the extreme end of this spectrum), and it can be useful when there is a bodemonstrated need to address specific muscles. However, approaching human movement with this mindset sometimes leads us to lose the forest for the trees. In many contexts, it can be helpful instead to think about the types of movement your body performs rather than taking a more narrow focus on particular muscles.

Your body functions as a wonderfully complex and interconnected machine, and viewing exercise through the lens of movement allows us to better appreciate the harmonious nature in which our body coordinates multiple muscles (and, for that matter, other structures and systems like our nervous system or cardiovascular system) to accomplish any given task. The list below of fundamental human movements is by no means all-encompassing, and in daily life we often combine these motions without thinking about it. However, from this simple list we can generate countless exercise possibilities. Perhaps most importantly, you can achieve tremendous efficiency in your training by developing coordination, strength, endurance, and power in these basic movement patterns. Here lies your foundation:

- Upper Body Push:

To paraphrase a definition given by strength coach and author Dan John, upper body pushing movements are those in which you separate yourself from something in your environment. In daily life, this might be pushing a door open or putting a box up on a high shelf. Common exercise examples include push-ups, bench presses, or overhead presses. Broadly speaking, these exercises strengthen the muscles of the chest, shoulders, and triceps (the back of the upper arm).

- Upper Body Pull:

Just as pushing exercises separate your body from something in the environment, pulling exercises draw them together. In daily life, this might be opening the refrigerator door or rowing a paddle on a boat. In the gym, this includes exercises like bicep curls, pull-ups, freestyle swimming or the rowing machine. Pulling exercises are generally used to strengthen muscles of the upper and mid back as well as the biceps (the front of the upper arm) and forearms, contributing to grip strength.

- Squat/Lunge:

Sometimes called "knee dominant" movements, squatting and lunging are lower body movements that generally involve a deep bend at your hips, knees, and ankles. You will usually maintain a more upright posture. Many different squat and lunge variations exist, using different foot positions, directions of movement, and equipment. Some machine-based exercises like leg presses can also be included here, since the basic mechanics and muscles involved are largely the same. These movements often rely on muscles of the thigh (especially the quadriceps, in front) and hips to create motion.

- Hinge:

These are lower body movements that primarily involve a deep bending and extending of your hips, with relatively less motion at the knees and ankles; for this reason, many people refer to hingeing movements as "hip dominant." While hinge and squat exercises generally share many characteristics, most standing hinge exercises feature a less upright posture. The most obvious instances of hip hingeing in daily life are present in moments of bending over to pick things up from the ground. Example exercises include deadlifts or kettlebell swings, as well as glute bridges or hip thrusts (which are generally done lying on your back). Like squats and lunges, hinge exercises challenge muscles of the lower body including the thighs (often biasing the hamstrings, in back) and hips.

- Core Stability:

Ask ten different coaches which muscles belong to the "core" and you might well get ten different answers. As before, all the muscles and tissues of the human body function in such an interconnected manner that it is truly difficult to consider the muscles of the midsection in isolation from the rest of the body. Indeed, "core" is kind of a nebulous term, but for our purposes here we are speaking of the area around the midsection, perhaps between the hips and the ribcage. When stable, the core helps transmit force between the upper and lower body.

This doesn't mean the muscles of your midsection (and, with them, your lumbar spine back) shouldn't ever move through their natural range of motion; context matters! A dancer's core can and should move much differently from someone lifting hundreds of pounds; the "core training" that each of these individuals performs may differ substantially as a result. That said, when we refer to core strength, we can generally think of creating stability in three planes of motion: front-to-back, side-to-side, and in rotation. Stability, as we'll discuss later, is not an absolute lack of movement; it is the capability to prevent unwanted motion.

Front-to-back stability means preventing excess forward and backward bending of your spine. Planks are a simple but useful example of an exercise that develops this type of stability. Side-to-side stability involves preventing your body from tilting sideways (think of walking with a heavy bag of groceries in one hand), and can be developed with exercises like side planks or suitcase carries. Rotational stability involves the prevention of unwanted twisting of your body; it is essential to many sport movements like kicking, throwing, or swinging a club/racket; rotational stability can be developed with many exercises that only involve one arm or one leg working at a time, such as single leg deadlifts or one arm rows, or exercises that rely on opposite arm and leg working together, like crawling.

- Locomotion:

Locomotion broadly refers to transporting your body through space. While any of the fundamental movements listed above can be performed in such a manner, we often perform them in a relatively stationary fashion in the context of structured exercise; locomotion is therefore deserving of separate mention. Walking and running are the most obvious examples; so easily taken for granted, they are incredibly complex motions that involve coordinating all major joint systems of the human body.

Blurring the line between general physical activity and exercise, walking deserves particular attention. Special circumstances aside, walking is the lowest hanging fruit to pick for developing general physical fitness, especially for those who have been highly sedentary for many years or have numerous training limitations. While we cannot pretend that walking 10,000 steps a day will prepare you to be an Olympic champion, the benefits (improvements of cardiovascular health and circulation, respiratory health, strength of muscle, bone, and connective tissue, etc.) of general activity are innumerable.

External load can also be added to locomotion with excellent results. Exercises such as suitcase and farmer carries (which involve walking around holding weight in one or both hands, respectively) challenge the strength of one's grip, balance, and postural integrity while moving through space.

- Breathing:

To speak of breath as a fundamental movement may seem obscure, and yet it is the only movement within this list that is truly essential for survival. Everybody alive breathes; we all participate in the act of drawing in oxygen and expelling carbon dioxide. If you're reading this book, be proud—without question, you're already doing one of the fundamental movements. Good on you!

Among this list of basic movement patterns, breathing is unique in that it can be performed involuntarily (unless you, unlike most of us, are routinely doing squats and bicep curls in your sleep). However, great benefit can be had from bringing conscious attention to how you breathe. By consciously controlling the rate and mechanics of breathing, you can substantially impact both your health as well as physical performance.

Try this experiment: set a timer for 2 minutes; breathe in for 5 seconds through your nose, then out through your mouth for 10 seconds (try 2 in and 4 out if that is difficult). As you breathe in, imagine expanding your belly in 360 degrees like you're filling up a balloon; try to breathe into the waistband of your pants without actively pushing your belly out. As you exhale, allow this balloon to slowly empty as you breathe out as much of your air as possible. After two minutes, relax for a moment before moving on. When ready, set a timer, this time for only 30 seconds (possibly less); this time, breathe in through your nose for one second, and breathe out forcefully your mouth for one second. While as before you can try to fill your belly as you breathe in and empty it upon the exhalation, you may naturally find your chest expanding and shoulders lifting with the breath.

What differences did you notice during these two experiments? Most will find their heart rate and blood pressure lower (if you're able to measure) after the slower breathing cycle, and may even feel a sense of calm. The latter method is much more stimulatory, and will likely raise your heart rate. The first is more appropriate as a default manner of breathing throughout the day and can be useful when trying to shift into a more relaxed state, such as when trying to sleep, calm down from a tense situation, or as part of practices like meditation. Yawning in the middle of an important meeting, or getting ready to go do a hard workout? Try some cycles of the faster breathing and see if that doesn't light a fire in you.

MOVEMENT QUALITIES

After considering different fundamental types of movement, we can think about movement qualities. These are basic physical attributes that can be developed across the entire body and expressed through any and all of the different fundamental movements.

- Strength

Physical strength can be broadly thought of as the ability to exert or withstand force, generally in relation to something in your external environment. While we typically think of using strength to produce motion, it is also essential in the prevention of unwanted motion, which we call stability (more on this in a moment). It should also be noted that, while many of us associate "strength" with maximal strength (e.g., the most weight someone can use for one repetition of an exercise), strength is relative. Increasing the amount of weight you can use for five repetitions signifies an increase in strength just like an increase in a one-rep maximum.

Muscular development and strength increases often go hand-in-hand, but not always. Strength is also highly dependent on the nervous system, as your brain coordinates your body's efforts to maximize force and coordinate your muscular effort in the most efficient manner possible. Proper alignment is also critical to strength optimization (try holding a two-pound weight overhead as opposed to directly in front of you at shoulder height). Some people shy away from strength training if they are averse to gaining excessive amounts of muscle, but this need not be the case. While building muscle mass can benefit health, performance, and body composition, strength carries its own benefits and can be developed somewhat independently.

Strength is often referred to as the master quality—that is, generally speaking, increasing strength generally allows you more readily or thoroughly to develop the other physical qualities listed here. Put another way by Brett Jones, "Absolute strength is the glass. Everything else is the liquid inside the glass. The bigger the glass, the more of "everything else" you can do. This idea has obvious limits in practice. All of us are limited by both the amount of time we have to train as well as our physical ability to recover from training; past a certain point strength may not be what limits your improvement and time must be spent developing other qualities or refining technique. Otherwise, the strongest among us would also run the fastest, be the most flexible, and perform the best in all athletic endeavors.

What is important to understand is that strength often is a limiting factor in improving your physical well-being. Yes, you might be able to improve your posture with a lot of stretching and foam rolling, but the lowest hanging fruit might be strengthening muscles like those of your upper back, which can help prevent slouching. You can do all the fancy breathing drills you like, but your breathing mechanics will also improve if you strengthen your lungs, diaphragm, and other breathing muscles through consistent cardiovascular exercise.

Generally speaking, strength is optimally developed through multi-joint exercises that involve many major muscle groups at once and can be progressively loaded over time. Preferred choices include variations of squats, deadlifts, lunges, bench presses, pull-ups, rows, and loaded carries (e.g., farmers carries and suitcase carries). On a final note, most people don't ever need to test their maximal strength. If your workouts often involve banging your head against the wall to see how much weight you can use for one rep, just know that you can get extremely strong with much less risk. Performing lifts at or very close the limits of your strength is highly fatiguing and carries a greater chance of exceeding what your body can tolerate. Occasionally testing a one-rep max can be highly enjoyable (and, let's be real, stokes the ego), but just know that you can train to a high level of strength at lower intensities, in sets of three to eight reps, give or take.

- Mobility & Flexibility:

While these terms are often used interchangeably, and mobility and flexibility are highly related, they have some important differences. Think of mobility as the ability of your individual joints to move through a certain range of motion without external influence. Flexibility refers to the overall ability of a muscle to be lengthened (stretched), with or without external assistance. Mobility can be position specific; some people can lift their arms overhead if lying down on their back, but struggle to do so when standing up. Executing basic strength training exercises through a full range of motion can be a fantastic means of preserving and often improving mobility and flexibility in tandem with methods such as stretching, massage, and training methods that focus on flexibility development such as yoga.

Though almost all joints of the body have some capacity for mobility, many mobility issues can be addressed by tending to the shoulders, the thoracic spine (the upper part of your spine, in the same approximate range as your ribcage), the hips, and the ankles. Each of these areas is capable of motion in all three planes of motion (front to back, side to side, and rotation); issues can arise if a loss of mobility in these segments results in compensation from other areas of the body. Likewise, a well-balanced training routine should aim to maintain an amount of muscular flexibility appropriate to an individual's needs and goals (a gymnast needs far more hamstring flexibility than a sprinter, or most people for that matter). For those who spend significant amounts of time sitting, I highly encourage regular stretching of the calves, hip flexors (muscles at the front of your hips and thighs, chest, and lats (large muscles that run along your back, terminating near your armpit). These are, of course, generalizations and your individual needs may differ significantly. Find a trainer, physical therapist, or other movement coach properly certified (through systems such as FMS or PRI) to better understand your needs.

Whether due to past injuries, sedentary lifestyles, or other realities of getting older, many of us lose mobility and flexibility we took for granted when younger. Do not allow this to prevent you from training! Not all exercises are appropriate for all people; stick to exercises you are able to perform comfortably and safely with good technique ("perfect" technique does not exist!). Often, you can modify an exercise or your setup to train around any limitations you might have in order to still make progress toward your goals. For example, someone with very little available motion at their ankles will often be very bent over when squatting, which prevents them from training the muscles they intend to target and potentially causes discomfort over time. A barbell back squat (where weight is placed across the upper back) may not be appropriate. However, by elevating this person's heels and having them hold weight in front of their body, they may be able to squat with their body in a far better position and enjoy the wonderful benefits we typically associate with the squat movement. Always do what you can, where you are, with what you have.

- Coordination:

Coordination is the purposeful combination of movement and force to complete a desired task. Your brain and body are in constant dialogue, with sensory information sent to the brain and movement commands in turn sent out to the body. No different from learning to play an instrument or speak a language, movement can be approached as a skill to be learned and refined over time. Part of training involves strengthening your "hardware"—building up stronger bones and muscles, creating more mobile joints and resilient connective tissues, etc.—and part of it involves upgrading your "software" by learning and practicing progressively more complex movements (don't misinterpret this as encouragement to do the most awkward, convoluted exercises you can think of!). Although we've spoken of a small number of fundamental movements, remember that you can create almost infinite variety of specific exercises to expand your movement literacy over time. Showing up to the gym and trying to do Olympic weightlifting exercises or backflips can be a recipe for failure and humiliation: there's too much going on! Start simple, with exercises that you can confidently execute with clean technique, and build up to more complicated movements depending on the demands of your particular health and fitness goals. Machines can be a wonderful place to begin for many people, providing an opportunity to make progress toward their goals while developing confidence and basic physical capacity. To use a familiar cliche, mastery is generally defined not by the ability to do the complex, but rather by the ability to do the basics at an exceptionally high level.

- Stability & Balance

Stability pertains to the ability to prevent unwanted motion. People too often mistake stability to denote a lack of movement, especially with regard to core training. If you want a lumbar spine that does not move, vertebral fusion is an option, but not recommended unless truly necessary! Having a stiffened midsection is much more important if you're lifting hundreds of pounds off the ground than if you are lifting a feather. In training, many people struggle to prevent their shoulders from shrugging upward when doing upper body exercises; this doesn't mean the goal is to lock your shoulder down and back at all times. Look in the mirror and try lifting your arm overhead with your shoulder pulled down away from your ear the entire time; compare that to letting your shoulder shrug slightly when reaching your arm up. Which was more comfortable? Stability is not about eliminating motion entirely, it's about having appropriate amounts of movement. Relative to machines, free weights often require more effort to stabilize your body, the equipment, or both. Some equipment further increases these challenges by creating inherent instability or distributing the weight differently—to experience this, try lifting equivalently an equivalently heavy dumbbell, kettlebell, and half-full jug of water.

Balance relates to your body's ability to keep your center of mass over your base of support; more simply, we generally think of balance as your ability to remain upright or otherwise properly oriented for the task at hand (for example, not falling off the side of a bench when lying down to perform a bench press). Maintaining balance requires stability, especially through the midsection and lower body when standing. This entails having adequate strength in the tissues around the feet, ankles, knees, and hips to prevent postural collapse. Balance is also highly neurological, relying on proper coordination and rapid response to direct appropriate changes of body position in the face of disturbance.

- Power

Power introduces a time component to strength. If strength pertains to the ability to either produce force (acceleration) or absorb force (deceleration), power generally denotes the ability to do so quickly. If two people squat one repetition of 200 pounds, but one of them is able to perform the movement more rapidly, that person has demonstrated more power. Running requires more power than walking. Many exercises that are used for the purpose of power training are explosive in nature, and may thus require a greater amount of coordination and tissue resiliency (especially if impact forces are involved). For this reason, power training is generally not recommended for someone who is new to training or has not trained for a substantial period of time.

That said, the ability to express power is essential to almost any sport activity; think of swinging a racket or club, running and changing direction, or throwing a ball. It can also be critical for safety. Your ability to jump to safety or catch yourself and prevent a fall both rely on power (can you jump slowly, or trip and catch yourself slowly?). While absolute strength can be maintained to a surprising degree as we age, power and speed are among the physical qualities lost most rapidly. Wonderful progress can be made simply by performing basic exercises more rapidly at first, and later introducing explosive exercises and those involving impact when and if appropriate. To properly train power, you'll generally perform very few total repetitions and take relatively longer rest periods since the ability to produce maximal power fatigues you quickly. Approach each rep deliberately so as to maximize explosiveness.

- Endurance

While we will touch on cardiovascular health and fitness shortly, here we are referring to muscular endurance, the ability of a muscle (or muscles) to exert force consistently or repeatedly over a period of time. To illustrate the difference, an athlete who has spent many years swimming may have tremendous cardiovascular endurance, but may not have developed adequate muscular endurance in muscles like the calves should they decide to run a marathon on a whim. A powerlifter may be able to bench press more than double their own bodyweight, but it's quite possible they would lose a push-up contest to any number of group fitness devotees. Maximal strength and strength endurance are two different animals. Training muscular endurance can play a critical role in living life comfortably from a physical standpoint, whether that's having the stamina to play with your kids, maintain a good posture with less effort, or go backpacking with your friends and not feel like you need a rest every 30 seconds when going up a steep hill. In an exercise setting, muscular endurance is typically trained with moderate weight, higher repetitions, and shorter rest periods.

Energy Systems Development & Cardiorespiratory Fitness

Entire books are dedicated to speaking about the development of cardiorespiratory fitness and energy systems development; here we will attempt to provide a cursory understanding of their function and importance. Cardiorespiratory fitness relates to the body's capacity to circulate blood among various organs and tissues, delivering oxygen and other essential nutrients while removing metabolic waste products. Energy systems are the mechanisms by which your body creates the necessary energy needed for all bodily function, including but most certainly not limited to movement.

There are three energy systems, or pathways, through which your body can produce energy. The differences between them lie in their relative rates of energy production and capacity to sustain energy production. One system, referred to as the phosphocreatine system, produces energy at the fastest rate but has a limited capacity to do so. This system dominates in efforts of maximal intensity and minimal duration, up to approximately 10 seconds (it is common to see Olympic sprinters slow down even before the end of a 100 meter race!). An example workout might involve 8-10 intervals of 5-10 seconds apiece, with 3-5 minutes of rest between efforts. Possible exercises used might include sprinting, a rowing machine, jump squats, or a stationary bicycle.

The second system, referred to as anaerobic glycolysis or the lactic acid system, can still produce energy at a high rate, though not as high as the ATP-CP system, and can be the dominant pathway in efforts up to 1-2 minutes at high enough intensities. In track and field, the 400 and 800 meter runs are known as particularly brutal events due to the exceptional degree of fatigue and sensation of your lungs, heart, and muscles being on fire! Many CrossFit or high intensity style classes challenge this system. An example training session might involve 4 to 6 intervals of working for 1 minute at a high intensity and resting for 2 minutes.

Finally, and perhaps most familiar, the aerobic system has the slowest rate of energy production but by far the greatest capacity. As your body exerts effort for longer periods of time, your relative ability to produce force necessarily decreases and your body relies increasingly on energy production via the aerobic pathway. Classic examples might include long-distance runs or bike rides of 30 or more minutes at a low intensity, but can also include higher intensity workouts such as 12 to 15 intervals working for 30 seconds and resting for 30 seconds, or 4 to 6 intervals of 2 minutes work and 1 minute rest. In the latter two example, the relatively short recovery period and the high number of intervals dictate that the relative intensity of each interval must be lower and that your body must produce much of its energy aerobically.

It seems that, for a while, aerobic training fell out of favor in the fitness industry while high intensity interval training carried far more appeal (when people suggest that intense 7-minute workouts can deliver the same benefits as a lower intensity, 60-minute workout, it's understandable that many would opt for the 7-minute option). However, the foundation of cardiovascular fitness must be initially built with basic aerobic capacity. While lower intensity, long-duration cardiovascular exercise is likely overrated from a fat loss standpoint, it is enormously beneficial for the health of your heart, lungs, arteries, veins, brain, and nervous system. Moreover, your ability to recover is largely driven by the aerobic system, both during exercise and in between sessions. If you find yourself needing a lot of time to catch your breath between sets of squats, for example, you might find that spending some time improving your aerobic system helps you get more out of your sessions by allowing you to get more done in the same amount of time. This certainly does not mean that you need to become a triathlete if your goal is building muscle, only that cardiovascular strength and endurance do occasionally limit people's capacity to train more effectively.

Even brisk walking can be highly beneficial, but cardiovascular exercise can be as diverse as running, biking, swimming, dance, martial arts, or even just a trusty machine at the gym with a built-in TV to play Netflix for you. For most people, including two to three days of aerobic training (even lasting as briefly as 20 to 30 minutes) will be enormously beneficial and is highly recommended . . . and no, getting your heart rate elevated doing lunges is not the same thing. Many people now have access to heart rate data on their phones, smartwatches, or cardio training equipment at the gym; aerobic work will often involve a slightly lower heart rate, especially for longer intensity workouts (one guideline developed by Phil Maffetone uses a default range of 160 minus your age up to 180 minus your age, with some modifications available based on fitness level). Other options include regulating your effort by breathing in and out only through your nose or by ensuring that you can comfortably hold a conversation in full sentences as you exercise.

No one system ever functions independently of the others; you are never exclusively producing energy through any one pathway. Understanding these different pathways can be essential for directing your training in a manner best aligned with your health and fitness goals.

- Muscle Building and Fat Loss

Muscle development and fat loss may not be physical qualities, per se (both of these can be accomplished in the process of developing other physical qualities), but deserve to be addressed here since they are the desired outcome of many people's training. Many other factors outside of training will dictate muscle development and fat loss (such as eating enough or sufficiently few calories, respectively), but here are some brief training considerations.

Generally speaking, training to build muscle might involve slightly higher repetitions (and, consequently, slightly lower weight) than training purely to increase strength. This relates both to repetitions done in each set, but perhaps more importantly to the number of total repetitions done in a workout or even over the course of an entire training week. For example, performing a squat workout with three sets of five repetitions may be preferable for strength development, while a session of seven sets of five may better stimulate muscle growth. Although many classic training texts recommend sets of approximately six to twelve repetitions to focus on muscle growth (and this is a fine starting point), contemporary research demonstrates muscle being built in repetition ranges as wide as three to 30 repetitions per set, provided adequate intensity. Most beginner and intermediate trainees would still do well to focus on some of the basic exercises previously discussed. This generally means focusing more on multi-joint exercises that involve many large muscle groups, especially if training time is limited (for example, selecting chin-ups rather than bicep curls, even if you want bigger arms). Incorporating other exercise variations, machines, or isolation movements can be highly useful to address any gaps and increase the total stimulus to your muscles with lower cost on your ability to recover.

Training for fat loss need not include endless hours of cardiovascular training; although exercise will certainly burn calories, your nutrition is far easier to manipulate. Orient your training to maintaining muscle mass so that, as you lose weight, you lose as little lean body mass as possible and maximize fat loss (this also makes it easier to keep the fat off after the fact). As such, training during fat loss will often resemble training to build muscle: the style of training that will optimally stimulate muscle growth during periods of higher calorie intake is, unsurprisingly, the style of training that helps maintain muscle when food intake is decreased. Other minor differences might include incorporating more general physical activity throughout the day (and perhaps a bit more cardiovascular exercise as needed), and you might progress your workouts by taking less rest rather than increasing the weight or repetitions from one week to the next.

PROGRAM ARRANGEMENT

Session Organization

Up to now, we have spent this section of the chapter discussing different training considerations. We'll now turn our attention to laying these components out in a practical manner in the context of a training session. Important components of a typical training session include a warm-up, power and strength work, energy systems development (aka cardio), and the cool-down.

According to chiropractor, physical therapist, and strength coach Charlie Weingroff, a proper warm-up accomplishes four main tasks. First, the warm-up serves to increase core body temperature—literally, you are warming your body up. Merely body temperature and facilitating blood circulation can immediately improve measures of movement quality such as flexibility, strength, power, and muscle elasticity. Second, the warm-up helps to stimulate the central nervous system. You are preparing your body for the intense neurological demands of training, whether that involves producing high levels of force or coordinating complex movements. Third, warming-up allows you to express your current levels of mobility and flexibility. The goal is not necessarily to increase mobility; you're making sure you have access to what you need in order to perform well in that day's workout (if the goal is to increase range of motion in a movement, prepare to use much less load or force). Finally, the warm-up serves as a dress rehearsal for the main movements of your training session. Simply put, if you are preparing to squat, your warm-up can and should include movements that resemble squatting. This serves both to help warm-up the specific muscles and tissues involved in the exercises you'll be doing as well as to allow you to practice and refine technique, making any necessary adjustments as necessary before the stakes get higher with more weight, speed, etc. The warm-up period can also serve as an ideal opportunity to work on learning new movement skills. If the goal is to learn or polish technique on a relatively new skill, you will be better served to do this while you are mentally and physically fresh, rather than near the end of a training session when you are exhausted. You can also use this time to do any desired work to improve movement quality (sometimes called "corrective" exercises); these are generally low-intensity drills, sometimes passive, that aim to change movement behavior by increasing joint mobility, muscular flexibility, coordination, or muscular awareness (sometimes called "activation drills"). Both of these are fine things to spend time on; just be wary of dedicating so much attention and time to either of these that you forget to actually train with good effort toward your main goals. If you're working to lose

50 pounds, spending half of your time at the gym on a foam roller just won't cut it. Hips feel tight and deadlifting doesn't feel good that day? Skip the 20 minutes of hip stretches just so you can deadlift, and go do something else instead that doesn't need as much hip mobility. You can stretch your hips that night while you're watching TV and deadlift next time!

After warming up, you'll generally want to prioritize exercises that are more complex, involve a high degree of force production, and involve multiple muscle groups. As such, power exercises will typically come first if they are part of your program. From there, focus on bigger, multi-joint strength exercises, especially those which involve heavier weights in your particular session. A barbell bench press would likely precede a dumbbell bench press due to the greater capacity required to lift heavy weights using the barbell. Pull-ups and bicep curls both tax the muscles that bend the elbow; the pull-ups would likely precede bicep curls, since they involve more muscle groups and are more systemically taxing than the curls. Generally, as you get later into the workout and into a deeper state of fatigue, you can pick exercises that are simpler and create less overall fatigue. While you might still feel as if you're working hard on the leg extension machine in the 50th minute of a one hour workout, the overall challenge on your body is nowhere near what it would be if you were exerting an equal amount of perceived effort on a barbell squat. Loaded carries are another personal favorite—for the most part, I trust myself and my clients to walk with decent technique, even when fatigued.

There are numerous ways to organize and combine different exercises within this main portion of the workout. At times, you will perform one exercise in isolation and rest before performing that same exercise again. In other models, you might combine multiple exercises in a group (often called supersets or circuits depending on how many exercises are included in one group), sometimes working the same muscle group, in other instances working opposing muscle groups. When pure strength is the goal, it can be helpful to train at a relatively slower pace in which you allow yourself plenty of rest. This might look like performing a set of five repetitions in the deadlift with a relatively high weight, then resting 3 minutes before performing the deadlift again. For many people, however, time efficiency is maximized with circuit training where three or four exercises are grouped back-to-back. By combining exercises with relative overlap in the muscle groups used, a greater training density can be achieved while still allowing decent rest for any one muscle group along the way. An example of this would be performing a squat, followed by a push-up, followed by a chin-up, with relatively little rest between the individual exercises. Although it may feel fast-paced, the muscles powering each individual exercise rest while the other two are performed. This style of training can also carry value for fat loss training, where the goal over time may be to perform a greater total amount of work.

As per usual, how you choose to structure your workout depends entirely upon your goal as well as practical considerations such as how much time you have available to train. I'm sure this can all get overwhelming, and it can certainly be helpful to seek the help of a coach so that you can just dedicate your mental bandwidth to showing up and working hard, Don't be discouraged! Most any program can work for a while provided you show up and consistently put in a good effort.

After performing the main strength training of your workout, you may consider incorporating energy systems development (cardio training) toward the end of your workout. If your schedule allows, it can often be advantageous to perform cardiovascular work on a separate day from your strength training in order to produce more effort and thus experience greater benefits. However, if it's more practical and realistic to include cardiovascular work during the same session as your strength training, that is totally fine as well. Moreover, most forms of cardiovascular exercise (particularly those done using a machine) will also involve less complicated technique than many strength training exercises, and thus are still suitable to be performed after the rest of training.

Whether or not some form of cardiovascular training has been included, effort should be made to cool down after training. This may include such elements as deep breathing, stretching, foam rolling, using a steam room/sauna, or contrast baths/showers (alternating using heat and cold). Some of these focus on cognitive and psychological relaxation while others focus on physical aspects like promoting circulation. The general concept is to have some way to bring your body and mental state back down to baseline after the stimulation of your training session, thus facilitating the start of the recovery process.

Program Organization and Progression

The difference between merely working out and legitimately training is that training represents a purposeful approach toward exercise that is directed at accomplishing specific goals. By extension, a proper program organizes your individual training sessions in a cohesive manner so that you can make as much progress as possible given the constraints of your time, energy, and ability to recover. Programs commonly last between six to twelve weeks, though shorter and longer options certainly exist; this generally is enough time to allow adaptation while avoiding physical or mental burnout (generally, one or multiple parameters of the program will progress in difficulty as the program goes along, such that the end of the program represents a climax or opportunity to test performance).

Most training programs are organized week-to-week, since most people plan their lives this way naturally. As such, likely the most important factor to consider when laying out your training program is what's realistic given your other commitments. If you'd like to work out three days a week, we could argue all day long about how it's optimal to space your workouts evenly across the week—Monday, Wednesday, and Friday, for instance—but if you're more likely to sustain your commitment by working out on Saturday, Sunday, and Monday, that's entirely fine! As is often said, the science is in the compliance. Better to diligently execute a decent plan than half-heartedly execute a perfect plan.

In most cases, if you are working out three or fewer days per week, full body workouts will make the most sense and give you the greatest return on the time you invest. This does not mean you will perform the exact same movements in each workout, but rather that each workout will include exercises addressing each of the fundamental movement patterns. The collective amount of work any given muscle will be able to perform will increase when you spread the work out across multiple days. That said, in cases where you might have training sessions on back-to-back days, it may make more sense to split your efforts in order to better promote recovery. For example, somebody who can only train on Saturday and Sunday may choose to perform squatting, pulling, and locomotion exercises on Saturday, and dedicate Sunday to hingeing, pushing, and core training. These sorts of training splits can also make sense for people who train more frequently; training the entire body five or six days a week might hinder recovery and make it difficult to truly challenge any given movement or muscle.

Splits might be oriented around movement patterns, such as having a "push" day, a "pull" day, and a "leg" day; some people treat squatting and lungeing movements as lower body "pushing" exercises and hingeing or other hamstring-dominant exercises as lower body "pulling" exercises, such that the leg day could be subdivided into "lower push" and "lower pull" days in a four day weekly training split. Other programs organize the training week by focusing on specific muscle groups. One five-day per week example (I feel like every dedicated gym-goer I know has done some version of this at some point in their lives) might involve training the chest on Monday, the back on Tuesday, the shoulders on Wednesday, the legs on Thursday, and the arms and core on Friday. These days, I'm suspicious of people who only perform leg exercises once per week, but that's just me!

One way or the other, rest must be taken during the course of the training program. Ultimately, training presents a stress on the body from which it must recover. Training breaks the body down, and it's really through the recovery process— eating well, getting enough sleep, etc.—that we get bigger, faster, or stronger. Some people enjoy including some form of physical activity every day; there's nothing wrong with this, especially if some day's activities are of a much lower intensity or are actively focused on physical restoration. Indeed, rest and recovery aren't optimized by sitting on the couch sipping beer and eating nachos; rest days can provide a wonderful opportunity to focus on mobility work (such as stretching or massage), include extra walking or low-intensity cardiovascular work, or spend time on other things that facilitate progress toward your fitness goals (I love the notion that Sunday's "workout" is grocery shopping and meal prep if the goal is fat loss—time well spent!).

Over the course of a training program, change must be made to continue making progress. During the program itself, it is more common to change variables such as the weight being used (or speed in cardiovascular exercise), the volume performed (sets, reps, or duration) of a given exercise, or the amount of rest taken between exercise. Exercise selection may be varied within a program, but often is changed from one program to the next. Some of this depends on experience (a less experienced trainee will benefit from spending time getting more comfortable and skillful with a smaller variety of exercises) as well as personality (some people crave far more variety than others). Other variables such as training frequency or program emphasis (e.g. emphasizing strength development versus muscle growth) are generally adjusted in between programs, after any relevant assessments are performed. Ultimately, your body will adapt to stimuli and demands it experiences after enough exposure. According to a training principle known as progressive overload, you must continually challenge your body by shifting one of these variables (or more) if adaptation is to continue. Which variable(s) you choose depends on the goals you are trying to achieve and the progress that has been made. Indeed, the training program itself acts as a continual assessment process; every repetition, every set, every workout serves as a chance to evaluate progress, both objective and subjective. For a fat loss client, progress might be maintaining strength or cardiovascular stamina while losing weight (their relative strength has increased); for a strength-focused trainee, progress may simply be lifting more weight with the same perceived amount of effort. That said, the conclusion of one training program marks an important time to reflect upon the successes and/ or shortcomings of the work that has been performed and to use the data to make the best plan possible for the following block of training. If your goal is to run one mile in a faster time and you have made minimal progress but have succeeded in gaining muscle, this is valuable data! Certainly other lifestyle factors would need to be examined, but the training program can and should be revised in light of the assessment results.

Example Training Program
Below is an example of what a program could look like for somebody training three days per week. All of the workouts are full-body in nature and include a mixture of equipment; the strength exercises are organized into two circuits, each containing three exercises. This particular example may be appropriate for someone who has been training for a couple of months and does not have any substantial injuries or movement limitations, but adjustments could be easily made for someone who has less experience or needs to work around any sort of restriction. The cardiovascular training uses a variety of machines and incorporates different interval structures to allow development of capacity at different relative intensities.

3-DAY FULL-BODY PROGRAM

DAY 1
Warm-Up

A1) Kettlebell Goblet Squat (heels elevated on 10lb plates)
A2) Incline Dumbell Bench Press
A3) Lat Pulldown (palms facing toward each other)

B1) Side Lunge
B2) Farmers Carry
B3) Side Plank

C) Incline Treadmill Walk 15 Minutes at 70% effort

Cool-Down: foam rolling for legs and upper back, stretching for hip-flexors and inner thighs

DAY 2
Warm-Up

A1) Dumbbell Bench Press
A2) One Arm Dumbbell Row
A3) Hip Thrust with Upper Back on Exercise Bench

B1) Crawl in Place
B2) Lying Hamstring Curl
B3) Suspension Strap Row

C) Rowing Machine 3 minutes work, 1 minute rest x4

Cool-Down: Deep Tissue Massage

DAY 3
Warm-Up

A1) Assisted Pull-Up
A2) Kettlebell Deadlift
A3) Seated Dumbbell Overhead Press

B1) Alternating Reverse Lunge
B2) Turkish Get-Up
B3) Kettlebell 1-Arm Farmer's Carry

C) Airbike or Stationary Bike 30 seconds work, 60 seconds rest x 8-10

Cool-down: 5 minutes of deep breathing/meditation, 10 minutes in steam room

Training for Successful Aging
Having established a practical framework for setting training goals and understanding how to structure your training routine accordingly, we will conclude with some specific thoughts on how to train to facilitate successful aging. By this we mean training in such a way as to maximize function, independence, and vitality as you get older. Eventually, performance and fitness goals are pursued

in service of supporting general well-being (e.g., you might not want to irritate a cranky elbow just to do one more pull-up than the week before!). Regardless of your age, you can always train and improve your health and physical fitness; just make sure to start where you are, be patient, and progress appropriately. Examine your current routine for any sobvious gaps and consider training in a fashion that develops these attributes:

Strength, especially in the lower body and grip:
Basic strength training can do wonders for preserving lean body mass and preventing injury. Again, think of basic drills such as squats, deadlifts, lunges, rows, pull-ups/lat pulldowns, push-ups/bench presses, and farmers carries (am I sounding like a broken record yet?). While age-related loss of muscle mass (known as sarcopenia) is inevitable, it can be greatly mitigated through resistance training, promoting general function as well as metabolic health. Gradual degradation of bone mass can eventually result in osteoporosis (often of particular concern for women) and, as a result, increased fragility - a fall that wouldn't phase a 12-year old in the slightest may well break the hip of an 89-year old. Loading your body's tissues against the force of gravity may be one of the most important things you can do for injury prevention.

The lower body and grip may be especially important to prioritize for functioning independently through daily life. You need the strength to walk, go up and down stairs, and get up and down from the couch or toilet. Many of us have also seen commercials featuring an elderly person exclaiming, "Help, I've fallen and I can't get up!" While falls are extremely problematic as is, lacking the strength to recover and seek assistance can exacerbate an already dangerous situation. In addition to the fundamental movement patterns already outlined, training for successful aging should specifically include time spent getting up and down from the ground (with assistance, if needed). Grip strength will allow you to continue lifting heavy objects, open jars, and walk around holding your own groceries or luggage. Strength through the posterior chain (think hamstrings, glutes, and back) can also support maintaining a tall and upright posture. As alluded to earlier, strength is the master quality and will aid in maintaining joint mobility, muscular flexibility, and even power.

Coordination and Balance
We have spoken earlier about coordination and balance; in the context of training for healthy aging, these qualities can be especially important for safety. Training in

a reactive fashion –that is, being presented with a relatively unpredictable stimulus and responding accordingly—can be tremendous for preserving reflexes. This can be as simple as playing a game of catch, or performing exercise in a manner similar to the game "Simon Says" (heaven forbid training should be so enjoyable as playing childhood games!). Enormous portions of the human brain are dedicated to the constant problem-solving process of receiving sensory information and responding with an appropriately coordinated movement. Indeed, exercise is generally regarded as one of the single most important things a person can do for maintaining cognitive health.

Balance exercises may be as simple as single-leg exercises such as lunges, single leg deadlifts, or slow marching, but again require substantial strength as well as coordination. Falling presents a great risk to physical health and well being; sadly, almost everyone can relate to knowing somebody whose health and well-being were greatly compromised after a bad fall, and in many cases with the elderly these falls seem to mark the beginning of a decline toward death. Training balance in conjunction with fundamental strength can be essential in preventing a fall outright; coordination and reflex training can aid in prevention as well, or at least in mitigating the damage of a fall (if you fall in the shower, I'd much rather have you catch yourself with your hands and hurt your wrists than bang your head off the tile).

Power
As alluded to earlier, power involves the rapid production or absorption of force. Remember that power is relative. For a firefighter, the expression of power might involve kicking down a door and sprinting up a flight of stairs; for a grandmother, this might mean quickly stepping out of the way as her grandchildren come barreling down the hall and threaten collision! Jumping out of the way of danger on time is expressing power by producing force; tripping on a crack in the sidewalk and rapidly catching all of your bodyweight on one leg is expressing power by absorbing force (again, we see that rapid force absorption - the ability to decelerate - is critical for fall prevention). Power is one of the qualities most readily lost with age, but - as with muscle loss - this decline can be greatly mitigated through training. Earlier we noted that power is essential to most sport activities such as running, jumping, throwing, and swinging (a bat, club, racket, etc.).
If you strive to feel vital and enjoy these activities into your later years, train accordingly!

Cardiovascular Endurance and Aerobic Capacity

Cardiovascular and metabolic diseases are two of the most common health issues many people face during their lives. Excess body fat, high blood pressure, insulin resistance, and abnormal elevation of cholesterol and/or triglycerides elevate the risk of heart attacks, diabetes, stroke, and other metabolic conditions. While exercise alone is often insufficient, and these issues should be addressed through a combination of lifestyle factors in conjunction with any necessary medical care, cardiovascular exercise can be a critical component of prevention or treatment. Moreover, successful aging is not merely the prevention of these disease states - our goal is to help you thrive in your later years! Cardiovascular training should be an essential part of any long-term training plan so that you may enjoy being physically active without being out of breath.

Joint Mobility & Muscular Flexibility

Gradual decreases in your available joint mobility and muscular flexibility eventual limit your movement options. As before, performing fundamental movements through full ranges of motion may be your single best bet for maintaining comfortable movement. Seek appropriate treatment, rehabilitation, and training for any injuries you may encounter along the journey of a life well-lived. Over time, you may find yourself dedicating extra time to physical recovery and restoration - massage, foam rolling, stretching, and mobility-focused exercise practices such as yoga or martial arts.

Pelvic Floor Function

Pelvic floor training may be treated as a particular branch of strength training, but merits particular discussion for those wishing to age gracefully. While women may be more familiar with pelvic floor training through experience with pregnancy, childbirth, and menopause, both men and women can experience pelvic floor dysfunction as they age. Resulting issues can include pain or discomfort, bladder and bowel issues, and sexual dysfunction. As per usual, pelvic floor issues should be addressed through a combination of medical treatment, when needed, alongside lifestyle factors including exercise, healthy nutrition, sleep, and stress management. Thankfully, exercise and physical activity in general can be highly beneficial for the strength and function of the pelvic floor. Kegel exercises are specifically focused on strengthening the muscles of the pelvic floor - to perform these, try to replicate the sensation of stopping urination. Exercises specifically focused on strengthening nearby musculature (around the pelvis and hips) may also be of particular utility, though even low- to moderate-intensity physical activities such as walking can help. If you are currently experiencing pelvic floor issues, high intensity exercise, especially activities involving repeated impact forces, may be inappropriate; as always, make sure to consult with your physician regarding any medical issues that may impact your training.

CHAPTER SUMMARY:

PART 1

1. When establishing health and fitness goals, find clarity in the specific outcomes you'd like to achieve. One possible way to structure your goals is to make them SMART - specific, measurable, attainable, relevant, and time bound.
2. Determine whether your goals primarily relate to health, fitness, or body composition. These three categories largely overlap, but some goals may concentrate on one or two areas even at the possible expense of one of the others. The nature of your goal will be very important in shaping the choices you make with respect to exercise, nutrition, recovery, and other elements of daily life.
3. After clarifying your outcome goal, define your process goal(s) - specific behaviors and habits that are under your control. These behaviors, when executed consistently, should help you achieve your desired outcome goal. Pick 1-2 behaviors to focus on at a time in order to give yourself a high chance of achieving and sustaining success.
4. Periodically reassess your progress. Use both objective, quantitative measures that help you understand the relative progress you have made toward your outcome goal as well as subjective or qualitative assessments that might better reflect your experience of the change process. Also assess your consistency with the behavior(s) and habit(s) you are working on to best determine if they are sustainable and contributing positively to goal accomplishment. When you are ready, you can add additional layers in order to achieve additional progress. Use this continual
5. process of experimentation to learn about your preferences and what works well for you.

PART 2

1. Incorporate fundamental human movements into your training routine: squat, hinge, push, pull, core training, locomotion, breathing.

2. Begin training by establishing basic coordination, strength, and aerobic capacity while learning proper training technique. Develop and improve other physical qualities such as mobility, flexibility, balance, power, and endurance as needed depending on your specific training goals.

3. Arrange individual workouts to include a proper warm-up, power and strength training, cardiovascular work (aka energy systems development), and a cool down to begin the recovery process. Arrange the broader training program to fully train the entire body over the course of the training week (or some regular cycle of time); this can be done using full body workouts or training splits, which divide workouts by body part or types of movement.

4. Over time, progress variables such as the amount of weight used, volume (sets times repetitions), rest, training frequency, and exercise selection (using different exercises or veequipment - possibly, but not necessarily more complex). Which variables you change will be largely decided based on your goal.

5. Consider what it means to train in a way that supports long term well-being and allows you to thrive in your later years. Muscle mass and power are lost as part of the natural aging process, but losses of function and vitality can be greatly mitigated through training. Basic strength training, mobility and flexibility work, and cardiovascular exercise will work wonders for maintaining independence and physical well-being, and may help to prevent injury and other common health conditions.

www.ingramcontent.com/pod-product-compliance
Lightning Source LLC
Chambersburg PA
CBHW050339270326
41926CB00016B/3523

This compelling anthology of stories from academics who identify as having a working-class background offers new insights into our understanding of the relationship between academia and class.

Offering a substantial contribution to the body of research that uses autoethnography, the volume opens a platform for academic authors to reflect on their own lived experience through critical study of oneself and one's own socio-cultural context. The book is a useful resource for autoethnographic research and readers who want to understand the lived experiences of becoming a higher education professional; they will see farther and more clearly through the authors' lenses.

Although a working-class heritage underpins the autoethnography of each of the writers, the intersections of social class with race and gender are also explored, providing in-depth knowledge about personal journeys into academic life.

While the legacy of elitism remains in higher education, and with very little history or class culture in the field of higher education to identify with, the volume can give voice to and authenticate the authors' experiences, and more importantly, challenge the dominant discourses that maintain and perpetuate elitism and exclusion within higher education.

'The collection provides a solid foundation for students and academics, of important questions being asked about transitioning into academic life.'
Professor Giorgia Doná, Co-director of the Centre for Migration, Refugees and Belonging, University of East London

This book fully explores the developmental journey and experiences of working-class academics, using an affective approach which brings together class, race, ethnicity, gender and the intersection between them.

Class issues that have long been sidelined are finally foregrounded and examined through a critical conversation focusing on the lives of academics whose backgrounds diverge from the middle-class norm.

The Lives of Working Cl&

The book provides a platform for the authors to discuss who they are as academics, their family backgrounds and what it means to be a professional in the academy.

Burnell Reilly invites working-class academics to write about their careers in higher education. This use of autoethnography is important as it generates a profound understanding of the lived experiences of individuals.

The work is compelling and makes a significant contribution to our insights into the predicament of working-class academics. The book, therefore, has the potential to improve efforts to encourage more inclusive approaches to supporting the recruitment and advancement of those from less traditional backgrounds.

Dr Victoria Showunmi, Associate Professor, Institute of Education, University College London

This inspirational book critically analyses and reflects upon the journeys of colleagues from a working-class background into the perceived higher echelons of academia, using autoethnography as its methodology. The stories are honest and impactful as they describe the often not straight-forward routes into higher education. Instead, the routes meander through education, seizing opportunities as they arise. Many academics recognise the imposter syndrome and feelings of not belonging in a certain arena, with notions of class, race, gender, sexuality and identity firmly ingrained into the culture. However, the contributors to this book have demonstrated a tenacity and attitude towards learning that has led them to where they are now, warriors and champions of widening participation.

This book will be useful to academics to reflect upon their own journeys but mainly to all who think that higher education and the world of academia is 'not for them', based upon their views and experiences of class, etc. Being the first in one's family to attend higher education and then pursue a career in it may feel challenging and daunting and could be accompanied by a sense of loss (of identity) and betrayal (of background). This book acknowledges those feelings through its reflexive and often cathartic accounts while also demonstrating what can be achieved.

Dr Jodi Roffey-Barentsen, School of Education, University of Brighton

As a postgraduate student, I have found this collection of autoethnographic studies to be an enlightening experience when considering my approach to my studies. The format of these autoethnographic findings has shown that there is another way possible, a way that allows a deeper examination of a subject that is so close to me and that allows me the scope to delve into it intensely. This collection has shown me the importance of personal power when discussing issues relevant to the self and how utilisation of that power can be cathartic while creating a deeper understanding from the perspective of the writer.

This interesting compilation has been invaluable to me as I take my next steps along my educational path, giving a powerful insight into how others have used an autoethnographical approach to critically examine a variety of subjects. The book has been able to show the scope of this method and its possible uses within my work and I am sure it will be a helpful starting point for other students who are considering the possible structure of their studies.

Joanne McLeod, Post Graduate Research Student,
MA Education: Culture, Language and Identity,
Goldsmiths, London

The Lives of Working Class Academics: Getting Ideas Above Your Station

EDITED BY

IONA BURNELL REILLY

University of East London, UK

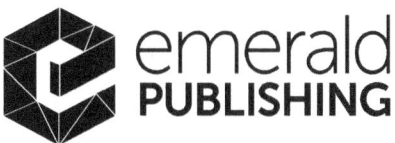

emerald
PUBLISHING

United Kingdom – North America – Japan – India – Malaysia – China

Emerald Publishing Limited
Howard House, Wagon Lane, Bingley BD16 1WA, UK

First edition 2023

Reprints and permissions service
Contact: permissions@emeraldinsight.com

British Library Cataloguing in Publication Data
A catalogue record for this book is available from the British Library

ISBN: 978-1-80117-058-1 (Print)
ISBN: 978-1-80117-057-4 (Online)
ISBN: 978-1-80117-059-8 (Epub)
ISBN: 978-1-80117-060-4 (Paperback)

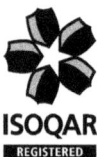

ISOQAR certified
Management System,
awarded to Emerald
for adherence to
Environmental
standard
ISO 14001:2004.

ISOQAR REGISTERED
Certificate Number 1985
ISO 14001

INVESTOR IN PEOPLE

In honour of my grandmothers:
Anna Teresa Byrd[1], née Reilly
and
May Beatrice Bridgman, née Loynds

---

[1]'Byrd', formerly 'Bird', is a pseudo-translation of the Irish surname 'MacEneaney' (MacLysaght, E., *More Irish Families,* Cambridge University Press, Cambridge: UK, 1996). Although many variations of the spelling exist, MacEneaney is an anglicised form of an original Irish Gaeilge name (according to my great-aunt), recorded as 'Mac an Éanaigh' (Woulfe, P., *Irish Names and Surnames,* published by M.H Gill and Son, Dublin: Ireland, 1922) in Ulster.

Anglicisation of Irish names was commonplace in Ireland and intensified during the seventeenth century, a period known as the 'Penal Laws' (Cusack, M., http://www.libraryireland.com/historyIreland/penal-laws.php), in a bid to reduce Irish identity and enhance British control of the country. This was Britain's attempt to oppress Ireland, the culture and the language. The Gaelic Revival movement of the nineteenth century caused many people to reclaim their indigenous names (Smyth, W.J., http://publish.ucc.ie/doi/atlas). The 1737 penal law, banning the use of Irish in the courts, was recently repealed following a community-led campaign for an Irish Language Act in the north of Ireland (www.irishlegal.com/articles/centuries-long-ban-on-irish-language-in-northern-ireland-courts-to-be-scrapped).

Table of Contents

About the Contributors

Khalil Akbar is a Senior Lecturer at the University of East London. He has completed a BA in Education Studies and an MA in Education (Leadership and Management). He has also completed teacher's training and held a number of strategic and transformational roles within primary schools. Khalil is currently undertaking a Doctorate in Education with research focused on how Primary school children experience and understand British values.

Professor Samantha Broadhead is Head of Research at Leeds Arts University and is interested in arts education and the work of Basil Bernstein (1924–2000). She serves on the *Journal of Widening Participation and Lifelong Learning*'s editorial board. Broadhead has co-authored with Gregson (2018) *Practical Wisdom and Democratic Education – Phronesis, Art and Non-traditional Students*, Macmillan Palgrave. She also has co-authored with Davies and Hudson (2019) *Perspectives on Access: Practice and Research*, Emerald Publishing Limited.

Dr Teresa Crew is a Senior Lecturer in Social Policy at Bangor University and a Senior HEA Fellow. In 2020 she published a book on working-class academics entitled *Higher Education and Working-Class Academics: Precarity and Diversity in Academia*. Her research and teaching interests centre around the broad area of class and social inequalities.

Dr Jo Finch is Professor of Social Work and Post Graduate Research at the University of Suffolk. Jo was formerly a children and families social worker, practice educator and play therapist, working in a number of London Boroughs. Jo has written extensively about practice learning and assessment and PRE-VENT. She is the author of *Supporting Struggling Students on Placement* (Policy Press) and co-author of *Share: A New Model for Social Work* (Kirwin Maclean Associates).

Dr Craig A. Hammond is Senior Lecturer in Education at Liverpool John Moores University; prior to moving to LJMU, Craig taught across further education and college based higher education (CBHE) for 18 years. His recent publications are *Hope, Utopia and Creativity in Higher Education: Pedagogical Tactics for Alternative Futures* (Bloomsbury, 2018), and *Folds, Fractals and Bricolages for Hope: Some Conceptual and Pedagogical Tactics for a Creative Higher* Education (Palgrave Macmillan, 2019). He is a Managing Editor for the journal *PRISM*, and Co-Vice-Chair of LJMU's Centre for Educational Research (CERES).

Dr Alpesh Maisuria (orcid 0000-0002-1787-8675) is Associate Professor of Education Policy in Critical Education, University of the West of England, Bristol, UK. Through underlabouring Marxism with Critical Realist philosophy of science, which is largely terra incognita, his work examines the ideological and political drivers of policy decisions to critique the role and function of education in (re)producing forms of inequality. He is the Editor of the first ever *Encyclopaedia of Marxism and Education* (published by Brill).

Dr Colin McCaig is a Professor of Higher Education Policy and works in an educational policy research centre at Sheffield Hallam University. His main research interests are the political economy of the English HE system, with a particular focus on policies designed to widen participation (WP), and he is the author of many books and research articles in these fields. As a researcher and evaluator he has also authored and contributed to many reports for HEFCE, OFFA and the OfS, and sits on the Effectiveness of WP Outreach Working Group of TASO – The Centre for Transforming Access and Student Outcomes.

Dr Michael Pierse is a Senior Lecturer in Irish Literature at Queen's University Belfast. His research mainly explores the cultural production of Irish working-class life. He is author of *Writing Ireland's Working-Class: Dublin After O'Casey* (2011) and editor of the collections, *A History of Irish Working-Class Writing* (2017), *Rethinking the Irish Diaspora: After the Gathering* (co-edited with Devlin Trew) and *Creativity and Resistance in a Hostile World* (co-edited with Mahn, Malik and Rogaly).

Dr Iona Burnell Reilly is a Senior Lecturer in the School of Education and Communities at the University of East London. Iona lectures in Sociology of Education. Her research interests are social class and inequality in education; widening participation in higher education; and the experiences of the working class in HE. Iona's teaching experience and background is in Further Education, where she taught English Language (ESOL) and Access courses at an inner London college for 10 years before moving into Higher Education.

Dr Carli Rowell is a Lecturer at the University of Sussex, as well as a sociologist, feminist and ethnographer and much of her work grapples with issues pertaining to contemporary social, spatial and geopolitical (im)mobilities particularly in relation to educational (in)equalities. She has conducted funded research on working-class students' experiences at an elite UK university (ESRC) and working-class early career researchers' experiences of moving through doctoral study into/and out of the academic workforce (SRHE). She tweets at: @carliriarowell.

Dr Peter Shukie is programme leader for Education Studies and Action Research lead in College Based Higher Education in East Lancashire. His PhD focussed on community engagement in technology through Community Open Online Courses, where everyone can teach and learn, for free. Dr Shukie imagined, then made real, the collective that led to the Working Class Academics Conference and continues to advocate for working-class voices in the ways we create a new academy.

Dr Hannah Walters is at King's College, London. Hannah is a feminist sociologist of youth with particular interest in girlhood and the intersections of class and gender. Her work uses participatory and creative methods underpinned by the principles of feminist research. She tweets at: @hanwalt.

Dr ML White is a Senior Lecturer in Teacher Education at Moray House School of Education & Sport, University of Edinburgh. She is interested in how we prepare beginner teachers to work in areas of socio-economic disadvantage, reaching and teaching students in poverty and exploring pedagogies that support a transformative and activist orientation. ML is also interested in civic media practices, social geography and how we experience space and place in education and learning.

Professor Marcia A. Wilson works at the Open University as the Dean for Equality, Diversity and Inclusion (EDI). She is responsible for embedding the EDI agenda across the institution. Her work includes equality projects with Universities UK, and she has an interest in racial trauma in sport. She is a multiple award winner and uses her platform to raise awareness about inequalities to generate institutional and sector-wide change.

Dr Steve Wong is a Senior Lecturer of Education Studies at the University of East London and Lecturer of Applied Linguistics at UCL Institute of Education in London. His research interests relate to the broad areas of language and social interaction, and cultures of hybridity arising from the intersection of language(s), race and ethnicities. His work is informed by cross-disciplinary understandings of sociology, sociolinguistics, cultural studies, anthropology and education studies. His research takes the linguistic ethnographic approach.

Foreword

> Academia has rarely developed complex understandings of working-class people.
>
> (Reay, 1997, p. 18)

This book is a collection of autoethnographically inflected accounts of what it is like to be working class and what it is to be a working class academic. Perhaps the most transformative aspect of this collection lies in its approach towards writing working-classness – through auto-ethnographies produced by working class academics. For some time, there have been problems in the way that class is applied in education research – there has been a tendency towards understandings that have ignored some of the significant and meaningful ways in which class is lived and class is done. There have been some major oversights such as the primacy often given to white male experiences and 'the possibility of a complex trajectory for people who remain working-class is often denied' (Reay, 1997, p. 19). In addition, there have been problems with the ways in which class has been theorised and analysed. Some time ago, Rosemary Crompton (1998, p. 114) warned that 'it is not possible to construct a single measure which could successfully capture all the elements going to make up social class – or even structured social inequality'. Nevertheless, work on class and education can sometimes seem inert and stuck, relying on proxies such as the receipt of free school meals rather than more powerful and complex approaches. The chapters in this collection include diverse and situated accounts from a set of academics who all identify as working class (in different ways) and whose various narratives challenge the sorts of shortcomings I have described here.

There have been some notable developments in class theory that have enlarged our critical horizons. Here I am thinking about the ways in which we recognise that there are 'very many different ways of being working-class' (Reay, 2017, p. 5). First, there are fractions of class, and these are fluid, shifting according to economic changes and individual experiences of turmoil and distress, where families edge out of being part of the 'respectable' working class and teeter haphazardly on the border of being 'rough'. There are emotional ambivalences, and sometimes high costs, attached to this shifting between being, and not being, respectable. Social class is also powerfully shaped by place – by attention and commitment to 'home' and where we come from, as well as where we may have settled in our journeys from our working-class origins to our jobs in the academy. Any work on class and education may be limited if it does not speak of space and place; from the recognition of access to privilege and limits to social goods, perhaps because of poor transport and high travel costs for example, space and place are strongly implicated in social reproduction and the ways in which class inscribes itself in the lives of us all. There are also other differences too – differences of accent and how we speak – differences in the language we use to speak and write of ourselves and others.

And then there is diversity and intersectionality. Social identities and our classed identities are sculpted out of the structural and material resources that are available to us. These resources that speak powerfully to us, about who we are and may be and desire to be, are amalgams of discourses from our gendered selves, our ethnicity, our embodied selves, our sexualities. They are also constructed out of our age, the times we live in, as well as the places where we live and the faith communities that we may belong to or come from. If this were not complex and complicated enough, aspects of our identities, and for academics of working-class backgrounds, our classed selves are interpellated by educational moments that may provide (sometimes) advantages, by luck and chance as well as by serendipity. So social identities are contingent, fluid and always in a process of emergence, matters that are addressed in this set of autoethnographies.

This book, *The Lives of Working Class Academics*, works as an important corrective to the common-sense notion of the academic being middle class. Here this notion is troubled – troubled by a set of arguments that recognises that working as an academic is generally regarded as a middle-class occupation, although things are changing. A report by the Social Mobility Commission (2017) found that while 58% of academics in the survey reported coming from a middle-class family, 14% were from a working-class background. In this diffuse, rich and emotionally authentic set of chapters, the voices of a range of academics speak to their experiences of this voyage from one class into another as well as into a very powerful motor of reproduction – the university. Yet, what of the university? Given its hierarchical and oppressive nature, and the importance of place/space, what role does the type of university, perhaps the subject discipline, as well as the academic positionality of the authors of these beautifully crafted pieces play in being working class in the academy? As Iona Burnell Reilly asks of these working-class academics in the preface to this collection, how have they become who they are in an industry steeped in elitism? How have they navigated their way, and what has the journey been like? Do they continue to identify as working class or have their social positioning and/or identities shifted?

Forewords are necessarily short in length and so they are limited in what they can express. What I can say from having read these chapters is that in their range they go a long way towards capturing the diversity of working-class academics' accounts and are all here in one place – something that has not been addressed for a long time. Some of these narratives privilege gender; others incorporate race/ gender into their stories. There are accounts that speak of micro-aggressions and introjected values that attempt to situate being working-class as a negative and demeaning identity, and there are others where being working-class is something shared and valued – an asset to be drawn on for solidarity and comradeship. In much of what passes for work 'on' the working classes, their voices are situated in the margins, their lives written out as if being working-class were somehow a homogenous experience to be retold by others. This powerful collection gives a lie to this violent act; it also works as a corrective to how we construct the subjectivity of 'the academic' from the written words and lives of working-class academics.

Meg Maguire
Professor of Sociology of Education
King's College, London

References

Crompton, R. (1998). *Class and stratification: An introduction to current debates.* Polity Press.

Reay, D. (1997). The double-bind of the 'working-class' feminist academic: The success of failure or the failure of success? In P. Mahony & C. Zmroczek (Eds.), *Class matters: 'Working-class' women's perspectives on social class.* Taylor & Francis.

Reay, D. (2017). *Miseducation inequality, education and the working classes.* Policy Press.

Preface

The Importance of Autoethnography as a Research Method

Byrne describes autoethnography within his own context as a 'tool with which to understand individual and shared experiences of class in higher education' (2019, p. 133). My intention for this book was to collect stories from academics who identify as having a working class background. These stories would be an account of their lives, their experiences and their journeys into becoming a higher education professional, including an in-depth look at their educative experiences along the lifespan. Rather than writing about working-class academics, I have asked working-class academics to write about themselves. McKenzie, writing about her own background, and experiences of the social class structure, comments that 'Narratives, and storytelling, are important in working-class lives. It is how we explain ourselves, how we understand the world around us, and how we situate ourselves in a wider context' (Mckenzie, 2017, p. 6).

One of the requirements of contributing authors for this book was to position themselves as being from a working-class heritage. Reay points out that 'To own an identity as "working class" is, among many other things, to accept one's social inferiority' (1997, p. 228). Crew explains this point further:

> What working class means to everyone looking in at the working class, and sometimes how working-class people see themselves, is that working class means failure, working class means at the bottom of everything. Working class means not being educated, not well read. It always has these really negative connotations. Everything that is about being at the bottom, not good enough.
>
> (Crew, 2020, p. 24)

Initially, my concern was that, for some, writing about one's social class may be a difficult, even painful, experience. Another concern was that people might feel uncomfortable about revealing themselves and their background. Crew recounts some of the challenges she faced while producing her book, including some uncomfortable conversations: 'Perhaps claiming a working-class identity, from the supposed advantaged financial and educational perspective of an academic, could be seen as pretentious. Or, as someone said to me during the writing up of this research, "wanting the best of both worlds"' (2020, p. 25). Geraldine

Van Bueren, chair of the Alliance of Working Class Academics, poses a different kind of concern[1]: 'In academia, people don't feel able to talk about their backgrounds freely because they think it will negatively affect their career' (cited in Wilby, 2019). Byrne presents a different view when he states 'Working-class people are, by definition, relatively uneducated, which exposes the link between class and academia, and the inherent dissonance in thinking about oneself as a working-class [person]… the academy is not just classist, it is the *source* of classism, and of the very concept of the working-class' (2019, p. 136).

These problematic factors are what make the lives of working-class academics all the more interesting, rich and powerful. How have they become who they are in an industry steeped in elitism? How have they navigated their way, and what has the journey been like? Do they continue to identify as working-class or have their social positioning and/or identities shifted? These questions and more will be addressed and answered through each author's fascinating account of their journey. Ryan and Sackrey comment on what instigated their journey into publication: 'we began to wonder if other upwardly mobile academics had experienced similar feelings of displacement or dissatisfaction, and perhaps more importantly, internalised conflict' (1984, p. 6). Thirty-eight years on and, having undergone my own journey, this very question is now on my lips.

Autoethnography is a fascinating method of research that allows the author to reflect on their own lived reality and explore their personal, professional and cultural experiences (in this case, their journey and experience of becoming an academic). 'Autoethnography in its most simplified definition is the study of the self' (Reed-Danahay, 1997, p. 9). However, unlike autobiography and autofiction, autoethnography is a critical study of oneself, and how we understand our relationships to socio-cultural contexts. Hughes and Pennington comment on autoethnography as 'critical reflexive narrative enquiry, critical reflexive self study, or critical reflexive action research in which the researcher takes an active, scientific, and systematic view of personal experience in relation to cultural groups identified by the researcher as similar to the self' (2017, p. 11). Simply put, the researcher is the subject of the study, critically reflecting and interpreting their own life, social background and personal experiences. Autoethnography, as all research methods, is driven by theory; different theoretical and conceptual frameworks can be used to frame and/or underpin the autoethnographer's story. Hughes and Pennington provide guidelines to writing an autoethnography and, among others, state that theories are the basis of the account (2017); they also remind us that using a theoretical framework can serve to 'protect the autoethnographer from accusations of narcissistic navel-gazing' (2017, p. 51).

Reflexivity is central to the process of rigorous autoethnography. Researchers are not free from assumptions and biases, and we all have different ways of interpreting the world. By describing, analysing and understanding their background, the autoethnographic process connects the writer's personal and self-narratives to a wider social, cultural and political context. Each of the authors

---

[1]The Alliance of Working Class academics is a UK-based organisation that supports faculty and students from diverse working-class backgrounds.

within this book has self-defined as being from a working-class heritage. The writer's social class may not be the only aspect of their lives that they reflect on and analyse; they might also draw on race, ethnicity, gender, religion and the intersections between them, in order to fully explore their experience, journey and development into becoming an academic in higher education (HE). Reflexivity, Hughes and Pennington remind us, is 'a central criterion of autoethnography [and] provides researchers with a forum for expressing their awareness of their integral connection to the research context and thereby their influence on that context' (2017, p. 93).

Lovett and Lovett (2016, p. 147) identify that 'An understanding of class is best achieved when studied in conjunction with other social identities like race and gender'. Although a working-class heritage will underpin the autoethnography of each of the writers, the interlocking sections between class, race and gender may also be relevant, possibly for some authors more than others, and this is because, Avis argues, 'analytically we cannot separate relations of class from those of gender and race, in practice they are intertwined. We are all positioned in relation to our class, gender, ethnicity, sexuality and so on' (2009, p. 14). One of the advantages of using autoethnography as the method of research is to reveal and authenticate the power relations, the oppressions, the subjugation and the privilege within and between the stories of people's lives.

Intersectionality, a term coined by Kimberlé Crenshaw (1989), is used to describe the ways in which one oppressive trait is interconnected with another; it is the cross-over between two or more distinct discriminations. When bell hooks (1982) referred to herself as a working-class black woman, she may well have been influenced by Claudia Jones, the American civil rights activist, who used the phrase 'triple oppression' to describe disadvantaged black women (cited in Lynn, 2014). Jones believed that black women's triple oppression, based on race, class and gender, preceded all other forms of oppression. hooks, entering HE in the 1960s, writes about her experiences of triple oppression – racism, sexism and class bias – in the academy. In her book *Ain't I a Woman* (1982), hooks challenges the view that race and gender are two separate phenomena, asserting that the struggle to end racism and sexism are inextricably interlinked. This early form of what we now call 'intersectionality' broadens the lens, identifying multiple factors of advantage and disadvantage, as well as race, class and gender; other factors may include caste, sexuality, religion, disability and physical appearance.

Why, we may ask, is any of this important? Hughes and Pennington (2017) have written about autoethnography as 'critical social research'. They cite Jupp (1993) as defining this as encompassing 'a broad range of social science studies that purposefully challenge existing understandings and foundations of knowledge' (Hughes & Pennington, 2017, p. 17). It is usual for social researchers to pursue topics that are close to their experiences of the social world, and this is certainly true for me. Critical research is the paradigm whereby researchers start with a criticism of the social world, that there is something wrong and needs to be fixed. The criticisms usually involve social inequalities and injustices; 'Critical researchers see the world as being divided and in constant tension, dominated by the powerful, who oppress the people and use the state and its institutions as tools to achieve their purpose' (Sarantakos, 2005, p. 51).

The critical research paradigm is a step further from interpretivism; not content at interpreting the social world, the critical social researcher aims to change it. Gray asserts that 'The assumptions that lie beneath critical inquiry are that: Ideas are mediated by power relations in society. Certain groups in society are privileged over others and exert an oppressive force on subordinate groups' (2020, p. 30). My objective was to give voice to working-class academics, a space to share their stories, and to situate their lived realities, in order that they can be acknowledged and understood. I do feel that not enough is known and understood about the lives and experiences of working-class academics, many of whom undergo unique and profound experiences. We all live in and experience the social world differently; having an understanding of each other's unique lived realities is not only very interesting but is necessary for the good of humanity, and for a progressive and inclusive society. Byrne notes that 'Autoethnography, writing ourselves into our work, is a way to give voice to marginalized groups and contribute to democratizing academic culture and writing' (2019, p. 146).

The legacy of elitism remains in HE, inequality and prestige have persisted, and with very little history or class culture in the field of HE to identify with, this can, for some working-class academics, make their experiences fraught and difficult. My aim for this book is to share those fraught and difficult experiences, give voice to and authenticate them, and more importantly, challenge the dominant discourses that maintain and perpetuate elitism and exclusion within HE.

Iona Burnell Reilly

References

Avis, J. (2009). *Education, policy and social justice*. Continuum Publishing.

Byrne, G. (2019). Individual weakness to collective strength: (Re)creating the self as a 'working-class academic'. *Journal of Writing in Creative Practice, 12*(1 & 2), 131–150.

Crenshaw, K. (1989). Demarginalizing the intersection of race and sex: A black feminist critique of antidiscrimination doctrine, feminist theory and antiracist. *Politics in University of Chicago Legal Forum*, 1, 139–167.

Crew, T. (2020). *Higher education and working-class academics precarity and diversity in academia*. Palgrave.

Gray, D. (2020). *Doing research in the business world*. Sage Publications.

hooks, b. (1982). *Ain't I a woman. Black women and feminism*. Pluto Press.

Hughes, S. A., & Pennington, J. L. (2017). *Autoethnography: Process, product, and possibility for critical social research*. Sage Publications.

Lovett, N., & Lovett, T. (2016). Academic alien: Portrait of a working-class man's higher education experience. *International Journal of Social Science and Humanities, 6*(2), 145–148.

Lynn, D. (2014). Socialist feminism and triple oppression: Claudia Jones and African American women in American communism. *Journal for the Study of Radicalism, 8*(2), 1–20.

Mckenzie, L. (2017). *Getting by: Estates, class and culture in Austerity Britain*. Policy Press.

Reay, D. (1997). Feminist theory, habitus, and social class: Disrupting notions of classlessness in women's. *Studies International Forum*, *20*(2), 225–233.

Reed-Danahay, D. (1997). *Auto/ethnography: Rewriting the self and the social*. Berg.

Ryan, J., & Sackrey, C. (1984). *Strangers in paradise: Academics from the working class*. South End Press.

Sarantakos, S. (2005). *Social research*. Palgrave Macmillan.

Wilby, P. (2019). The lawyer who wants more academics to 'come out' as working class. *The Guardian*, 9 July 2019. Retrieved from https://www.theguardian.com/education/2019/jul/09/lawyer-wants-academics-come-out-as-working-class

Chapter 1

Navigating the Relational Character of Social Class for Capitalism in the Academy

Alpesh Maisuria

Abstract

This chapter is a Marxist Critical Realist inspired discussion of my interest in, and experiences of, being a working-class academic from Indian/African heritage. I begin my autoethnography by problematising the limits of defining social class from a gradational approach, which is the most common way to make sense of social class in academia and beyond. I argue that neoliberal capitalism organises people into workers and owners of production and without this acknowledgement, discussion of social class in the gradational approach is limited. I then go on to critique the de-centering of social class, for which I used Critical Race Theory (CRT) as a case study. My intention is to promote the explanatory power of approaching social class as as an organisational relationship, which assimilates racism, in the service of capitalism. Throughout the chapter, I provide examples of the way that I navigate this intellectual standpoint in the classroom, specifically through utilising the concepts of *mystification* and *feasibility* that I developed through my PhD that focussed on social class in Sweden. Without dismissing the value of the gradational approach of understanding social class *in toto*, and also the importance of personal identities (indeed I have focussed on my ethno-racial identity), my basic argument is that without the centralisation of social class, and crucially its articulation with neoliberal capitalism, social class becomes a *descriptive* category rather than *explanatory*, rendering the possibility of radical social change as severely diminished.

Keywords: Social class; social status; Marxism; neoliberalism; critical realism; feasibility; mystification; inequality; inequity; racism

The Lives of Working Class Academics, 1–15
Copyright © 2023 Alpesh Maisuria
Published under exclusive licence by Emerald Publishing Limited
doi:10.1108/978-1-80117-057-420221001

Preamble

Referencing Ellen Meiksins Wood, Webber (2015) writes that 'There are really only two ways of thinking theoretically about class: either as a structural location or as a social relation'. The point being made is that gradational schemes that try and measure social class position actually measure *status* and socio-cultural *markers*, which may be interesting and useful points of departure, but, he goes on:

> ...there is a very long way to travel in order to identify how a class 'in itself' becomes a class 'for itself', to use Marx's terminology for the movement between an objective class situation and class consciousness, or from social being to social consciousness. In order to get there, we need to think of class as a social-historical process and relationship.
>
> (Webber, 2015)

Webber (2015) then cites a pithy comment by E. P. Thompson that '[t]he working class did not rise like the sun at an appointed time. ... It was present at its own making', thus making the point that E. P. Thompson was stating the importance of social class to be understood historically, dialectically, and materially emergent in/through social relationships. In other words, and more directly, social class is entangled in a web of relations that encompasses social relationships that are always conditioned by capitalism. The masses have been purposefully encouraged by the global ruling class to think of ourselves as individual agents acting freely as consumers and rational beings (homo economicus), rather than being socio-economically related *for* capitalism. There is a necessity to have consciousness of this reality, thus in order to create the modicum of possibility to progress to eudemonia – flourishing for all.

These words of preamble provide the sentiment for the three overarching objectives for this chapter: (1) problematise gradational approaches to social class, arguing that a focus on status does not hold explanatory power; (2) critique the de-centering of social class, for which I used Critical Race Theory (CRT) as a case study; and (3) promote the explanatory power of approaching social class an organisational relationship in the service of capitalism. My basic argument throughout this autoethnography is that without the centralisation of social class, and crucially its articulation with neoliberal capitalism, social class becomes a *descriptive* category rather than *explanatory*, rendering the possibility of radical social change as severely diminished.

Ways of Thinking About Social Class

During my undergraduate, in 1999, I vividly remember a seminar exercise led by my lecturer that involved an opening provocation – *What social class are you?* I had deliberated this question for many years, and so I was able pontificate – 'I'm at university *now*, so I must be middle class'! I was making the association between my educational status and my transient social class positionality. There were nods of agreement. Others in my classroom recognised social class as both reflecting, as well as causing, economic, social and cultural differences – the term inequality became a trope. These differences were described through differentials in income, wealth, status, education and lifestyle; mortality and health were mentioned too. Many of my fellow students pointed to *income* as the most significant *marker* of social class, and this was discussed as part of expressions of wealth indicated through private possessions. Income and wealth were perceived to denote social class but nobody explicitly discussed social structure, capitalism and social relations beyond superficial socio-cultural markers (e.g. house size/type/location, brand/cost/model of car and so forth). The discussion we were having was not *sui generis*. Education, employment and occupation, and other socio-cultural and consumption markers, are widely often used in this way to make sense of, and measure, social class. These markers are also used to argue that social class is either important (see neo-Weberians), or unimportant (for instance, as compared with ethno-racial identity), or that we live in a post-class society (including those who take up the dubious promotion of Post-Humanism/New Materialism). In that seminar during my undergraduate, we were far from being a class for itself – we did not see the connection we had to each other and the economic system, as is the case in society more generally.

During my teens, this point about contemporary society being post-class was a focus for former Conservative Prime Minister John Major in 1990 through claiming he would propel us into a 'classless society', and then in 1999, and giving ballast to this post-class zeitgeist, Tony Blair claiming 'I want to make you all middle class'. Both Major and Blair were seemingly promising the expansion of the middle segment of the social structure. These promises were framed by the unavoidable need to address social inequality after almost two decades of the aggressive pursuit of neoliberalism with its concomitant market policies, promotion of self-interest and individualisation, with a heavy dose of laissez-faire governance (Maisuria, 2022). This environment commenced with the fundamental political antipathy to working class issues, solidarity, empathy and comradeship. This antipathy was so stridently promulged by Thatcher in her now infamous 1987 statement that clearly placed individuals at the centre of social ills, rather than the government's pursuit of neoliberalism. On society, Thatcher stated:

> There is no such thing! There are individual men and women and there are families and no government can do anything except through people and people look to themselves first. It is our duty to look after ourselves and then also to help look after our neighbour and life is a reciprocal business …
> (Thatcher, 1987)

For Thatcher, even a rhetorical 'pursuit of equality' by the government 'itself is a mirage' (Thatcher, 1975). The notion of a caring and sharing society was being cultivated as an anathema during the 1980s by Thatcher's dominant ideology.

Against this political backdrop that I was living through and learning about via osmosis, there was a shift away from thinking about the role of the State and its institutions, such as education, and this made common understandings of social class to be about differentiation with socio-cultural markers of status. This is now the most common way that social class is understood by those within and beyond academia. For instance, the titles of the presentations at the 2021 Working Class Studies conference are a strong indication of the diminution of a relational approach to social class – none of the papers had Marx, only five included the word neoliberalism (four were in the same Panel), and one had the word capitalism. This shift in definition can also be seen more widely, including in the design of official/popular class schemas, such as the Registrar General, Goldthorpe and the Great British Class Survey that places people in a grade ranging either five or seven 'classes' – a gradational approach.

Grades of Social Status Versus Social Class as a Capitalist Relation

But by the time I embarked on my third year of university, I came to realise that there were fundamental problems with this gradational way of thinking about social class. At best it is superficial (for instance where does the Royal Family fit? Or the super-rich?), and at worse it absents the objective reality of the world, which is structured by capitalism to satisfy its reliance on social class relations in its system of value production. In Hill and Maisuria (2022), we discuss efficacy of both the *gradational* model and also the *relation* model of understanding social class and its lived reality. While popular class schemas (like the ones mentioned above) and mainstream responses to the question *What social class are you?* elicit responses that refer to social class, they are actually measuring status in *gradational* way of thinking. Thus, we make the point in Hill and Maisuria (2022, p. 627) about grades of social status:

> ... they are actually not classes, but rather they are gradational categorisations based on the sociologist Max Weber's theory of status. Importantly they are not articulated as part of a relationship of social groups, so it is unclear how one 'class' relates to another – these gradational schemas hide the essential connective economic relationships between groups. .... in these [neo-Weberian] schemas, people are graded in a hierarchy but they are missing the essential relation, the Capital-Labour Relation.

My co-author for that chapter, Professor Dave Hill, was also my tutor at university more than two-decades ago. In my second year at University, Dave had an enormous impact on the way that I began to understand social class as a relationship in capitalism between two classes – this is what is called the Capital-Labour relation in Marxism. Knowledge of this was a revelation. I grew up in the city of Bradford and wool mills from a bygone era of a distinctive capitalist ruling class were everywhere, some mills were being repurposed, such as for my college education, but many remained derelict. These mills represented a time when the dominant mode of production was visibly *industrial* capitalism.

With Dave's intellectual resource, I began to become conscious of my background and the way that society was organised then, but has now become invisible (see my discussion of mystification below). This social organisation took the form of workers and also those who owned the means of production in capitalism. My interest in social class was piqued by a significant problem with finding out about the way that workers were the ones who produced *value* through their labour to produce things and provide services (commodities), but the fruits of this labour (profit) was disproportionately taken by the those who owned the means of production (proprietors of factories, companies, equipment), this is clearly an *exploitative* relationship. I have come to realise that nobody can escape this organisational structure, and there is a place for everyone and everyone has a place to service capitalism in this epoch of globalisation.

My academic career and teaching have been based on exposing this fundamental truth with capitalism, which is now in its neoliberal form and being augments by technological developments (including, AI and the 4th Industrial Revolution).

Neoliberalism

Neoliberalism is a term that is regularly used by those who are interested in education. For example, Stephen Ball's work on the marketisation of education over many years has been rightfully celebrated, but his work does not adequately make the articulation that neoliberalism is about the essence of the social relations of production. His work is maladroit for showing that the relationship between the workers and the capitalists is exploitative and based on value creation through the production of commodities. If this organisational relationship is not recognised with/through education, then the role and function of education for neoliberalism cannot be fully grasped and status quo will endure.

My research, teaching and general scholarship utilises Marx to have an account of social class that tries to capture objective reality. In the three volumes of *Capital*, Marx and Engels explained that society has an objective reality that is organised by the capitalist mode of production (see Maisuria, 2022). Exempting capitalism and the way that it arranges people into two antagonistic groups in society means that discussions of social class, inequality, inequity, poverty, injustice become *descriptive* rather than *explanatory*. For many years, my teaching has tried to enable students to understand that social class is *more* than merely private possessions, consumption, lifestyle choices and embodied subjectivities, which are the markers of social and positionality success (or lack of). Rather it is about the centrality of the labouring class (my students, me, us!) who get paid for their labour and this is used for survival, today this means paying for food, bills and debt – including tuition fees. The commodity produced by the labour of the worker is sequestered for market-place exchange by the capitalist class for more money than the total cost of production. This means value produced by the worker's labour (the output/service provided) must be greater than the sum total cost of production, including raw materials, buildings and materials, and crucially the wage (Maisuria, 2022). Wage labour, as it is termed in the Marxism, is dehumanising and alienating in neoliberalism. I ask my students whether their job (all my students work) is satisfying, fulfilling, paid appropriately and makes them feel human. Suffice to say the valuations are rarely positive, and we draw conclusions from this about the status quo.

My teaching practice is framed by a Critical Education approach (see Mathison & Ross, 2022), and the entry point is always to begin with the following pivotal provocations:

What the world is like in your perception? What do you perceive the world to be like for others? How do you think they perceive it? Why do you think in this way?

What would you like the world to be like? What do you think others want the world to be like? Why do you think in this way?

How do we get there? What role can you/do you play for this vision to become feasible? How can you work in solidarity with others? Why do you think in this way?

This approach to navigating issues of social class and capitalism in the classroom is how I characterise Marxist pedagogy and praxis that is based on the reality and experiences of students and their perspectives. At the foundation of this approach is Joyce Canaan's counsel to me that we must work *within* and *against* neoliberalism (see Canaan, 2005; Canaan & Singh, 2013; Asher, Cowden, Housee, & Maisuria, 2022). I have found this idea incredibly profound as a maxim for life as an academic where I am servicing the very problems that I identify by labouring for a neoliberal university. In the words of Canaan:

> Teachers who engaged in a dialogue that focused upon and took seriously students' thoughts, and considered them agents capable of expanding their limited understandings, could empower students to develop active thought, which they could then use to help themselves and other oppressed groups.
>
> (Canaan, 2005, p. 163)

In provoking these questions, my navigation of social class as a topic of dialogue is animated by a material base. For instance, the British government in 2020 provided an excellent teaching opportunity for this when it issued 'guidance' that revealed an insight about how the capitalist ruling class are frightened of the ever-present possibility of revolutionary momentum building. It said: 'schools should not under any circumstances use resources produced by organisations that take … a publicly stated desire to abolish or overthrow democracy, [and] capitalism' (Department for Education, 2020). Using the real-world examples like this to think about social class and associated ideas of democracy in capitalism places the objective reality of world at its centre, rather than circumnavigating it like so much discussion of social class does in the academy. Understanding that, we as, individuals working in collective symphony, organised through Trade Unions, and other ways, can effect the unfolding of history. To demonstrate this, I tell students that people-power forced the Government to remove this overtly ideological repressive diktat from its guidance.

So in the classroom, we progress discussion about the direction that history is travelling – are things getting better for us individually and humanity as a whole? In Maisuria (2022, p. 486), I wrote that:

> Marx foresaw the development of a society under capitalism where the ruling class would gradually become enormously wealthy through the work of the labouring class. In this historical evolution, the profits of those who own the means of production (see any rich list for names – every year this will include: Jeff Bezos and Mark Zuckerberg, Warren Buffett, Carlos Slim and Bill Gates) will exponentially become greater, while workers' wages will remain stable, decrease, or only marginally increase. The increasingly exploitative relationship between the two classes was described as a continual source of struggle by Marx in the following terms: 'The history of all hitherto existing society is the history of class struggles'
>
> (Marx & Engels, 1848)

The Critical Education-based pedagogy inevitably entails discussions that are filled with indignation, deflation, depression. But nevertheless, these are important discussions about social class, which not only expose social class but also connect it to neoliberal capitalism. Only with this pre-requisite understanding can resistance be mounted for a better existence for us all. The important message that my students take away is that pessimism and nihilism is not an option if change is desired. Only people working in solidarity can make history, but conditions are deliberately made difficult for us because it threatens the capitalist ruling class dominant hegemony (Marx, 1852; see also; Mayo, 2015; Maisuria, 2020).

These existential and material discussions of life and history are designed to lead to *good sense* about who we are in the system that we inhibit (Maisuria, 2020). Bhaskar (2016, p. 173) describes the value of this process for finding unity and developing collective (class) consciousness:

> … the process of basic human interaction, including the swapping of life stories, gets underway, then gradually the move to more difficult topics can begin. However, there may be a surprise here. For it may often transpire that what the other whom we are fighting wants is something very similar to what we want. Thus probably the overwhelming majority of soldiers fighting in the First World War wanted 'bread, peace and land'. Discussion of shared or similar objectives may point the way to the isolation of the real constraints on the attainment of these objectives. … the other is often merely developing a part of oneself that one has chosen not to develop or to see; so that the other is merely showing us a repressed, denied or forgotten part, aspect or possibility of oneself.

The key point is that there is a pulse of freedom when we talk and discuss what the world is like, and what we want, and how we can get there (Bhaskar, 1993).

As part of these stories, with my students, I contribute a brief exchange that I had with my father. Soon after finishing my undergraduate degree in 2002, I decided that I wanted to follow-up on my emerging interest in policy with a Master's degree and do this in London – some three hours away from my birth city, rather than return home. I sought permission from my father, who tersely stated: 'Why'! This is symbolic. My family were immigrants settling in Bradford having arrived from Kenya (with Indian heritage), and 1960s Britain was no place for people like my father to be getting above their station, or encouraging others like him to do so, including his children. Social and education policy was about assimilation – 'leave your funny foreign stuff behind and be more like the British' was the tenor of the moment, and my father had been inculcated into the zeitgeist and this stayed with him throughout his life. The whole system and the culture had been designed to stabilise the status quo through promoting individualism. The working class were actively trained to be the agents of their own oppression. I was living Paul Willis's *Learning to labour: How working-class kids get working class jobs* (Willis, 1979). This story and my wider biography of being the outsider in many different ways (see Maisuria, 2017, pp. 90–93) finds echoes with the experiences of my students. We are all in search of that pulse of freedom (Bhaskar, 1993).

De-Centring Social Class

This chapter has so far dealt with inadequate ways of dealing with social class by those who claim to take social class seriously but use a gradational approach, which I have argued lacks explanatory power. I will now provide some commentary on those approaches that attempt to de-centre class and concomitant problems and the threats that these poses.

Over the last 4 decades, various alternative intellectual and ideological trajectories have emerged to negate the Marxist approach of social class as relational in a capitalist world. Prominent among these, are those that focus on centring either: 'race', gender, sex, religion, disability, democracy, either to exclude social class or de-centre it.[1] I point out to my students that social class is conspicuously missing from the radar of many people, which is problematic because class conditions the way they can access opportunities, and how these opportunities materialise. In other words, there is an absence of consciousness of social class an objective social relation with real consequences. In Hill and Maisuria (2022, p. 625), we point out that:

> ... it is therefore striking that in the UK, social class is not a protected characteristic as part of the Equality and Human Rights Commission's Equalities Act 2010. Unlike age, disability, gender reassignment, marriage and civil partnership, pregnancy and maternity, race, religion and belief, sex, and sexual orientation, it is legal to discriminate against a person based on their perceived

or ascribed social class. Social class protection and equality is not a
human right
(see Equality and Human Rights Commission, 2021)

In my experience of navigating social class in the classroom, this is a profound
revelation to students and colleagues with whom I teach. Pointing out that social
class discrimination matters but is legally permissible becomes even more
powerful when I explain the exploitative nature of neoliberal capitalism, and that:

> ... this exploitation is irrespective of identity and personal
> characteristic of the workers, put another way, capitalism does
> not care for ethno-racial background, sex/gender, and cultural/
> lifestyle preferences of the individual. At different moments
> different groups of people will face differing levels of
> exploitation (a convenient way to create social antagonism
> within the labouring class taking the focus away from systemic
> exploitation).
>
> (Maisuria, 2022, p. 486)

Critics of my centring of social class have in the past have remarked, 'but you're
not working class'. Even in the form of banter, the provocation is not hollow. The
assumption is that, academics have a comfortable existence and they should have
drifted away from their youthful and misguided commitment to class struggle. One
senior staff member told me that I would 'grow-out of' my 'obsession with class',
and there have been similar comments about my take-up of Marxism. I have taken
this to mean that they want me to pipe-down and worry about my future prospects,
come-in from the margins, and generally settle with the status quo, perhaps offering
suggestions to reform neoliberalism rather than get rid of it.

I have learnt that my promoting of social class, particularly from a Marxist
position, is perilous, especially when visiting the United States (I elaborate on this
below), and generally it is not a good career move to 'do' social class in a radical
way. My fellow-Marxist and collaborator Grant Banfield profoundly expresses this:

> Just like you, from my earliest days as an academic I had been
> advised again and again not to concern myself with Marx or issues
> like social class. Both were considered intellectually passé and
> definite career killers. In terms of the latter, that advice has
> probably been proven correct. However, I never entered
> academia for a 'career'. I was motivated by the opportunity
> academia provided me to research, think and teach.
>
> (Maisuria & Banfield, 2022)

With the newer generation of Marxist academics, my advice has been simple –
be strategic about when you pipe-up, do not believe that you can win all battles,
and find pockets of solidarity with fellow intellectual travellers. For me the
network of people associated with *Journal for Critical Education Policy Studies*

(JCEPS) and the *International Conferences on Critical Education* (ICCE) has been an invaluable source of inspiration in an otherwise solitary existence in university departments. It is for these sources that, some two decades on in the academy, I'm penning this chapter about social class and Marxism.

During my PhD, I published and spoke at events about the way that the then-burgeoning popularity of Critical Race Theory (CRT) could be counter-productive to attempts at rectifying historical injustice if they excluded class and capitalism as the roots of racism (see Cole & Maisuria, 2007; Maisuria, 2011). One of my contentions was that a blanket operationalisation of the organisational concept of *White Supremacy* was a blunt tool to describe and *explain* racism in all its forms. This critique (with Mike Cole) offered *xeno-racism* as a more efficacious alternative for explanatory power (see Cole & Maisuria, 2007). Crucially we connected manifestations of racism with capitalism calling it *xeno-racism*, which we said was a toxic conflation of xenophobia (fear of foreigners) and traditional racism (based on skin colour/heritage). We did this to incorporate the experiences of workers from Eastern Europe. The Brexit vote that seemed to mobilise a high-tide of xeno-racism unfortunately seems to have vindicated our argument that we made 10 years before the referendum on the United Kingdom's membership of the European Union.

Perhaps more importantly in our critique, the *White Supremacy* concept *prevents* action that would be created with a united front of all those concerned with racism because it seems to blame White people, *in toto*, for racism. The crucial point here is that it removes the focus on the *system* of capitalism, which does not care about the skin-tone of the worker that it wants to exploit to extract value from. Of course all workers are exploited for neoliberalism, some more than others (e.g. disabled workers). As opposition to my critique of *White Supremacy*, I have also had a different version of the 'but you're not working class' ad hominem levelled at me – 'you're from a BAME background, how can *you* argue that social class/capitalism is more important than race!'. Along the same lines, I have encountered: 'you're a race traitor', 'you are a coconut' (that trope amused me), and even been told that I have been granted 'enhanced standing' (see Maisuria, 2011, p. 89) all because of my problematisation of *White Supremacy* and promotion of Marxist understanding of social class and neoliberalism as the basis for racism. This latter 'enhanced standing' criticism came at the 2010 *American Educational Research Association* (AERA) annual conference where I received a very angry response from a group of individuals in the audience to a critique of CRT that was presenting. I must admit to being rather surprised, both at the pro-CRT audience who found my Marxist critique unconscionable to even intellectually reason with and also with a couple of White people who had been quiet in the heated reaction during the presentation but afterwards, during a reception, sidled-up beside me and whispered – 'thank you, we can't say those things' – then slipping-off into the crowd before I had a chance to reflect. This really struck a chord and was demonstrative of the all-so common de-centring of social class and attempts at consigning it a shibboleth.

My response to those who resent my promotion of social class/capitalism for explaining racism rather than the *White Supremacy* concept has been that I have been physically attacked on three occasions because of the colour of my skin, I certainly do understand and feel racism. My critique is rooted in the fact that I am a non-White person, not despite it, and it is from this position that I perceive the fundamental primary importance of class, and recognise the way that the *White supremacy* concept counterintuitively divides the working class for capitalism to operate most smoothly. In my publications, I have promoted the centrality of capitalist relations of production that acknowledges the way in which particular groups in society have historically, and continue to be, made to be *more* exploitable. This is a much more efficacious and comprehensive way to understand racism (see Cole, 2017, for developments of this work). To dismiss this account of reality is folly, my PhD study was instrumental for me arriving at this position.

Mystification and Feasibility

My PhD focussed on social class consciousness and practices in Sweden. I set-out to explore social class in a social democratic country that provided the conditions for historic and comparable low levels of inequality. Of course, in a country where egalitarianism and humanitarianism has been the governing objective, my study on social class inequality elicited interest, and, importantly, it helped me navigate the complexities of its material manifestation. What I got to be most valuable was the discovery of deep mechanisms that elided equity (distribution of opportunities) and equality (outcomes) that I used to develop an explanatory framework (see Maisuria, 2017, pp. 183–191). This framework focussed on the interdependent mechanisms of *mystification* and *feasibility* (see Maisuria, 2017, pp. 183–191). The former was about the way that neoliberalism was made to be being confusing and veiled (what I called *mystified*), and as a result largely negated in consciousness and explanations of social class (and racism). This was facilitated by claims such as 'equity exists for all' in Sweden – this argument can be observed beyond Sweden in the form of social mobility hubris. Moreover, when the mystification was unveiled and the feasibly of claims about equity were shown to be fallacious, then feasibility claims were redeployed to be about the *un*feasibility of an alternative to address inequality (see Maisuria, 2017; Maisuria, 2023).

As an academic, I have devoted much time to critiquing and disseminating these manoeuvres to deflect away from class inequality and neoliberalism. Using Critical Realism, I elaborate on these points in Maisuria (2022, pp. 493–494), here is a glimpse:

> Working against mystification and promoting a belief in the feasibility of alternatives to the neo-liberal class-based status quo is probably the greatest task for critical educators and activists for social justice. In Western and economically developed countries, the struggle is hard because neo-liberal capitalism is deeply established in the ideological, political, social and cultural realms that are enmeshed in creating the conditions in which a mass *common sense* is manufactured. This *common sense* that has prevailed, since the fall of the Berlin Wall, emerges through

some identifiable mechanisms. These are oscillating in degrees of intra-dependency between:

- Neo-liberalism best serves the economy through talented individuals being rewarded:
  - Self-interest is key for us all to individually prosper.
  - The investment in the concept of *society*, rather than *self*, promotes social loafing and laziness. Selfishness is good because it incentivises and motivates.
- *There is no alternative* (TINA) to the status quo.
- The alternatives to neo-liberal capitalism that may/do exist are not feasible because:
  - They are less desirable because they promote reliance on welfare – those who scrounge from the State or rely on productive others,
  - On balance, the status quo is *as good as it gets*. The problems of inequality are outweighed by the good stuffs (i.e. the availability of commodities),
  - In the end, the communist/socialist alternative is not feasible because it is idealist and utopian, not practically realistic and will end with brutality and barbarism.
- Inequality is natural. It has always existed in human relations, and always will. It is nature and part of the history of past, and will be the history of the future.
- We are genetically wired to be competitive and neo-liberalism facilitates this most inner urge. Self-interest promoted in political economy and socio-culture (i.e. education policy that focuses on personal investment and return in the labour market) aligns with our nature.
- Neo-liberalism advances civilisation through advancement in productive technologies. AI and robotics as part of the 4th Industrial Revolution is great for efficiency, and if it means workers become dispensable because machines can do their jobs, then the company will become more profitable and the worker will try to up their productivity and/or opt for reskilling.

Over my teaching career, these have been incredibly productive points of discussion with students about social class and capitalism (and subsidiary discussion about identity, social mobility etc). The next stage comes organically when we discuss *what can be done* (to paraphrase Lenin), and the difficulty of struggle:

These messages are spread ubiquitously and they are the mechanisms that generate the *appearance* of the narrative that a) nothing *needs* to be done and/or b) nothing *can* be done for serious change. This latter point is effectively symbolised in the popular British cultural slogan: *keep calm and carry on* with suffixes such as *shopping, drinking tea,* and so forth. While these narratives and slogans may seem benign, they actually represent a deep mechanism that generates mystification that in turn generates a tendency for the maintenance neo-liberalism in every auspice of lived reality that is almost inescapable. The point here is that the dominant hegemonic ideology cannot exist without the infrastructural apparatus that supports it in lived reality, these include: schools, media, and popular culture, which seeks to establish the consciousness for its *consent*. The strategy for struggle needs to include educating about class relations and neo-liberalism. Along with the belief in social mobility and meritocracy, people have been conditioned to get-on with life with the message *be a striver rather than a moaning skiver*. In addition, very few people would want to risk themselves against the very powerful State apparatus for fear of reprisal and negative consequences. The continued successes of these apparatuses mean that there is relative stability – an equilibrium despite some knowledge of injustice.

(Maisuria, 2022, pp. 494–495)

I ask my students to contemplate: what is the masses' tolerance level of injustice and what are the mechanisms that create this level? The answers to this dual question can be the pressure points to strategically locate activism for the working class to be 'for itself'. I always maintain a note of optimism by asserting that even in the state of general and mass acquiescence to the status quo, spaces always exist for struggle because the twined narrative of 'neoliberalism is best' and 'there are no alternatives' are difficult mystifications to maintain by the ruling neoliberal class while gross inequalities and inequities are very evident.

Conclusion

I have argued that taking the gradational way of seeing social class as possessions and lifestyle choices that indicate social status grade negates the way that capitalism organises us into related but antagonistic classes. Possession of a comparably big house or flashy car may indicate a 'middle class' status, but this has little association with neoliberal capitalism, its social relations and production of value. Moreover, middle class status is likely to be built on borrowing and debt, and so this status is very temporary and/or precarious. In addition, gradational classification of class by status is denoted by relativity in temporal terms, and by geography too – one could be middle class in Bradford but not in the Cotswolds. And this is why I pivot understanding of social class to questions of wider social structure – neoliberal capitalism. However, I have not argued that socio-cultural status and gradational markers of social class (and also ethno-racial identity) are unimportant, of course they have an impact on people in a multiplicity of ways, especially in respect to disempowerment. Only recently, I was invited for interview at an elite university, and it struck me how the whole nature of the event was purposefully designed to intimidate those who were not schooled in buildings with oak panelled walls.

Finally, to reiterate, I have had three overarching objectives for this chapter: (1) to problematise gradational approaches to social class, arguing that a focus on status and socio-cultural markers denoting lifestyle choices does not hold explanatory power, (2) to critique the de-centering of social class, for which I used CRT as a case study, (3) to promote the explanatory power of approaching social class as an organisational relationship in the service of capitalism that subsumes and accommodates racism and other identities and personal characteristics. I have been settled on navigating class through a Marxist Critical Realist lens because of its ability to power explanation of the condition of modern society, and importantly provide a bellicose attitude for struggle.

Note

1. I have used 'race' with inverted commas to recognise the socio-political and ideological nature of this particular term. See Maisuria (2011, pp. 80–81) for an extended discussion.

References

Asher, G., Cowden, S., Housee, S., & Maisuria, A. (2022). *Critical pedagogy and emancipation: A festschrift in memory of Joyce Canaan*. Oxford: Peter Lang.
Bhaskar, R. (1993). *Dialectic: The pulse of freedom*. London: Verso.
Bhaskar, R. (2016). *Enlightened common sense – The philosophy of critical realism*. London: Routledge.
Canaan, J. (2005). Developing a pedagogy of critical hope. *LATISS: Learning and Teaching in the Social Sciences*, 2(3), 159–174. doi:10.1386/ltss.2.3.159/1
Canaan, J., & Singh, G. (2013). Joyce Canaan on the neoliberal university, critical pedagogy and popular education. In S. Cowden, G. Singh, S. Amsler, & S. Motta (Eds.), *Acts of knowing: Critical pedagogy in, against and beyond the university* (pp. 145–161). London: Bloomsbury.
Cole, M. (2017). *New developments in critical race theory and education: Revisiting racialized capitalism and socialism in austerity*. London: Palgrave MacMillan.
Cole, M., & Maisuria, A. (2007). "Shut the f*** up", "you have no rights here": Critical race theory and racialisation in post-7/7 racist Britain. *Journal for Critical Education Policy Studies*, 5(1).
Department for Education. (2020). Guidance plan your relationships, sex and health curriculum. *Information to Help School Leaders Plan, Develop and Implement the New Statutory Curriculum*. Retrieved from https://www.gov.uk/guidance/plan-your-relationships-sex-and-health-curriculum
Equality and Human Rights Commission. (2021). Protected characteristics. Retrieved from https://www.equalityhumanrights.com/en/equality-act/protected-characteristics

Hill, D., & Maisuria, A. (2022). Social class: Education, social class and Marxist theory. In A. Maisuria (Ed.), *Encyclopaedia of Marxism and education* (pp. 624–643). Leiden/Boston: Brill.

Maisuria, A. (2011). A critical appraisal of critical race theory (CRT): Limitations and opportunities. In K. Bhopal & J. Preston (Eds.), *Intersectionality and race in education* (pp. 76–97). London: Routledge.

Maisuria, A. (2017). *Class consciousness and education in Sweden: A Marxist analysis of revolution in a social democracy*. London: Routledge.

Maisuria, A. (2020). Hegemony. In S. Themelis (Ed.), *Critical reflections on the language of neoliberalism in education: Dangerous words and discourses of possibility* (pp. 84–92). London: Routledge.

Maisuria, A. (2022). Neoliberalism and revolution: Marxism for emerging critical educators. In A. Maisuria (Ed.), *Encyclopaedia of Marxism and education* (pp. 483–500). Leiden/Boston: Brill.

Maisuria, A. (2023). Mystification of production and feasibility of alternatives social class inequality and education. In M. Cole (Ed.), *Education, equality and human rights* (5th ed.). London: Routledge.

Maisuria, A., & Banfield, A. (2022). Working with critical realism: Stories of methodological encounters (A. Maisuria & G. Banfield, Eds.). Routledge.

Marx, K. (1852). *The eighteenth Brumaire of Louis Bonaparte*. Retrieved from https://www.marxists.org/archive/marx/works/download/pdf/18th-Brumaire.pdf

Marx, K., & Engels, F. (1848). Manifesto of the communist party. *Marxists Internet Archive*. Retrieved from https://www.marxists.org/archive/marx/works/1848/communist-manifesto/

Mathison, S., & Ross, W. E. (2022). Critical education. In A. Maisuria (Ed.), *Encyclopaedia of Marxism and education* (pp. 129–146). Leiden/Boston: Brill.

Mayo, P. (2015). *Hegemony and education under neoliberalism. Insights from Gramsci*. London: Routledge.

Thatcher, M. (1975, September). *Let our children grow tall*. Speech to the institute of SocioEconomic Studies.

Thatcher, M. (1987). Interview for woman's own ("no such thing as society") in Margaret Thatcher foundation. *Women's Own*.

Webber, J. (2015, July). E. P. Thompson's romantic Marxism. *Jacobin*.

Willis, P. (1979). *Learning to labour: How working-class kids get working class jobs*. Farnborough: Saxon House.

Chapter 2

Mr Airport Man and the Albatross: A Reverie of Flight, Hope and Transformation

Craig A. Hammond

Abstract

This chapter is an autoethnographic account of my journey from a working-class childhood and youth to becoming an academic in a large UK university. Using the techniques of poetics (Bachelard, 2004), the chapter focuses on several pivotal periods in my life, where I encountered a sequence of events that were to influence my journey towards transformation. Back in my early 20s, I knew that I wanted to change and to grow in new directions; however, infused with a particular heritage, set of experiences and cultural values – none of which embraced, recognised or understood learning and university as a possibility – I struggled to make sense of my feelings of frustration and being stranded. This is where my strange fascination with the airport, music, daydream and the notion of flight emerged (see Bachelard, 2011; Seres, 1993). Here, the nebulous and seemingly futile ache for an alternative and better future emerged as a potent hope and journey towards transition.

Keywords: Gaston Bachelard; dynamic imagination; flight; reverie; Albatross; memory

This is a story about two angels. You may be similar to Michel Seres's character *Jacques* in *Angels: A Modern Myth* (1993) and think that the notion of angels is either childish or naïve, and that people shouldn't believe in such '[s]imple-minded stories for kids!' (Seres, 1993, p. 115). But I urge you, bear with me, and think about what I have to say; the two angels that I wish to tell you about initiated a powerful journey of transformation back in the 1990s, and enabled me to transgress an ascribed life of working-class childhood and youth. I have retrospectively given them the following names: *Zaphkiel* and *Israfel*. *Zaphkiel*, as he is a ruling angel of the planet Saturn (Guiley, 2004, p. 374), and in angel lore is

The Lives of Working Class Academics, 17–28
Copyright © 2023 Craig A. Hammond
Published under exclusive licence by Emerald Publishing Limited
doi:10.1108/978-1-80117-057-420221002

recognised as being a special guide – or preceptor angel – to Noah (Davidson, 1971, p. 227). This is an important heritage, and one that has relevance for my story, as the *Book of Jubilees* notes, Noah received guidance on the building of the ark, was bestowed knowledge of redemption, and given restorative secrets of healing (Segal, 2007, p. 171).[1] *Zaphkiel's* connection with the planet Saturn is also relevant, as Rudolf Steiner notes in *Rosicrucianism Renewed* (2007), the planet Saturn is powerfully symbolic where the principles of liberation and renewal are concerned. The other angel messenger in this story is *Israfel*; so chosen because in Arabic folklore, he is referred to as the angel of music, song, and resurrection (Davidson, 1971, p. 151). Hence, where *Zaphkiel* represents the mediation of escape and redemption (Davidson, 1971, p. 147), *Israfel* is associated with music and its cipheric ability to encode transformative messages of hope and change.[2]

Etymologically the word angel derives from the Greek term angelos, itself a translation from the Hebrew word *mal'akh* – both terms mean messenger or envoy. As Seres tells us, angelic messengers usually remain invisible, however, they also have the ability to make themselves 'appear and then disappear ... [and] move through space at the speed of their own thoughts' (Seres, 1993, p. 7).[3] As my story unfolds, *Zaphkiel* and *Israfel* will hopefully come to be understood as important envoys for another character that I wish to introduce here, that of *Mr Airport Man*. A literary leitmotif, *Mr Airport Man* is a historiographic version of me, back in the 1990s; at this time, I was a 22-year-old weaver, working on a rotating 8-hour shift pattern at a local textile mill.

I first started to encounter the alter ego of *Mr Airport Man* when I caught the train from my hometown of Blackburn to Manchester Airport, every third week – on a Monday, which was the first day of my 22.00 to 06.00 night shift (and a day that was relatively 'free'). Sometimes my airport visits would need to be quite brief, so I would buy a coffee, sit in the café and runway viewing area of *Terminal One* and listen to music. Occasionally, if weather and time permitted, I would walk around the periphery of the airport to the outdoor viewing area, to get a closer view of the runway, and experience the aircraft landing and taking-off in proximal and visceral detail.

I must point out that all of the details relating to *Mr Airport Man* are now lodged in the annals of my distant memory; as such, I can only recall – and recollect – elastic fragments. Chronology and details relating to the minutiae of these everyday events are now long gone; after all, their memorial and rever-berative traces extend and refract across an almost 30-year period. As such, I am not able to specify the precise number of times that I ventured across to Man-chester, to reunite *Mr Airport Man* with *Zaphkiel* and *Israfel*. However, over the 5-to-6-year period that these events relate, I would suggest that they accumulated to at least double-digit figures. My traces of *Mr Airport Man's* pilgrimages are therefore a mismatched patchwork of registered instants; some tinged with coldness and rain, and some with a backdrop of warm and pleasant sunny weather. The above points are important, and worth emphasising, as they are a key aspect of the style – and methodology – adopted to shape and structure this piece of autoethnographic writing. What follows is a reflective accumulation of aphoristic fragments, loosely sutured texts that, as a whole, build a montage of personalised, asynchronous and *nostalgic* insights.[4] Non-chronological in sequence, they connect and relate as a subjective trove of memorial debris, as well as an array of allegoric experiences, and replete with a retroactive symbolism, which I have developed and applied to aid emphasis and relevance.

I also use the term nostalgic here purposefully; as Boym (2001) tells us, it is akin to, 'a mania of longing'; as such, my memories harbour a nostalgic capacity, 'for remembering sensations, tastes, sounds [and] smells' (Boym, 2001, p. 4). *Mr Airport Man* is therefore – and always was – a nostalgic character; a private expression and manifestation of personal longing, the symbolic start point of an embarkation on a grail-like quest, in search of socio-economic escape, and the discovery of a new homeland never previously experienced. Further borrowing from Boym's typological analysis of nostalgia, my selection of recollected experiences should be considered as creative and restorative stories, rather than factual statements that relay fixed details as historical accounts. The resultant segments are therefore an attempt to, 'make sense of [my] seemingly ineffable homesickness' (Boym, 2001, p. 41) as a pre-destined and emplaced working-class 'conscript', and the subsequent search for hope, escape and transformation – as an undergraduate student, and later as an academic. The nostalgic stories contained here are therefore dislocated palimpsests, memorial texts repopulated with hindsight, academic enculturation in the form of a Bachelardean philosophy, and a malleable approach to content and time.

As Gaston Bachelard tells us in *Dialectic of Duration* (2000), the mind is an ultra-sensitive time detector, with an ability to conjoin discontinuities that characterise the shifting nature of archived time; as we listen inwardly to its segments, they morph, interpenetrate and cascade within us (Bachelard, 2000, p. 81). In *Intuition of the Instant*, Bachelard reinforces this and tells us that the seductive malleability of memory means that we do not encounter its re-emergence as a unified set of in-tact details. As a receptor of myriad incidents, the mind performs alternative manoeuvres by subjecting remnants to the processes and impact of daydreaming – or within the context of a Bachelardean theoretical framework reverie. As such, originary details become smashed and reconstituted as infusive sets of discrete instants (Bachelard, 2013, p. 10). He thus reminds us that:

> ...the asymmetry between past and future is radical. In us, the past is a voice that has found an echo. We thus attribute a force to what is no more than a form – or better yet, we assign one sweeping form to a plurality of forms. It is through such a synthesis that the past begins to take on the weight of reality.
>
> (Bachelard, 2013, p. 31)

In this domain of mutations, the creative act of memorial recounting takes place through a punctuated terrain of creative instants (Bachelard, 2013, pp. 9–10). Full of lacunae, these irruptions merge along their peripheries, and develop as a dust of novel emergences (Bachelard, 2000, p. 112). Bachelard would therefore have positively recognised my memorial malleations and regarded them as affirmative permutations, as he notes,

...we realize that the deformation we impose on things always means actively acquired information. And so it is a question of taking shape, often with great difficulty, rather than losing shape. Thus, we come to experience deformation as dynamism.

(Bachelard, 2018, p. 17)

Language and Childhood

Basil Bernstein (2003) tells us that particular social groups organise around common principles of socio-economic communication; as part of this, they produce particular forms – and patterns – of language and inter-subjective speech codes. Such differences within and across particular social groups extend far beyond styles and nuance in dialect; they 'occur in the normal social environment and [are] ... distinguished by their forms of speech' (Bernstein, 2003, p. 46). In my own immediate and extended family environment, I recall hearing conversations about winning the *Littlewoods Football Pools*, and what we would do with the money; unsavoury monologues about the alleged perils of immigration; and the immediacy of not being able to afford things due to constant and lingering money problems. I also recall heated exchanges about the precarity and aftermath of being made redundant; and to 'just do the best that you can at school' (which overall, was pretty terrible – as it just didn't make sense or seem relevant to me). Slang, dialect, idiosyncratic and staccato peculiarities very much characterised the style and content of these conversations. A distinctive, colourful and in some ways quite unique heritage, but one that wasn't embraced, recognised or accepted by middle-class standards (characteristics which, of course framed and communicated the cultural milieu of the school environment). At home, foundational and pivotal skills associated with successful schooling, such as academic progression, critical reading, debating balanced arguments, seeking out evidence etc., did not feature at all. I carried this void of purpose relating to the alien environment of the school and wider educational knowledge throughout my entire compulsory schooling experience.

In a complementary sense, Pierre Bourdieu (1996) identifies the *habitual* cultural styles and influences cascaded and perpetuated as part of class-based environments; again, within the working-class environments of my childhood and youth, these aspects were really quite distinct and socio-economically particular. I recall that as a family we considered popular music and mainstream cinema (and in the late 1970s/1980s the emergence of video), package holidays to Spain, sport, second-hand cars, clothing fashion and home décor of particular relevance and importance. However, this was always situated against the backdrop of a habitus tinged with financial precarity and debt, and the increasing realisation that the socio-economic horizon of a working-class future had been ingloriously and systemically predestined. All of this was bluntly reinforced by several flattening and ultimately rather pointless meetings in my final year at school with a peripatetic career's advisor. Based on two meetings and conversations, it was summarised for me – in descending order – that I had the 'dole' to look forward to, but only if the other slightly more appealing options of: labourer, factory worker, or soldier in the army didn't materialise.[5] Thinking back, I was vaguely aware that some of my school peers – those who had consistently populated the 'top sets' – were going to college to do A-levels; however, again, the meaning of this didn't really register, as I had no immediate or extended reference points to guide me, through either dialogue or lived experience.[6] I just didn't know what this all meant; the notion of college, A-levels, pathways to university, studying towards and reading for a degree etc. had never featured as part of our everyday family discourse. For all of the points of criticism levelled at Bernstein and his theory of linguistic codes, within the microcosm of my own lived experience, his analysis seems to have been largely correct.

However, what I did have – and frequently engaged with – was an important form of escape facilitated by the music that I listened to. Through the abysmal schooling experiences, the tribulations and traumas of socio-economic precarity, and the realisation that as a consequence of my working-class positionality (in the late 1980s), my opportunities were to be somewhat limited; I sought – and found – solace in an unconquerable and private world of music-hued reverie. This deep relationship with music had always been with me – or so it seemed. One of my earliest recollections was getting permission to play records on my parents' turntable. I guess the year will have been circa 1978, when I was only 7 or 8 years old; on this occasion, one record in particular intrigued and resonated with me: It had a painted scene on the sleeve, a solitary bird hovering over the sea; this was set against a beach, and beyond this was a forest that seemed to stretch into and beyond the horizon. The record was *Albatross* by Fleetwood Mac, and I was entranced.

I recall listening to this over and over and gazing *in*to the picture on the record sleeve. I had no words to articulate, but reflecting back on this formative moment, I experienced a profound sense of emotion; whilst this seemed tinged with an emerging melancholia, it also harboured hope and beauty. I imagined soaring and escaping as a bird to a deserted tropical island; the warmth of the sun, and the unbridled possibility of having the freedom to do anything – liberated from the bleak constraints of my everyday life – was quite wonderful. Whilst I hadn't named him at this early age, I got a sense that somehow *Israfel* was making an initial appearance, transcribing the tentative beginning of a hidden code in my mind, and registering the initial outline of a map of future escape. Bachelard would suggest that this encounter uncovered a special type of flight, one of dynamic imagination. The whole aesthetic associated with evocative music, the image of the bird and the sky, situated against a limitless ocean and forest, prompted an early awakening of imaginary flight. For the unspecified duration of a few fleeting moments, I was mesmerised by the visual beauty of the bird in its solitary flight, and my young imagination was liberated beyond the ordinary course of everyday things. Far from being a gentle take-off, the experience resonated as a 'gushing forth of being', and a fleeting experience of 'new life' (Bachelard, 2011, p. 155).

Excursus 1: The Albatross

The albatross belongs to a taxonomic group of birds called Procellariiformes; this name comes from – and is associated with – the Latin word *procella*, which means 'violent wind' or 'storm' (Lindsey, 2008, p. 4). Traditionally, two species of albatross are seen as belonging to this group: the royal albatross and the wandering albatross (Lindsey, 2008, p. 13). The name albatross has been through a number of iterations and permutations and is derived from the term *alcatrace*, a term that Spanish and Portuguese navigators adapted from the Arabic word *alcatraz* or *al-gaṭṭas*' which identified a kind of sea eagle. With reference to the bird itself, two characteristics in particular appear to have captured the public imagination, these being its great size, and also its seemingly miraculous ability to navigate enormous seafaring distances with graceful ease, over relatively short periods of time (Lindsey, 2008, p. 7). The most influential taxonomist where the albatross is concerned is probably the Swedish scientist Carl von Linné (1707–1778), known commonly by his latinized name, *Linnaeus*. In 1758, he included the first formal scientific description of the bird in his influential text *Systema Naturae* (Barwell, 2014, p. 26). Introducing the albatross to Western science, *Linnaeus* attached two additional epithets: Diomedea and exulans. Exulans is a Greek word that translates as 'exile', and Diomedea relates to *Diomedes*, a character from classical Greek legend. Diomedes was a prominent figure in Homer's Iliad; serving with Odysseus and Palamedes as a naval commander, they sailed with Agamemnon to lay siege to Troy, and recover the abducted Helen. However, Diomedes later offended the goddess Athene, an offence to which she responded by conjuring a ferocious sea storm, which ultimately wrecked and sank his fleet. A vengeful goddess, she drowned his men, turned them into large birds, and prevented Diomedes from returning home by committing him to exile on a deserted island (Barwell, 2014, pp. 26–27).

The *wandering albatross* or Diomedea exulans is therefore a lifelong and homeless wanderer. There is evidently something metaphorical, powerful and evocative about this; public and poetic fascination with the albatross maybe as a result of its size, or its graceful stature and demeanour, or the way that it permanently travels and roams across oceans – by utilising the up drift of ferocious storms – or maybe a combination of all of these things. Lindsey (2008) confirms this, and notes that it is 'not easy to be entirely unmoved by' this wanderer, the albatross as storm-rider and ultimate flying machine (Lindsey, 2008, p. 3).

Bachelard suggests that the *flying* creature is imaginatively profound because it seems capable of escaping its immediate environments, and utilises an invisible ether to transcend gravity and ground; as such it is a conscious visualisation of our latent freedom (Bachelard, 2011, p. 8). Provoking an aerial imagination, it becomes a winged seed, 'which, at the slightest breath of air, is seized with the hope of rising' (Bachelard, 2011, p. 157). Aerial imagination thus asserts itself when we encounter images that soar upwards and vanish. However, to extend this beyond mere personal story, requires us to learn how to rise up, to imagine and fly without hesitation, 'whithersoever we are impelled – we free-born birds! Wherever we come, there will always be freedom' (Bachelard, 2011, p. 158).

I feel that through music and daydream I learned to imagine and explore as a Diomedea exulans, and this has served me well. My wandering has meant that I have been able to drift beyond earlier storms into new adventures, and with this a range of unexpected discoveries. Experiences that I would never have encountered had I not set-off in search of a strange and little understood (on my part) land of academic mystery. Certainly, time spent battling my fears and inadequacies in different universities as an undergraduate and postgraduate, and later as an academic, has required intense study, dedication, sacrifice and a committed work ethic. But the strength and belief to leave my previous positionality, to mutate my identity and enter into, participate, and grow as an academic exile, has been undergirded by the important experience of imaginative flight and aerial escape. Now, as a working-class exile in the territories of academia, I am proud of my heritage, and of the distance that I have travelled. But I do not mourn my exile; I do not miss it or the terrain of my heritage – with confining limitations. I do still have a working-classness, and this will always be a part of me; but I am no longer working class.

Mr Airport Man

It is summer 1993; there is a slight breeze, but the sun is warm enough to make it pleasant; I've gotten to the airport nice and early, and so walk around to the outdoor aircraft viewing area. I am surrounded by plane spotters, uniformly bedecked with binoculars, *Airband scanners* and zoom lens cameras; a veritable band of butterfly collectors. I have got my *Walkman*, pen and notepad; equipped with these, I start to scribble random thoughts, words and ideas; embryonic hopes, distant and seemingly unrealistic possibilities; bad poems and unfinished lyrics for never-written songs. Somehow, I just know – and sense – that through *Zaphkiel* (as he fleetingly takes on the form of an ascending aircraft) that I need to gaze into and imagine beyond his skyward messages of longing. That with *Israfel*, as he mediates a music-hued cipher through my Walkman, that I have to translate and annotate their meditations as talismanic echoes. I also know that somehow I need to believe that I can escape from the constraints of the life that is crushing me.

A *British Airways* 747 jumbo jet reaches the end of the taxiway and turns on to the runway, and I find that once again, almost 20 years later, I am listening to the song *Albatross*. Beyond the throttle and thrust of the accelerating aircraft, I am reminded that this is no ordinary fascination with flight; it is something more than – and quite unrelated to – the strange practice of butterfly collecting.[7] Beyond the musical traces and jet engine vapour trails, I discern my messengers' codes, and start to refibrillate the sputtering belief and possibility that a new journey can be travelled. In a memory whorl, excavated by the beautiful music, I am enveloped by a powerful reminiscence; through the visual wonder of flight and dynamic imagination, the ascending aircraft pinches my breath. I somehow know – and sense – that *Zaphkiel* is a silver metal albatross, and *Israfel*, a muse, and that they want me to follow and embark on a journey of ascensional longing and personal change, and hunt for jettisoned and discarded traces of hope. I see pulsing lights on the undercarriage of the mechanical albatross, and they shimmer throughout its graceful ascent. About four or five miles in the distance, they glint and blink one last time before finally disappearing into a thin cloud blanket; with this, seated at the edge of the aeroplane viewing area, I start to recognise myself as *Mr Airport Man*; equipped with imaginative and transformative possibilities, I start to pursue a very different and alternative journey.

Bachelard reminds us that the notions of *wing*, *cloud* and imaginary flight evoke the dreamer to mutate into whatever they wish; they can incite visions or sketches of something beyond the limitations of a lived life (Bachelard, 2011, p. 13). In doing so, the dreamer, 'that twin of our being' opens up the adventures of reverie, and, accepting the help of great dreamers, enters into the world of the poets (Bachelard, 2012, p. 8). In this potent state of reverie, dreamers dream of what they could have been and in rebellion against themselves, dream of what they could and should be. But to start to establish an alternative future beyond the realm of its internal idea, requires that the values and principles of flight find a physical channel to facilitate release (Bachelard, 2011, p. 10). As a result of the shaping function of time, year by year, 'we end up resembling ourselves. We gather all of our beings around the unity of our name' (Bachelard, 2004, p. 99); but to move beyond the folded threads of our history, shaped and told to us by others, we need to activate the power of ascensional escape, by discovering and pursuing a forgotten childhood that becomes hidden within us. We need to learn to activate the latency of internal rebirth, through the power of reverie of flight beyond our own past; by searching for the pre-established building blocks of malleable childhood, we can engage in renewal. In doing this, learn how to reconstruct an alternative childhood beyond the one of the existing person, and to grow and soar in place of groundedness and disappointment. My meditations on the new child that I could become, beyond the existing constraints of family and socio-economic history, with its zones of regret and defeat, meant that I could search for a new and reanimated life (Bachelard, 2004, p. 126). By activating an imaginative reverie, using my new name – Mr Airport Man – notions of my old self were gradually ridded of prior labels and assumptions. With this, my potent reveries as a solitary child rose again as a forgotten fire, which 'can always flare up again within us' (Bachelard, 2004, p. 104).

Excursus 2: Back to the Future

It is December 2021, I'm away from home on a research trip, and things are a little bit strange down here in Oxford (but in a good way I think). As I start to write my autoethnographic piece, I rediscover *Mr Airport Man*, and I'm reminded of how I used to daydream of becoming something and somebody else. I absolutely didn't know who – or what; I just knew that to survive I needed to change, and to find a way of liberating my ache to be, do and give so much more. Memory work obviously necessitates the revisitation and confronting of past events (and permutations of oneself) that are forgotten; well, still there, but embedded beneath the surface, and blanketed by layers of later and more comfortable memorial material. Having excavated down and through to those earlier layers tonight, I've felt so desperately sad for the traces of that lost young man. I'd forgotten just how unhappy, barren and almost defeated he was.

As seems to be the case when I start writing something fresh, a new song serendipitously emerges and attaches itself to me. When I first hear it, I intuitively know that the song somehow harbours an unfolding message that I need to creatively decipher. Tonight, that song is *Dreaming of You* (Gonzalez, 2012). Irrespective of what the songwriter intended, tonight it has helped me resolve *Mr Airport Man's* lingering sadness; it has become a nostalgic love-song from the past, and transmorphed into a message from the 22-year-old me to a 50-year-old me. Through a strange quantum portal, *Mr Airport Man* is looking through to the future, and seeing a mirage of me as an albatross, and sending a message of longing out to me. In return – I don't know if he can hear me – but I'm calling back to him, and telling him to just hang-on because one day he'll be in the Bodleian libraries in Oxford as an academic; and he will have a beautiful, strong and loving wife; five of the most fantastic, funny, intelligent children; and six of the most enchanting grandchildren …

I'm glad that he held on …

I'm glad that he listened to the coded ciphers of hope from *Zaphkiel* and *Israfel*, and learned how to soar, travel and wander on the gales and uplifts of his storms. I'm glad that he resisted the urge to not get on the train for his first Open University class in 1994 (as he didn't feel that he was intelligent or good enough). I'm glad that he made friends with a *Hazey* anarchist at university in 1996, who helped him to discover a philosophical home in the works of Bloch, Benjamin, Buber and Scholem, and to recognise that some voids can only be filled by love; and that structural working-class wounds can't be healed through violence and anger. I'm glad that he listened to his wife, to use his passion and ideas to pursue a PhD. I'm glad that he became an *albatross exulans* and chose wandering over his structural positionality. I'm glad that he hoped, reached for and discovered an alternative childhood and subsequent transformed life as *Mr Airport Man* …

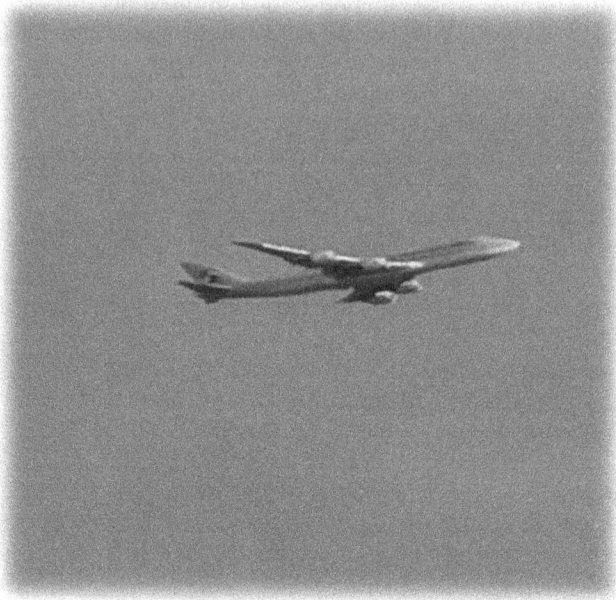

Personal Photograph Taken by the Author.

Notes

1. A related note of interest here, the word Jubilee refers to a year of emancipation or restoration. Segal further notes that the angel told Noah, 'the remedies for the afflictions of mankind and all kinds of remedies for healing with trees of the earth and plants of the soil and their roots. And he sent the princes of the remaining spirits to show Noah the medicinal trees with all their shoots, greenery, grasses, roots and seed, to explain to him why they were created, and to teach him all their medicinal properties for healing and for life' (Segal, 2007, p. 171).

2. Edgar Allan Poe's poem *Israfel* attests to the redemptive power of this angel in relation to music and song (Poe, 2005, pp. 273–275).

3. Seres in *Angels: A Modern Myth* suggests that airports and aircraft present us with 'angels of steel, carrying angels of flesh and blood, who in turn send angel signals across angel air waves ... Aircraft carry letters, telephones, agents, representatives and the like: we use the term communication to cover air transport as well as post. When people, aircraft and electronic signals are transmitted through the through the air, they are all effectively messages and messengers' (Seres, 1993, p. 8).

4. The notion of text is again purposeful here, and worthy of further elaboration. Its etymology is texere (which means 'to weave'), and texo (which means 'I weave'), therefore, my ruminations on memory and meaning should be read as nomadic, autonomic and unique offerings; the usurpation of the presence, legacy and coherence of the original context (Barthes, 1989). This renders the reception and transmission of biographic history as a fertile process, as its echoes resound and

malleate between the historical source and the contemporary receiver, in an open space of parallax and fracture. The lacunae between the event and the subjective recreation of memory does not perpetuate a trammelled or predictable form of unimpinged and unchanging material (Barthes, 1973).

5. I did join the army at 16 and have written about aspects of this in Hammond (2017); see Chapter 6, *Bye Bye Badman: The Redemption of Hope through Popular Culture.*

6. At secondary school, I did find geography and especially social geography fascinating, and during my options year (year 3 in 1985), I constantly came top of the class in tests. I recall asking to speak to the teacher, and almost pleading with them to allocate me a place in the GCE O-level group. But his response was, 'based on your low achievement in other subjects, I don't want to give you false hope'.

7. Walter Benjamin notes that: 'butterflies with superbright wings ... so often had lured me away from well-kept garden paths into a wilderness ... the more I strove to conform ... the more butterfly-like I became in my heart and soul ... in the end, it was as if [...] capture was the price I had to pay' (Benjamin, 2006, pp. 50–51).

Acknowledgement

The author would like to thank the Philosophy of Education Society of Great Britain (PESGB) for a small grant that supported the production of this chapter as part of the funded project: *A Catechism for Oedipus: A Critical Approach to Pedagogic Practice in Higher Education.*

References

Bachelard, G. (2000). *Dialectic of duration* (M. M. Jones, Trans.). Manchester: Clinamen.

Bachelard, G. (2004). *The poetics of reverie: Childhood, language and the cosmos* (D. Russell, Trans.). Boston, MA: Beacon Press.

Bachelard, G. (2011). *Air & dreams: An essay on the imagination of movement* (E. R. Farrell, & F. C. Farrell, Trans.). Dallas, TX: The Dallas Institute Publications.

Bachelard, G. (2012). *The flame of a candle* (J. Caldwell, Trans.). Dallas, TX: The Dallas Institute Publications.

Bachelard, G. (2013). *Intuition of the instant* (E. Rizo-Patron, Trans.). Evanston, IL: Northwest University Press.

Bachelard, G. (2018). *Atomistic intuitions: An essay on classification* (R. C. Smith, Trans.). New York, NY: SUNY.

Barthes, R. (1973). *The pleasure of the text* (R. Miller, Trans.). New York, NY: Hill and Wang.

Barthes, R. (1989). The death of the author. In *The rustle of language* (pp. 49–55). Los Angeles, CA: University of California Press.

Barwell, G. (2014). *Albatross*. London: Reaktion Books.

Benjamin, W. (2006). *Berlin childhood around 1900* (H. Eiland, Trans.). Cambridge, MA: Belknap Press.

Bernstein, B. (2003). *Class, codes and control: Volume I theoretical studies towards a sociology of language.* London: Routledge.

Bourdieu, P. (1996). *Distinction: A social critique of the judgement of taste* (R. Nice, Trans.). Cambridge, MA: Harvard University Press.

Boym, S. (2001). *The future of nostalgia.* New York, NY: Basic Books.

Davidson, G. (1971). *A dictionary of angels.* New York, NY: Free Press.

Gonzalez, G. (2012). *Dreaming of you.* On cigarettes after sex. Partisan Records.

Guiley, E. R. (2004). *The encyclopedia of angels* (2 ed.). New York, NY: Visionary Living, Inc.

Hammond, C. A. (2017). Hope, utopia & creativity. In *Higher education: Pedagogical tactics for alternative futures.* London: Bloomsbury Academic.

Lindsey, T. (2008). *Albatrosses.* Collingwood, VIC: CSIRO PUBLISHING.

Poe, E. A. (2005). *The collected works of Poe* (Vol. V). San Diego, CA: ICON Group International, Inc.

Segal, M. (2007). *The book of Jubilees.* Leiden: Brill.

Seres, M. (1993). *Angels: A modern myth* (F. Cowper, Trans.). Paris: Flammarion.

Steiner, R. (2007). *Rosicrucianism renewed* (M. Post, Trans.). Great Barrington, MA: Steiner Books.

Chapter 3

Power, Corruption and Lies: Fighting the Class War to Widen Participation in Higher Education

Colin McCaig

Abstract

Education is, or should be, a gateway to a better life, a better understanding of ourselves in a complex and hierarchical social world. As a political scientist from a working-class mature-student background I have been fortunate enough to build a career that not only celebrates and embodies the possibilities provided by educational access but also aims to highlight the staggering lengths the socially advantaged go to in their denial of educational opportunity for the vast majority of people from my background. Like all autoethnographies, I guess this contribution may seem an idiosyncratic take on working-class life and academia; it is at once a primal scream against ingrained classism we have to confront every day, but also a recognition of the intellectual pluralism and tolerance of academia that allows and rewards even members of the 'awkward squad' like me if we stick it out long enough. It is a rage against the machine, but hopefully, also a small step towards changing the definition of academia.

Keywords: Workers and bosses; supply–demand nexus; private versus public sector work; mature students; market differentiation; mythology of meritocracy

> I do not approve of anything that tampers with natural ignorance.
> Ignorance is like a delicate exotic fruit; touch it and the bloom is
> gone. The whole theory of modern education is radically unsound.
> Fortunately in England, at any rate, education produces no effect

The Lives of Working Class Academics, 29–40
Copyright © 2023 Colin McCaig
Published under exclusive licence by Emerald Publishing Limited
doi:10.1108/978-1-80117-057-420221003

whatsoever. If it did, it would prove a serious danger to the upper
classes, and probably lead to acts of violence in Grosvenor Square.
                    –Lady Bracknell, in *The Importance of being Earnest*,
                                              Oscar Wilde (2016)

Background – Early Life and Schooling

I was born at the very end of the 1950s in Luton, Bedfordshire. My father was a
Scottish apprenticed engineer and my mother a 'housewife' from a Scottish-Irish
background, although born in Kent. They had met in South East London in the
1950s and moved out to Luton (then an expanding London satellite town) in 1957
after the birth of my elder brother. A younger brother was born in 1964. We lived
in a council house, one of thousands built to accommodate the new influx of
migrant workers, especially after the opening of the first phase of M1 motorway
and the new Vauxhall Motors plant where my father was employed as a maintenance fitter, keeping the assembly line or 'track' running. He was also the
branch secretary for the AEU, the engineering workers' union, and a Labour
Party activist.

Holidays were almost always to Scotland where we stayed with relatives on my
father's side in Coatbridge and Airdrie, small industrial towns in the coal and steel
belt of Lanarkshire (to the east of Glasgow) with days trips to the Ayrshire coast,
lochs and Edinburgh (where my mother had lived during the war), with boat trips
to some of the inner islands. Although my father was a skilled worker who
worked all the overtime he could and we were never especially poor, we did
qualify for 'meal tickets' (FSM as it would be known today) when attending the
local comprehensive school, Icknield High, and were definitely aware of our
relative financial position because the school served both our small council
estate – Runfold – and private housing, including large detached houses in the
affluent Bedford Road area. While I was clearly aware that our family and those
of most of the estate kids were financially worse off than some of our peers,
friendship groups didn't usually form along class lines; it was more about football,
music, TV and movie tastes and personality. I had mates whose parents were
lawyers and doctors as well as builders and factory operatives and we all hung out
in each others' houses (ours was on the school cross-country route and groups of
us would routinely dive in there to dry off while mum made us sandwiches).
Living in a council house in the 1960s and 1970s didn't attract the opprobrium it
did in later decades – we weren't considered 'chavs' and 'pram faces' living as a
bovine underclass in 'sink estates' until *Shameless* and *Benefits Street* came along
to tell the middle classes just how underserving we were. Cheers, Channel 4, a
Tory invention to promote diversity but which cemented the trope that the only
skills the WC have are the ability to 'fiddle the benefits system'.

At school I was only ever good at English, History, Art and Geography and
won prizes for 'composition' and art at Junior School. I was rubbish at maths and
the sciences and was routinely in the top sets for the subjects I liked and the

bottom sets for those I didn't. I was always a bit of a 'class clown' (and was caned for larking about too much, a genuine badge of honour) and was quite popular, having mates on either side of the 'clever/funny' vs 'tough guys' divide. I was smart enough to talk myself into, and out of, trouble on a regular basis, a trait I seem not to have fully shaken off. I left school in 1976 with two GCE O levels (English language and History) and took up a job with WH Smith as a floor walker, though within months relegated to the store room for having hair judged to be too long, flares too wide and platform soles *way* too high.

What Class Means to Me and My Upbringing

While nobody I knew talked about class, even in a political household where I used to help my dad with his branch secretary paperwork, we all knew where we sat on the workers v bosses scale. The 1970s were politically tumultuous: strikes that brought down a Tory government; coal shortages that led to national power outages and homework by candlelight (luckily we had a coal-fired central heating system and a gas cooker); and the Yom Kippur War that led to a quadrupling of oil prices in the West and consequent food and petrol shortages. After 1975, with the Labour government reliant on minority support from the Liberals and the Ulster Unionists, the Tories with a strident new female leader who everyone just knew were going to win the next election. In 1979 they put duly Labour out of office, determined to destroy union power and go for high unemployment as the 'acceptable price to pay to tackle inflation' as Geoffrey Howe, the Tory Chancellor, noted at the time.

I continued in a series of low/no skilled jobs from the age of 16 to 31, with two periods of unemployment in the early 1980s, my only brush with educational self-improvement a Sociology A level at night school in 1983/1984; my first child, a son, was born between the two parts of the exam and I still (half-jokingly) blame him for only getting a D Grade. I enrolled on A level courses in Politics and Economics over the next couple of years but each time I had to drop out due to changing shift patterns at work (night shifts paid better and by 1986 we – married since 1978 – had two children and a mortgage to service); by this time I had seriously begun to regret leaving education at 16 and taking on ever more boring jobs with no intellectual stimulation and never enough money to do anything about it. In total I had 31 jobs over 15 years, my most valuable qualification a Fork Truck Driving Licence. None of those jobs, should they still exist, would be at the level of the minimum wage today.

Years later, as an academic I am not 'in the research' in the same way that a sociologist focussing on class or cultural identity might be, so class is not central to my work; however as political scientist focussing on HE policy, I know social class is absolutely central to the educational life chances of the poor and otherwise marginalised communities. Looking back, I suffered from the lack of such opportunities, what I now see as the systematic denial of educational opportunity by, and on behalf of, the middle and upper classes desperate to restrict wider entry to the professions they wanted to reserve for their own offspring.

Accessing HE was never on the radar for people like me (when I was 18 only about 10% of young people attended any kind of higher education), but that is probably more about working-class values back in the 1970s and my own family's relationship with the world of work. My father hoped I would end up working, maybe in an office rather than out in the cold, for a decent firm or one of the public utilities, but none of that was assumed to depend on education, and at 16 I had had enough of education anyway. Quite a few of my peers went on to FE college to 'learn a trade' (which you could access with two O levels), or even 6th Form College to take A levels (entry was 3 O levels or above) and thus get an office job; still others entered the Armed Services, all of which had excellent trade training, and one strange, quiet lad I was at school with was clearly destined for University (his dad was a stockbroker, whatever that meant) but I was happy just working for a living and having a bit of money and independence. I was envious of no one. It was a tough world with casual violence, drug taking and petty crime close to the surface, political and financial turmoil on every new bulletin, but it was 'our normal' and nobody I knew thought about it as class war until 'punk rock' entered our consciousness around 1977, and even then that seemed to be more about individual self-expression and anarchic rage against adulthood and conformity than about challenging economic inequality.

I didn't 'feel' particularly working class even as I raged against the Thatcher era and how it increased exploitation of people in low-paid, low-skill work like us. I knew people from my council estate that had gone on to work in the city and I knew old school mates from bigger houses and posher families that were working 'on the track' at Vauxhall or doing other low-status work, given the volatility of the labour market: in 1978–1979 I worked on the track alongside an airline pilot with a cut-glass accent who couldn't find work as oil price inflation and the consequent recession devastated the tourism industry. I always knew, however, that in general the rich exploit the poor/the powerful exploit the weak and the rationing of educational opportunity for those that 'deserve it', disguised as meritocracy, was central to the entrenchment of elites. During the Thatcher years the poor and minority ethnic groups were increasingly demonised, blamed for their own failure to succeed in this meritocracy, this 'class-less society' as John Major portrayed it. The Victorian morality concepts of 'deserving' and 'unde-serving poor' re-entered the discourse along with the return of charities and voluntary societies to the public feeding troughs. It was like Beveridge was never a thing, and Michael Young's *The Rise of the Meritocracy* wasn't a scathing satire.

I guess Lady Bracknell was right, education in England had no effect and it clearly suited the elites that we were so dis-educated that we were no threat to the toffs of Grosvenor Square.

Meanings of Working-Classness

For me the working classes were people who worked in the private sector of the economy for (not much) money – and that, to my consciousness, included routine office workers and those in retail, however smart they dressed, however warm, clean and comfortable their working environment compared with those I worked in. This kind of work context led to an awareness that if whatever your company made didn't sell enough units, or you weren't good at your job, you would be out of work regardless of what your 'permanent contract' said. The working classes, in this reading, are defined by their relationship to the supply–demand nexus within capitalism – as Marx and Engel realised – and I think that sometimes gets forgotten in sociological analyses that focus on WC culture. For me and my peers, working on the track at (US owned) Vauxhall Motors in the late 1970s or (Swedish owned) Electrolux making fridges and freezers in the early 1980s, it would be absurd to be calling for the overthrow of capitalism; we needed our employers to be better at the global economic rat race of capitalism so that we could (in theory) command higher, or at least more secure, wages.

Decisions made in Detroit and Stockholm determined our standard of living and state of the clothes our kids wore to school, and it wasn't uncommon for us to know of and comment about relative share prices in the works canteen. Of course, this was in those halcyon days when rising share prices accompanied the opening of more factories and the employment of more workers; from about the mid-1980s, improved share prices began to be linked to factory closures and the replacement of workers with automated manufacturing processes; often production was off-shored to places where labour was cheaper.

So we, the 'actual working classes' were necessarily very attuned to the changing basis of demand for labour in a way rarely acknowledged by middle-class academic sociologists (at least since Goldthorpe's Black Coated Workers studies, Goldthorpe, 1980). Consequently, the unwillingness of the working classes to call for the overthrow of capitalism was often branded as 'false consciousness' by the commentariat and academic sociologists. The longer I exist in the middle-class world of academia, the more ingrained I realise these beliefs are among my peers, even today. It is why I fight daily for higher education opportunities for all; I want to *change the definition of academics*, not just tritely theorise why the working classes are really better off getting 'back in their box'.

Mainly because of the auto-association between capital and labour in my mind, I would never, during those decades of factory/warehouse employment, have considered public sector workers as 'working class' in the same way as those that worked in the productive private sector. Even the lowest-paid council employees were protected from the vicissitudes of supply and demand: society would always need bin-men and park-keepers, (council) house painters and rent collectors; equally, well-respected professions made up of teachers, nurses, social workers and career advisers were protected from the harsh realities of the business cycle. They may not have earned much more than us, but they were (in those days at least) relatively protected from the precarity of life on the capitalist front line.

Class and My HE Journey

Entering the world of higher education at 31 in 1991 I had the same values I had as a teenager and was still poor, but I had long left the council estate I grew up in.

The dislocation from old school friends had already happened; we all grow physically apart (though often stay friends) as we age and enter other relationship through the normal processes, unless we stay in the same community (and that would likely apply to 'stay-homers' of any social class). Eventually, going to a Polytechnic at the age of 31 didn't feel like any kind of class departure to me, but I knew studying was different from (and a lot more rewarding than) working for a living, and given the level of pay in the kind of jobs I was giving up for a student grant, it wasn't even a financial sacrifice. My wife, who hadn't returned to full-time work after our children were born, also became a student at the same time, taking a four-year BEd degree; two grants plus some part-time work during the holidays brought our income up to what we had to live on when I worked 40 hours as a fork truck driver. Both graduating in 1994, we were pretty much instantly transferred into a much higher income bracket, even with my wife's primary teachers' entry-level salary supporting my postgrad studies (funded by ESRC for both the MA and PhD).

On enrolment at Huddersfield back in October 1991, I found a supportive environment where around 40 out of 150 on our BA degree (Historical and Political Studies) were mature students. Therefore I didn't feel the sense of class outsider-ness that many WC academics feel (e.g. Byrne, 2019; Mckenzie, 2015), certainly not the sense of being the only 18-year-old council-house kid from a Comprehensive at an elite university, surrounded by posh Grammar school kids. Being a mature student is also unusual in the literature – what coming from a working-class background means to someone like me with my work history (factories, warehouses, cold stores, security guard, aircraft cleaner, parcel delivery driver) is different to the deracination often noted by 18-year-old working-class school leavers when they progress to HE (any HE but especially selective HE). The confusion of going 'back home' at holidays and struggling to adjust with their former peers that never entered HE – the kind of social dislocation often reported by sociologists – never happened for me (for one thing, like most mature and most working-class students I was a commuter student and never lived in halls). Before I went back into education I had left home, married was on the 'property ladder' (i.e. mortgaged to the hilt), had two young children and had relocated to the north of England in 1989 to avoid financial penury. Cashing in on the huge difference between southern and northern house prices at that time, we sold our three-bedroom terraced house in Luton, paid off the mortgage and thousands more in credit card and other debts and bought a former council house in a West Yorkshire pit village for cash – and banked £15,000 on the deal. All of this long before even thinking of studying for a degree. By moving to Yorkshire we had bought ourselves options and a better lifestyle for our kids (aged two and four in 1989), even if I had remained a fork truck driver the rest of my working life.

Even among the mature student cohort at the Poly a couple of years later my 'actual working class' background was unusual – many of my peers had worked at respectable levels in office jobs and/or come from more comfortable back-grounds than I did, and often became mature students to try something different, do something more intellectually stimulating and worthwhile. It should be noted that between 1988 and 1992 the Conservative government encouraged growth in the system by slashing the unit of resource (funding per student) and most Polytechnics responded by expanding numbers. Participation among young people more than doubled in five years: from 15% in 1988 to 33% by 1993, as I realised later when I began to seriously research access to the HE system as part of my PhD. I and hundreds of thousands of my peers – mature students, 'women returners' (which in Huddersfield and Kirklees included many Muslims) as well as young people who would never have made it into the 40 universities that existed prior to 1992 – inadvertently benefitted from this early Conservative move to encourage competition and create a HE market (Further and Higher Education Act, 1992).

Much of my published policy analysis work across the last two decades has focussed on how system expansion necessarily *widened* participation and diversified the student body, how the ideas of expansion (in the name of human capital) and diversity (in the name of social justice) would not have been possible if left to the autonomous universities. These, in turn, accepted successive Conservative and Labour government's marketisation of the system which allowed them to remain at the apex of the hierarchy of newly unified system which had expanded to around 133 institutions in England alone by 1993 (McCaig, 2018). This institutional schism (pre-1992 vs post-1992 institutions) in many ways reflects social class divisions and plays out daily in the ways that these very different types of institutions aim to widen participation, indeed much of my academic work has explored the way that widening participation policy plays into our understanding of the differentiated HE marketplace (Bowl, McCaig, & Hughes, 2018; McCaig & Taylor, 2017; McCaig, Rainford, & Squire, 2022).

So, back in 1991, for me progressing to HE wasn't about class consciousness and that is in part because I wasn't surrounded by braying, self-confident children of the elite. Many of the 18-year-olds I came across over 5 years at Huddersfield's School of Music and Humanities (I taught Modern European History modules as an associate lecturer for two years after graduating) were only there because they had done less well in their A levels than they expected. Some of the young working-class students had chosen Huddersfield because it was local and allowed them to stay in the family home because they had little money to waste on rent and/or they had family responsibilities. It was their stories that formed my initial awareness of the differential experience of WC students, in particular the way that the WC (of any age, gender or ethnicity) embraced HE as pretty much the only route out of minimum wage and low-skill futures. Their life experiences were a million miles away from the 'rite-of-passage' procession of typical middle-class students at more prestigious institutions; for one thing, it seemed we were much more likely to actually enjoy the opportunity and – crucially, given the state of debate about access to HE today – to benefit from upward social mobility as a result.

That widening HE participation to people from our backgrounds has been a good thing and essential to the longer-term aim of creating a more socially just society is axiomatic for me, and I have always championed the concept in everything I do as an academic. This often involves wading through the weight of resistance to the expansion of the system that enabled (a tiny few) people like me to break into the system. Unfortunately, even post-1992 universities employ a large amount of academics that think (1) there are too many people in the system; (2) too many people in their classrooms; and (3) too many of them don't have the necessary educational credentials. Some of them have drunk the meritocratic kool-aid and apparently wish their own jobs and two-thirds of the HE sector away.

Social Class and the Confounding of the Mythology of Meritocratic Social Mobility

So where did we get the ridiculous idea that higher education – a publically funded service, remember – should be rationed in this way? As opportunities expanded to fill the human capital demands of the changing economy, it became important to social elites to differentiate the widening world of higher education. The first response to the Robbins Report (Committee on Higher Education, 1963) was to establish a set of Polytechnics without the ability to award their own degrees, and under the control of Local Education Authorities – with the effect that necessary expansion of higher skills provision would leave the autonomous universities unmolested and unreformed (to be fair, Robbins himself never intended to see a 'second division' of higher education created. It took an Oxford-educated Labour Secretary of State, advised by Oxbridge-educated civil servants to do that!). The public sector of HE – and the new Open University after 1970 – could do the widening participation work while the children of the aspirant middle classes finished their education – and developed their personalities (Gellert, 1991) – in residential universities based on the public school model. Meritocracy – the social 'sorting of the wheat from the chaff' – had to be maintained at all costs, and there was plenty of intellectual justification to draw on.

Mallock in his *Aristocracy and Evolution* (1898) employed social Darwinist arguments to suggest that the 'intentional few' (rather than random opportunity) showed an evolutionary survival of the fittest: Mallock 'yoked animal evolution as applied to society with Christian providentialism, in which the part of God was replaced by the "superchargeable few"' (Fawcett, 2020, p. 209). Here we see how easily the social control of organised religion (based on the acceptance of a rigid social order) was replaced in a more secular epoch by the social control of assumed meritocracy, in which the rich quite rightly rule the roost: Willian Graham Sumner was another influential social thinker who promoted the benefits of laissez-faire competition which sorted people into the 'fit' and 'non-fit', the 'more capable' (with attendant 'personal and social value') and the (valueless) 'non-capable'. Needless to say it fell to the more capable to lead: 'Only the elite of any society, in any age, think' (*Folkways*, Sumner, 1906, cited in Fawcett, 2020, p. 212). Oh, let us weep for the rich man's burden.

Schumpeter, in his hugely influential *Capitalism, Socialism and Democracy* (1942), similarly believed that capitalism (the natural order of things in competitive societies) could only survive the democratic pressure if led by 'an authoritative upper class … and institutional breakwaters against majority pressures'

(Fawcett, 2020, p. 216). Order – the rule of the deserving rich over the unde-serving poor – was essential to stable social functioning, and the hegemonic discourse of merit and meritocracy was essential to the subjugation of both the weak (who could be persuaded they were merit-less) and the aspirant middle classes, who were encouraged to become socially mobile by accumulating merit in the form of (rationed) educational opportunities.

Historian Selina Todd has recently produced a demolition of the *The Great British Social Mobility Myth* in her detailed social history *Snakes and Ladders* (Todd, 2021). Todd reserves especial ire for the charities and other lobby groups that consist the social mobility industry that disseminates the 'message that per-sonal aspiration and ambition can overcome "disadvantage"' (Todd, 2021, p. 339). Anybody actually working in the field knows that the working classes don't lack aspiration (Rainford & Harrison, 2020), but we certainly recognise a deficit discourse when we see one. It's the same 'blame the poor' game we have been reading for 150 years, yet we see it trotted out in supposedly critical sociology (much of it based on the theoretical works of Bourdieu and Sen's 'capability theory') that, somehow, transfers seamlessly into Conservative government pol-icies aimed at diverting the working classes away from HE access in successive White Papers (DBIS, 2011, 2016) and the more recent Leveling UP' agenda HE Act (HMSO, 2017; DLUHC, 2022; DfE, 2022).

Hardly surprising, given the focus of the social mobility industry is merely access to the most restrictive elite institutions, those who use the social class proxy of high A level entry grades to maintain the position of Russell Group institutions at the apex of league tables. These organisations have no intention of actually 'widening participation'; protected by legal autonomy over entry requirements, they only have to worry that they are not accused of contravening the anti-discriminatory clauses of the Equality Act (2010) which, notably, doesn't feature social class background among its protected characteristics.

The social mobility industry – much of it in the form of entrepreneurial voluntary 'third sector organisations' (TSOs) mainly reliant on state funding – merely services a charade that reinforces inequality of access. Dorling notes that 'there is no evidence that any initiatives run by social mobility charities and lobby groups has increased upward mobility or even working-class people's entry into higher education' (cited in Todd, 2021, p. 340). Not only do the elites of the Russell Group fail to widen participation, they and their acolytes actively prop up the system that systematically drives further access inequality:

> The social mobility industry claimed – in the words of the Speakers for Schools website – to shake up the current system to change the status quo. But in the 2000s and 2010s, none of those in this industry sought to remove the obstacles that prevent children from realising their ambitions. They offered no criticism of the ways that the Russell Group or private schools hoarded resources. They did not campaign against the preservation of wealth by the country's richest people.
>
> (Todd, 2021, p. 339)

Long before coming into the world of higher education as a student and then an academic, I had read enough history to know that restricted access to education is central to the deliberate entrenchment of social inequality, where only the achievements of the comfortable middle classes are valorised as meritorious. As a researcher and scholar of the relationship between power and ideas I remain convinced that only a relentless critical focus on the venal mechanisms of policymaking in the neoliberal HE market can cut through the hegemonic cultural mythology surrounding the notion of social mobility based on 'merit'.

My HE Journey, Student to Staff

Has being working class impacted my HE progression and career? Once in the system, I honestly don't think it has. From first temporary post at 39 (2 years fixed term, the first of 3 fixed term posts in 5 years), first permanent research post at 43 to Professor at 58 was quite rapid, and I am not conscious of being blocked or prejudiced against in interviews because of my class background; I am even more sure I have never been unjustly promoted as a 'token'. Focussing on politics and political economy I have been successful by most measures and I can only assume that I am good (enough) at what I do. I did well enough as an undergraduate to achieve a First Class Degree, and later secured ESRC funding for both my Master's and PhD at a Russell Group university. Since entering academia as a Research Associate (at the same RG institution), I have managed to do enough important research work with influential colleagues, then later bring in enough research income and produce enough research articles/book chapters and books to satisfy the promotion criteria, hopefully without treading on anyone's toes or even being overly ambitious.

However, my progression from undergraduate to post-graduate was affected by the fact that my BA Hons. (First Class) was from an ex-Polytechnic, and the University of Sheffield offered me a (funded) place on a Master's in Political Economy rather than take me straight onto a PhD. The significance of this only became clear to me when I started my PhD in Politics as part of a cohort including some that progressed directly from undergraduate 2:1s at pre-1992s.... with no need to have achieved a First or taken a Master's. That is where class bias comes in, in the minds of RG academics and managers, who, it seems, simply couldn't accept that somebody from my background could ever be as meritorious as somebody whose family background enabled them to achieve sufficient A level grades as teenagers. As a mature working-class student, you can bet this lesson was doubly noted. There never was any evidence that post-1992s were handing out Firsts more readily than pre-1992s, but they wouldn't take someone like me on a PhD on trust. Classist thinking undermines our HE system to an almost unique degree; first it denies access, then it denies progression, e.g. into post-graduate research, the gateway to academic careers; and then it reappears in the hiring practices of FTSE 500 employers who only deign to peruse applications from certain 'elite' universities (i.e. universities that only select from the social elite in the first place).

Class bias is everywhere, and if you are WC, you don't have to look for it, it is there in every ministerial speech (regardless of party) and every policy document, and in every patronising mission statement from the members of Todd's social mobility industry.

Working in the field of WP policymaking and employing critical policy discourse analyses (Fairclough, 1993; Fairclough & Fairclough, 2012) affords me the opportunity to highlight class-based rationing through the mechanism of institutional autonomy over admissions to the system. In this way my work exposes the venality of meritocracy and the mythology of social mobility discourses, prescribed as a way out of the poverty trap but in reality just intellectual cover for the reinforcement of social hierarchies. So my class war is based on what I have seen of the development of the HE system in my time, including the development of system differentiation as part of marketisation, and designed to restrict opportunities from the great unwashed.

Summary

For me, the benefits of being more politically than class-aware in the first 30 years of my life, and being an academic that analyses policy and policymaking rather than a sociologist focussing on culture and identity, are that I never felt I was abandoning a class identity to enter higher education. I was and am a student of politics and policy, and I'll remain a student of politics and policy so long as I am interested in them as subjects, or until I get told by colleagues and employers that I am no longer any good at my job. I note Byrne's (2019) point that he only became aware of becoming working class in academia, but I never saw the transition let alone thought that becoming aspirational was in some way a rejection of working-class identity. Nobody I grew up with was more aspirational than those that followed their dreams and abilities, whether that was to play football or cricket for England, be on stage or TV or make millions in the City; the fact that most of them may well have had their chances blocked by structural barriers is irrelevant to their, or their families', aspirations. If you are at the bottom looking up, what else can you do but aspire?

References

Bowl, M., McCaig, C., & Hughes, J. (Eds.). (2018). *Equality and differentiation in marketised higher education: A new level playing field?* Palgrave. Palgrave Studies in Excellence and Equity in Global Education. ISBN 978-3-319-78312-3. ISBN 978-3-319-78313-0 (eBook). Retrieved from https://www.palgrave.com/de/book/9783319783123

Byrne, G. (2019). Individual weakness to collective strength: (Re)creating the self as a 'working-class academic'. *Journal of Writing in Creative Practice*, *12*(1–2), 131–150.

Committee on Higher Education. Higher education. (1963). *Report of the committee appointed by the prime minister under the chairmanship of Lord Robbins* (pp. 1961–1963). Her Majesties Stationary Office.

DBIS. (2011). *Students at the Heart of the system*, higher education: Students at the heart of the system. In Presented to Parliament by the Secretary of State for Business, Innovation and Skills, By Command of Her Majesty, June 2011. CM8122 Crown copyright 2011.

DBIS. (2016a). Success as a knowledge economy: Teaching excellence, social mobility and student choice. White Paper Presented to. In Parliament by the Secretary of State for Business, Innovation and Skills by Command of Her Majesty, May 2016 Cm 9258 Crown Copyright 2016.

Department for Levelling Up, Housing and Communities. (2022, February 2). *Levelling up the United Kingdom*. White Paper. HM Government. Retrieved from https://www.gov.uk/government/publications/levelling-up-the-united-kingdom.

Department for Education. (2022, February 24). *Higher education policy statement and reform*. HM government. Retrieved from https://www.gov.uk/government/consultations/higher-education-policy-statement-and-reform

Fairclough, N. (1993). Critical discourse analysis and the marketization of public discourse: The universities. *Discourse & Society*, *4*(2), 133–168. Retrieved from https://www.jstor.org/stable/42888773.

Fairclough, I., & Fairclough, N. (2012). *Political discourse analysis*. London: Routledge.

Fawcett, E. (2020). *Conservatism: The fight for a tradition*. Princeton and Oxford: Princeton University Press.

Further and Higher Education Act. (1992). *Her majesty's stationary office 1992*. Retrieved from https://www.legislation.gov.uk/ukpga/1992/13/contents

Gellert, C. (1991). *The emergence of three university models: Institutional and functional modifications in European higher education*. Florence: University Models.

Goldthorpe, J. (1980). *Social mobility and class structure in modern Britain*. Oxford: Clarendon Press.

HMSO. (2017). Higher education and research act (HMSO, 2017). Retrieved from https://www.legislation.gov.uk/ukpga/2017/29/contents/enacted

McCaig, C. (2018). *The marketisation of English higher education: A policy analysis of a risk-based system*. Bingley: Emerald Publishing Limited. ISBN: 9781787438576. Retrieved from https://books.emeraldinsight.com/page/detail/The-Marketisation-of-English-Higher-Education/?k=9781787438576

McCaig, C., & Taylor, C. A. (2017). The strange death of Number Controls in England: Paradoxical adventures in higher education market making. *Studies in Higher Education*, *42*(9), 1641–1654. Published online 7th December 2015. doi:10.1080/03075079.2015.1113952

McCaig, C., Rainford, J., & Squire, R. (Eds.). (2022). *The business of widening participation: Policy, practice and culture*. Emerald Publishing Limited. ISBN 9781800430501.

Mckenzie, L. (2015). *Getting by* (1st ed.). Bristol: Policy Press.

Rainford, J., & Harrison, N. (2020). Why are we still so hung up on raising aspirations? *BERA Research Intelligence Special Issue*, *43*. Summer 2020.

Todd, S. (2021). *Snakes and ladders: The Great British social mobility myth*. London: Chatto & Windus.

Wilde, O. (2016). *The importance of being earnest and other plays*. London: Penguin Random House.

Chapter 4

'Friends First, Colleagues Second': A Collaborative Autoethnographic Approach to Exploring Working-Class Women's Experiences of the Neoliberal Academy

Carli Rowell and Hannah Walters

Abstract

Scholars have made important inroads to theorising and understanding working-class people's experiences of higher education (HE), as well as the broader complexities of navigating overlapping and sometimes competing middle- and working-class spaces.

In this chapter, we hope to add to this body of literature through examining the experiences and histories of two working-class women currently in the early stages of academic careers. Through the use of 'experimental autoethnographies' (Read & Bradley, 2018) and based on an assemblage of autoethnographic artefacts, we trace our journeys from undergraduate to post-PhD employment, picking up on key moments of pain, disconnect and isolation on the one hand, and celebration, support and pride on the other.

Through the tracing of these key moments in our recent academic trajectories, we make visible the difficulties of navigating elite spaces of academia as women with no family history of HE participation, exploring the ways in which we take on the role as 'academic translator' for those around us when discussing the labyrinthine meanings of academe. At the same time, and reflecting on these experiences from the perspective of navigating the margins of academia, we reject the pathologising narratives of working-class people and communities as uninterested in or hostile to HE through the unpacking of joyful moments shared with those around us related to our academic successes.

Finally, we point to ways in which we, as academics – however early career or precariously employed – are now in the position to support

The Lives of Working Class Academics, 41–55

Copyright © 2023 Carli Rowell and Hannah Walters

Published under exclusive licence by Emerald Publishing Limited

doi:10.1108/978-1-80117-057-420221004

marginalised students or colleagues, ending our chapter with a series of practical suggestions for making academia 'thinkable' for future generations.

Keywords: Autoethnography; collaborative autoethnography; experimental autoethnography; higher education; social class; working-class women

Introduction: Working-Class Journeys Into and Through Academia

Education for the working classes has been, and continues to be, about being found out, about not being good enough. Thus, education represents something to 'get through', something to survive, and then eventually leave behind (Reay, 2018). An array of sociological literature has long sought to explore working-class relations to education. Overwhelmingly, there has been the tendency to focus upon the educational failure of the working classes. However, in a time of expansion of HE, widening participation and a perceived need for university-level credentials to compete in a highly skilled global economy, sociological research has, only recently, begun to focus its attentions on working-class academic *success* (Ingram, 2009, 2011; Lehmann, 2013; Lehmann, 2015; Reay, 2001). Research highlights the manifold ways in which class backgrounds shape educational experiences and studies from across the global north continue to illustrate that social class remains a key factor with regard to access to university (Lehmann, 2007; Reay, 2001; Reay, Crozier, & Clayton, 2009). Sociological research has extensively recognised that institutional culture has long placed students from working-class backgrounds as the 'other' within HE (Lynch & O'neill, 1994; Tett, 2000) highlighting, that often, working-class students accept such dominant discourses, overwhelmingly envisaging HE as 'an unthinkable lifestyle option' (Archer, Hollingworth, & Halsall, 2007, p. 231), the preserve of those that are '"posher", "cleverer" [...] "people with money"' (Archer et al., 2007, p. 231). But what, then, of the working-class born women who journeyed to HE? What of the conflicts and contradictions? As well as the pleasures and possibilities of being working class in the contemporary university?

As working-class, early-career researchers, our journey(s) into, and through, academia were unforeseen, unexpected, risky and marked with uncertainty. Yet, we both pursued doctoral study and then later, academic careers, in spite of the sector's turbulence (Taylor & Lahad, 2018), our individual self-doubt and feelings of imposterism, and academia as a sector being cloaked in mystification. As women who come from family backgrounds where university education, let alone an academic career, is somewhat alien; seldom have we found ourselves in situations in our home and family lives where we might gain advice pertaining to the academic career ladder. In reflecting upon, and sharing, our experiences of being working-class early career women in academia, we unpick these turbulent journeys to, and through, the academy, and in this chapter, highlight key moments that capture these experiences. In doing so, we reflect on many of the feelings and emotions that are elicited as a result of being a working-class woman in UK academia, echoing, and building on, what our working-class women predecessors have so eloquently written about elsewhere (Crew, 2020; Hey, 1997; Hoskins, 2010; Lucey, Melody, & Walkerdine, 2003; Reay, 1997) and whose work has guided and comforted us during times of isolation and confusion.

Working-Class Women Aspiring to and Working in Academia

The contemporary era of HE is marked by increasing neoliberalism, as modern-day university education is being transformed from public ownership to that of private investment (Holmwood, 2014). Privatisation, casualisation, consumerism, marketisation and academic capitalism are all pervasive within UK HE, which is increasingly subjected to measures and metrics, through frameworks such as the Research Excellence Framework and Teaching Excellence Framework. This means that the daily practices and priorities of contemporary academics are continuously contested, defended and fought for (most notably through the recent national strike action). Despite the sector's turbulence, academia remains, for working-class academics, aspirational or otherwise, a seductive endeavour (Taylor, 2013) – a cohort that often engages in a 'labour of love' (Cannizzo, 2018) out of 'an ethic of service to others less "lucky" than them' (Mahony & Zmroczek, 1997, p. 5). Reay has written of how working-class women academics 'have the potential of subverting dominant discourses' and 'highlight the intricate psycho-social process of class experienced by the still working-class' (Reay, 1997, p. 26), and it is this that compels them to pursue an academic career. This sentiment has been recently echoed in the work of Wilson et al. when, reflecting on their experiences being feminist working-class academics within the contemporary academy write that 'we need to fight for the working-classes in academia' (Wilson, Reay, Morrin, & Abrahams, 2021, p. 38).

Whilst academia is often conceptualised as a 'dream space' among the imaginaries of working-class women (Archer, 2008), it also functions as a site of exclusion and marginalisation. Many working-class women in the academy have written of their experiences of navigating and existing within the middle-class space of academia. This is, arguably, nowhere more movingly articulated than in *Class Matters: 'Working Class' Women's Perspectives on Social Class* (Mahony & Zmroczek, 1997). This is an edited collection of emotive, reflexive and raw accounts seeking to engage with and theorise the complexities and tensions of social class, passionately exploring what it means to be a working-class, educationally successful woman. Highlighted within the literature are the ways in which pain, ambivalence and emotion are elicited as a result of both coming from a working-class background, and of now occupying a role previously the preserve of the middle classes (Mahony & Zmroczek, 1997). As Lucey, Melody, and Walkerdine (2003) note:

> Not only are working-class girls who do well at school and go on to higher education moving into intellectual and occupational spheres traditionally seen to be masculine, they are also moving out of their class sphere, beyond the wildest dreams of anyone in their families, into clean, professional, interesting jobs. Just

moving into the intellectual domain is a massive shift for them, requiring a complete internal and external 'makeover'.

(p. 297)

Of the working-class women who commit themselves to the academy, qualitative sensemaking accounts of their academic and work life uncover much revealing information. For example, the ways in which they actively seek to manage their working-class self in order to fit, such as through dress and speech (Hey, 1997); how they are often passed over for promotion (Reay, 2000); and how, as a result of their 'approachableness', they are often overloaded with what Wilson et al. (2021) refer to as the 'guilty burden' of pastoral care. As the authors write, this is work that they choose to do, yet which is seldom acknowledged, rewarded or formalised (Wilson et al., 2021). Rickett and Morris highlight how working-class women in the academy experience 'contemporary academic work as care-taking work' (2021, p. 95) and are called upon to deliver the emotion work of United Kingdom Higher Education (UKHE) under the guise of 'pastoral care'. This, Rickett and Morris (2021) argue, is rooted in classed and gendered histories of working-class women's work as being service work. It represents the pathologisation of working-class women within academia to the detriment of career progression.

In what follows, the chapter aims to contribute to this rich body of work and unpack the experiences of two working-class women early career academics – friends and collaborators with shared and overlapping experiences of negotiating the neoliberal academy.

Methods

When planning what to write for this chapter, it was important to us to approach it in a way that spoke to our complex experiences as working-class women in academia, while also reflecting the kind of solidarity and connection our collaboration has fostered. We, thus, decided to collect data via a co-interview, arranged around a series of, what we refer to as, 'autoethnographic artefacts' that were used as prompts to spark conversations around shared experiences (inspired by Read and Bradley's (2018) use of a similar approach to explore themes of time and waiting in the neoliberal academy). We both collected these artefacts over the course of a few weeks, and by the time our co-interview was scheduled, we had a collection of photographs, screenshots from WhatsApp messages, and a piece of creative writing. Artefacts were used as prompts, one-by-one, with the owner/author of the artefact introducing the piece and providing some context (as well as why they selected it), followed by a discussion between the two of us.

Our use of autoethnographic artefacts was inspired by arts-based and creative methods using elicitation techniques, such as photo elicitation and autoethnographic fictions (like those used by Taylor and Breeze (2020)). We were also inspired by Robards and Lincoln's (2017) 'scroll back method' for capturing longitudinal data from digital platforms (in our case, WhatsApp). Not only did WhatsApp messages feature as autoethnographic artefacts during the co-interview, but throughout this chapter we include snapshots from our text conversations with each other as part of the broader autoethnographic project. We do so both to provide insight into the nature and character of class and gender solidarity in the neoliberal academy, as well as part of broader political goals of making visible those modes of academic labour that often remain hidden (especially, as noted above, for working-class women).

Methodology

In order to work together on this chapter, we needed to expand our understanding and use of autoethnographic approaches – typically the work of a single researcher – in order to capture both of our experiences as part of one over-arching project. We came to 'collaborative autoethnography' (Chang, Ngunjiri, & Hernandez, 2013), a means of combining both group and solo work as part of a single piece, a process that allows researchers 'to benefit simultaneously from self and collective analysis' (p. 25). We began considering the ways in which such an approach might help us, as researchers, to push the boundaries of autoethnographic work to incorporate multiple experiences and lenses – i.e. 'multisubjectivities' (Chang et al., 2013) or 'multivocal'/'multivoiced' approaches (Lapadat, 2017).

Gannon et al. (2015) point to the radical potentials in, what they refer to as, collective biography work for exploring the politics of the academy. In particular, the authors highlight the ways that collaborative memory approaches allow for 'volatile and generative' discussions whereby stories carry the potential to '[spin] off [...] in unexpected directions' (p. 192). In turn, this allows for the 'collective production of meaning' (p. 192) and the generation of 'a new imaginary of academia that disrupts and critiques neoliberal discursive regimes' (p. 191). More broadly, scholars have positioned collaborative autoethnography as a method with the potential to generate deeper understandings of both the self and others, thanks to its dialogical nature – allowing collaborators to 'interrogate others' experiences intimately and deeply' (Chang et al., 2013, p. 28).

In the current project, the benefits of our collaborative ethnographic approach became clear when, during our co-interview, important/relevant themes and ideas, which may have remained hidden from the self (as would be the case in traditional autoethnographic work), were visible to the other and could, therefore, be probed in a deeper way. For example, during our interview, one of us revealed that she had approached a supportive lecturer to ask about the process of applying for a PhD and, off the cuff, mentioned that she had cried during the conversation. *When asked why,* a rich conversation *ensued* about the pain to a rich conversation about the pain and isolation of being the first person in your family to go to university, as well as the embarrassment of being thought to be getting 'ideas above your station'. Without the collaborative element here, this topic would have been lost to the flow of the single-lens autoethnographic project. As Chang et al. (2013) note, this kind of collaborative meaning-making makes individual stories richer, while simultaneously 'uncovering those hidden assumptions and elaborating on previously taken-for-granted events that were perhaps critical incidents impacting our identity formation' (p. 28). To push this idea further, this might be an example of how incorporating multiple perspectives might carry the potential to provoke themes of 'enduring or pragmatic social value' (Lapadat, 2017, p. 598) – particularly, as Ganon et al. suggest, in terms of generating a shared imaginary of the academy which transgresses neoliberal discourses of individualisation and hyper-competitiveness.

Our project also allowed for a deeper connection between us as collaborators and friends, generating a specific mode of solidarity that can only come from sharing these kinds of experiences. As our WhatsApp messages at the time reveal:

> Did some work in our chapter today really enjoyed it. Plenty left to do but I think it will be good
>
> Love our collaboration and more importantly you as a friend ♡
>
> You too babe, feel so lucky to know youuuuuu! ♡

Finally, we recognise the social construction and relational nature of social class (as well as, in our case, its intersections with gender), along with the partiality and contingencies of our stories here; indeed, that our work belongs to a 'particular time, place, discursive frame and present self of the writer[s]' (Davies & Gannon, 2006, p. 13). We do not claim our work speaks to objective truths about academic experience, and recognise that the memories and artefacts on which we draw belong to us/our situated knowledges/experiences. That said, and following the long tradition of autoethnographic work to 'gain an understanding of society through the unique lens of self' (Chang, 2008), we hope the following makes some contribution to our shared (scholarly and otherwise) understandings of the functions of class and gender, isolation and solidarity, and pain and pleasure within contemporary academia.

The Co-Interview

We scheduled and re-scheduled our co-interview a number of times, a fact which, in itself, reveals something important about the nature of contemporary class politics in the neoliberal academy. In trying to make time for our collaborative work, we both offered to work during our annual leave and even, surreptitiously, during strike action (i.e. on days we were not paid). Both of us were dealing with health issues at the time, but neither of us took sick leave – instead choosing to continue to work (or 'power through'). Our WhatsApp messages around this time clearly reveal both the ways in which we were struggling, as well as some of the pressures we felt from the university. The below are some excerpts, shared here in no particular order:

> "just in pain not like terrible but [...] my brain isn't that sharp tbh"

"I'm on leave but can do early like 9–11?"

"I will power through this afternoon"

"I also don't have as much time as I have other deadlines"

"My mental health has been wobbly lately so I'm not as reliable as I'd like to be"

Importantly, alongside these experiences of pain, distress and feeling squeezed by neoliberal academic regimes, our WhatsApp conversations also reveal moments of support and solidarity (again shared in no particular order):

'We'll get it done I'm sure'

'Please take good care of yourself'

'Your health comes first'

'U are top of the pile when it comes to making it in academia. Just got to 'ride the wave of precarity''

'Let me know if I can help with anything'

'you're like my therapist lol'

It was following a few rearrangements and a lot of 'powering through' that we eventually found time to sit down together and complete our co-interview. The below is an excerpt from our chat just prior to beginning the interview:

'Making a cuppa tea! Be with you 2ish x'

'OK I'm gonna get 1 too x xx x'

'I've got my dressing gown on because I feel fucking freezing by the way, just to let you know'

'Bet you look cute. Yeah it's cold innit'

We began our Zoom call; both of us sat at home wrapped up in warm clothes (including the aforementioned dressing gown!). During a chat about automated captioning on Zoom, we discussed the importance of being very clear with our speech in order that accurate transcripts were generated:

'Okay best RP accent' (in a joking voice)

'Just comes up afterwards, like it simply captions it so hopefully it understands <u>what I'm saying</u>' (underlined text in exaggerated clearly projected voice and RP accent)

(Do middle-class academics have these worries when conducting research? Are all of us this aware of our accents, speech patterns, clarity and so on?)

At one point during the interview the internet connection became unstable. We eventually reconnected, with one of us now tethering using her phone's data:

"My Internet went down. I connected it to my phone. [...]"

"Your data? Is it costing loads of money?"

(Is this another window into our epistemologies as working-class academics?)
We then began to chat about our experiences, using the autoethnographic artefacts we gathered as prompts for discussion. What follows is a discussion of two of the key themes that emerged from this process: of pain, disconnection and isolation on the one hand, and celebration, support and pride on the other.

On Pain, Disconnection and Isolation

"Is this a proper job or are you still a student?"

We are socialised to believe educational achievement to be a straightforwardly positive process and, for working-class people, one sometimes coded as escape or even 'bettering oneself'. But, building on the work of others (such as Lawler's (1999) discussion of pain and estrangement associated with this class movement, or Lucey et al.'s discussion of internal/external 'makeovers'), we hope to complicate these narratives, and engage with the ways in which the pursuit of HE, doctoral study and academic careers can also produce feelings of pain, disconnection and isolation for working-class people. In particular, we explore these feelings through the process of *translating* our academic lives and achievements to those around us.

When discussing our autoethnographic artefacts, one theme that emerged was the 'solo journey' through academia as a working-class person. Indeed, we both felt that our educational and academic journeys were ours alone and, in spite of support from our families (explored later), there were issues of *translating* these experiences to those around us. Early on in our conversation we realised one of the most basic ways this manifested was through questions from family members about being a 'perpetual student,' and asked 'when are you going to get a proper job?' – these comments were often wrapped up in jokes, but also speak to a disconnection between the worlds of our family and academic lives.

As one of her artefacts, Hannah shared a screenshot of a message she sent to her Whatsapp family group on the day she passed her viva. Though this is a piece of happy news, and Hannah said during the co-interview that her family were all celebratory about it, we also discussed how these kinds of achievements can require some explanation to our families. In the message, Hannah had written: 'I passed my viva' followed by an explanation of what that is – 'the oral defence of your thesis' – followed by what this means – that she was 'now Dr Walters'. We reflected on the ways these kinds of translations were likely not required of our middle-class peers and, indeed, how rare it seems to meet other academics who are first-generation university graduates.

We discussed how taking on the role of 'academic translator' can be part of a painful process associated with success in academia as a working-class person: we noted how '...there's almost a sadness that... and it's not a sadness... I'm not saying that they've done anything wrong [my family] and it's anything like that, but there's almost a sadness that your achievements never quite translate fully to your family'. We discussed how this sometimes led to us purposefully choosing not to share these successes with those around us. In part, this was because of the amount of labour – emotional and otherwise – these kinds of translations required. But also, given our positionality, it sometimes felt insensitive. During our interview, Carli noted on a recent piece of good career news she'd received that: 'Given the context and the climate, I just didn't share it with anyone...I was very mindful that a lot of people were struggling in their careers, losing jobs on furlough, let alone...making progress'. These kinds of negotiations – decisions around when or whether to share positive career news – we felt were the specific burden of working-class academics, whose achievements were often positioned in relief against their friends, families and communities; we agreed that these kinds of successes are rarely felt in straightforwardly positive ways, and are often wrapped up in feelings of guilt, and feeling like one of the 'lucky ones' (Mahony & Zmroczek, 1997).

By contrast, we noted that other kinds of achievement were, perhaps, more celebrated or understood by our families – we spoke about how this was both classed and gendered, and we had both observed family members being more comfortable celebrating what we noted were 'more understandable forms of achievement' such as getting married, having babies or buying a house. Similarly, there were moments where our achievements 'burst out' of academia and into 'the real world', a process which also helped with this process of translation. For example, Carli shared a story of when her nan discovered she'd written a chapter in an academic book. Her nan was excited and eager to see the piece, so much so that she badgered Carli for weeks until she finally took the book round to her nan's house. During our co-interview, Carli shared an image of her nan reading the book; though her nan commented that 'it's a bit technical isn't it?', the fact that she had a physical manifestation of her academic work clearly meant something to her family, and helped inform their view of what Carli's career entailed. Echoing this, Hannah noted that she had shared with her family times when her work had been picked up by more mainstream outlets, such as news media. She felt this ratification of a more mainstream publication (compared to academic publications) supported her efforts to explain her academic experience. At the same time, this was a way of sharing academic work in a way that is more accessible than the, often elitist, world of academic publishing (a world of pay-walls, labyrinthine metrics and filing systems, and often impenetrable language – as Carli's nan says, writing that is 'a bit [too] technical').

Indeed, it is important to point out that we see these issues of translation not as 'failures' on the part of our families, but rather as a complex entanglement of structural inequalities and, on our parts as working-class academics, personal anxieties around these wider relationships and what our careers mean to those around us. Working-class people have long been locked out of HE, and both of us recognise the complex web of circumstance – such as shifts in education policy, school peer groups, supportive teachers and luck – which led us to academic careers. At the same time, our own anxieties about our lives as academics – especially when considered in relief against our families' experiences – might mean we 'hold back' more than necessary when it comes to these discussions. Taken together, we feel this experience speaks to the dual identities carried by those of us navigating academia as first-generation, working-class academics: experiences of pain, disconnection and isolation.

On Celebration, Support and Pride

> "A doctor? You're going to study to be a Doctor of Medicine now?"

During our co-interview, both of us spoke early on about the support that we received from family members, and how this support manifested itself in different ways when compared to the support offered by the families of our more middle-class peers. As noted above, we had shared experiences of how our family members had little, if any, knowledge of what a PhD was prior to us commencing doctoral study, and the mystification of what exactly a PhD required remained throughout our time as postgraduate researchers and persists into our present-day lives as early career researchers. 'A doctor? You're going to study to be a Doctor of Medicine now?' – building on the discussion of Carli's nan reading her book chapter, Carli shared the story of when, upon graduation from her undergraduate, she told her family she would not be progressing into the world of work but instead would begin study for her doctorate. The image sparked a memory of her nan's confusion as to what a doctor, in this context, was.

However, in spite of these kinds of confusions, we both felt we had been supported by our families in relation to our pursuit of doctoral study, and later, of academic careers. The theme of familial support was central to much of our co-interview discussion, despite our family's lack of direct experience of HE. Reflecting on the collection of photos that Carli had chosen, she noted that, 'all capture, kind of, this moment of finishing the PhD, of it being over. Graduation and, also, you've got, like, the picture of me handing it in, like, my oral viva'.

Indeed, the majority of Carli's photos included her and her family. One of the photos was a close-up of her and her mum, looking directly at one another, hands in the air, faces scrunched up, both crying. In this image, she was reminded of the pride that her mother carried and, when asked what was going on in the photo, Carli shared with Hannah the following:

I think I chose those photos to kind of show, I guess like the first picture of me and my mum like was quite intentional to kind of show that her happiness and support. And just bursting with pride and like crying because at that moment, I was on campus early on to go and get my picture taken and then my nan, mum and dad joined me and my mum was the last one to join, because she was like busy like sorting out my nan and she just walked down the stairs and started crying. I asked her 'why are you crying?' she said something like 'I forgot that you would have like that funny hat on, I forgot that it means that you know you've got a PhD and not just an undergraduate degree' and she started crying and then I started crying and I just said, 'you're going to make me cry, my makeup'.

We began to talk about the ways in which our family had expressed support, pride and celebration. This led us to reflect upon the process of pursuing doctoral study and of the support that we received from our families. For Carli, support manifested itself in the form of encouragement, help with the domestic chores, such as making dinner, doing laundry and general day-to-day maintenance as, during the end of her PhD, she was living in her family home. For Hannah, this came in the form of domestic advice (from cooking tips to home remedies when she was unwell), as well as encouragement during times of stress. This included the advice, as one family member put it, to make sure you 'don't work yourself to a frazzle'. Where middle-class families might have offered support in the form of editing or proofreading the thesis, our own families showed support for our education through care and service work, reflecting working-class women's traditional and historical roles as caregivers or service workers (Taylor, 2012). By contrast, there exists a long history of sociological research that highlights the ways in which middle-class mothers deploy cultural and economic capital in order to secure educational advantage for their children (Kimelberg, 2014; Reay & Ball, 1997; Yemini & Maxwell, 2018).

Hannah noted how some of the support she received took the form of pride and celebration that her family expressed upon good career news. Reflecting on one of her autoethnographic artefacts, Hannah noted that though she can tell her family are proud of her, their expressions of pride contain 'none of that technical knowhow [of the mechanics of academia] that goes along with' these kinds of celebrations (such as insider knowledge of academic processes). We agreed that even these moments of joy can require some translation work. But that said, though complex, we both felt our families had celebrated our academic successes, in spite of the distance between these experiences and their own, and both of us felt these celebrations were rooted in deep pride and love from those closest to us. Importantly, we both expressed the ways these feelings were key support mechanisms for navigating the ups and downs of academic journeys – a working-class mode of social capital which became a key resource for surviving in academia. It is important for us to highlight these moments as part of this chapter, and to emphasise that this kind of support and celebration is deeply valued by both of us.

Conclusions

Working-class women within academia have written of the way in which they modify their language, speech and accents when shifting between a working-class and middle-class field of home and the university (Hey, 1997). But what about the way(s) in which we navigate an explanation of what we do as part of our job? How do we present our academic selves to our working-class family and friends? How are we able to 'translate' our academic success to them? Importantly, what is lost in this process of translation?

Through the tracing of key moments in our recent academic trajectories, we hope we have made visible the contrasting experiences of working-class academics of pain, disconnection and isolation on the one hand, and celebration, support and pride on the other. In doing so, we aim to contribute to and complicate long-standing narratives of academic success as straightforwardly positive experiences, while simultaneously rejecting narratives that pathologise working-class families and communities as anti-education. We reflect on these experiences from the perspective of 'navigating the margins' of academia, and of the plural identities carried by those of us from working-class backgrounds.

Finally, and drawing on our own trajectories, we close this chapter by pointing to ways in which we, as academics – however early career or precariously employed – are now in the position to support other marginalised students or colleagues, and outline some ideas for others to do the same:

• Where comfortable and safe to do so, make visible your working-class identity when teaching or interacting with students. Speak about being the first in your family to attend university. Make clear the ways university can be a complex, confusing space to navigate, and struggling with this speaks not to a deficit in students' abilities, but of a deficit on the part of the university to make these experiences more inclusive; speak and write in accessible ways.
• Be mindful of spaces in academia where class is missing from the conversation. Social class is not covered by equalities legislation in the United Kingdom, so is often left out of initiatives aimed at improving educational experiences for marginalised students. Where possible, bring up social class, pointing to it as one of a constellation of intersectional experiences students and colleagues might be navigating.
• Reject problematic confluences of working-class and whiteness. Firstly, because although class is complex and lived out by different communities and identities in different ways, working-class experience is not the exclusive preserve of white people. Secondly, because this is a tactic of white supremacy and the United Kingdom has a long history of positioning white working-class communities in opposition to communities of colour, as well as to migrants and refugees. Most recently, this can be seen in the current government's Education Committee report, *The forgotten: how White working-class pupils have been let down, and how to change it* (2021) (for discussion of how this is problematic, see Treloar's (2021) piece for The Runnymede Trust).

- Look for initiatives that might support this work (such as internal pots of funding that might bolster working-class students' CVs). For example, Carli was recently awarded institutional funding in order to pay working-class students within the department of Sociology to help co-design the curriculum for the module 'Class, Conflict and Culture: A View from Within'. The module aims to teach issues of class inequality from the viewpoint of the working class, and does so by drawing upon working-class academics, artists, activists, lyricists, writers and other non-academic material.
- Note that you're interested in supervising work concerned with social class on public-facing profiles, social media and throughout your teaching work.

Of course, this list is far from exhaustive, and we do not claim expertise in this particular space. Simply, we feel the above represents a good start for making academia more inclusive of working-class people and, in tracing our own journeys to academic careers, have both benefited from others' use of these approaches.

References

Archer, L. (2008). Younger academics' constructions of 'authenticity', 'success' and professional identity. *Studies in Higher Education, 33*(4), 385–403.

Archer, L., Hollingworth, S., & Halsall, A. (2007). University's not for me—I'm a nike person': Urban, working-class young people's negotiations of style', identity and educational engagement. *Sociology, 41*(2), 219–237.

Cannizzo, F. (2018). 'You've got to love what you do': Academic labour in a culture of authenticity. *The Sociological Review, 66*(1), 91–106.

Chang, H. (2008). *Autoethnography as method.* Abingdon, OX: Routledge.

Chang, H., Ngunjiri, F. W., & Hernandez, K.-A. C. (2013). *Collaborative autoethnography.* Walnut Creek, CA: Left Coast Press.

Crew, T. (2020). *Higher education and working-class academics.* Cham: Springer International Publishing.

Davies, B., & Gannon, S. (2006). *Doing collective biography.* Maidenhead: Open University Press/McGraw-Hill.

Gannon, S., Kligyte, G., McLean, J., Perrier, M., Swan, E., Vanni, I., & van Rijswijk, H. (2015). Uneven relationalities, collective biography, and sisterly affect in neoliberal universities. *Feminist Formations, 27*(3), 189–216. Retrieved from http://www.jstor.org/stable/43860820

Hey, V. (1997). Northern accent and southern comfort: Subjectivity and social class in class matters. In P. Mahony & C. Zmroczek (Eds.), *'Working-Class' women's perspectives on social class* (pp. 140–151). London: Taylor & Francis.

Holmwood, J. (2014). From social rights to the market: Neoliberalism and the knowledge economy. *International Journal of Lifelong Education, 33*(1), 62–76.

Hoskins, K., (2010, March). The price of success? The experiences of three senior working class female academics in the UK. *Women's Studies International Forum, 33*(2), 134–140. Pergamon.

Ingram, N. (2009). Working-Class boys, educational success and the misrecognition of working-class culture. *British Journal of Sociology of Education, 30*(4), 421–434.

Ingram, N. (2011). Within school and beyond the gate: The complexities of being educationally successful and working class. *Sociology, 45*(2), 287–302.

Kimelberg, S. M. (2014). Beyond test scores: Middle-class mothers, cultural capital, and the evaluation of urban public schools. *Sociological Perspectives, 57*(2), 208–228.

Lapadat, J. C. (2017). Ethics in autoethnography and collaborative autoethnography. *Qualitative Inquiry, 23*(8), 589–603. doi:10.1177/1077800417704462

Lawler, S. (1999). 'Getting out and getting away': Women's narratives of class mobility. *Feminist Review, 63*(1), 3–24. doi:10.1080/014177899339036

Lehmann, W. (2007). I just didn't feel like I fit in: The role of habitus in university drop-out decisions. *Canadian Journal of Higher Education, 37*(2), 89–110.

Lehmann, W. (2013). Habitus transformation and hidden injuries: Successful working-class university students. *Sociology of Education, 87*(1), 1–15.

Lucey, H., Melody, J., & Walkerdine, V. (2003). Uneasy hybrids: psychosocial aspects of becoming educationally successful for working-class young women. *Gender and Education, 15*(3), 285–299.

Lynch, K., & O'neill, C. (1994). The colonisation of social class in education. *British Journal of Sociology of Education, 15*(3), 307–324.

Mahony, P., & Zmroczek, C. (1997). Why class matters. Class matters: 'Working-class' women's perspectives on social class. In P. Mahony & C. Zmroczek (Eds.), *Class matters: Working class women's perspectives on social class* (pp. 1–7). London: Taylor & Francis.

Read, B., & Bradley, L. (2018). Gender, time and 'waiting' in everyday academic life. In Y. Taylor & K. Lahad (Eds.), *Feeling academic in the neoliberal university: Feminist flights, fights and failures. Series: Palgrave studies in gender and education* (pp. 221–242). Cham: Palgrave Macmillan. doi:10.1007/978-3-319-64224-6_10

Reay, D. (1997). The double-bind of the 'Working-Class' feminist academic: The failure of success or the success of failure? In P. Mahony & C. Zmroczek (Eds.), *Class matters: Working class women's perspectives on social class* (pp. 18–29). London: Taylor & Francis.

Reay, D. (2000, January). "Dim Dross": Marginalised women both inside and outside the academy. In *Women's studies international forum* (Vol. 23, pp. 13–21). Pergamon.

Reay, D. (2001). Finding or losing yourself?: Working-class relationships to education. *Journal of Education Policy, 16*(4), 333–346.

Reay, D. (2018). Miseducation: Inequality, education and the working classes. *International Studies in Sociology of Education, 27*(4), 453–456.

Reay, D., & Ball, S. J. (1997). 'Spoilt for choice': The working classes and educational markets. *Oxford Review of Education, 23*(1), 89–101.

Reay, D., Crozier, G., & Clayton, J. (2009). 'Strangers in paradise'? Working-class students in elite universities. *Sociology, 43*(6), 1103–1121.

Rickett, B., & Morris, A. (2021). 'Mopping up tears in the academy'–working-class academics, belonging, and the necessity for emotional labour in UK academia. *Discourse: Studies in the Cultural Politics of Education, 42*(1), 87–101.

Robards, B., & Lincoln, S. (2017). Uncovering longitudinal life narratives: Scrolling back on Facebook. *Qualitative Research, 17*(6), 715–730. doi:10.1177/1468794117700707

Taylor, I. (2012). Close encounters of the classed kind. Again.... *Social & Cultural Geography, 13*(6), 545–554.

Taylor, Y. (2013). Queer encounters of sexuality and class: Navigating emotional landscapes of academia. *Emotion, Space and Society, 8*, 51–58.

Taylor, Y., & Breeze, M. (2020). All imposters in the university? Striking (out) claims on academic twitter. *Women's Studies International Forum, 81*(1), 102367.

Taylor, Y., & Lahad, K. (2018). *Feeling academic in the neoliberal University: Feminist flights, fights and failures.* Cham: Palgrave Macmillan.

Tett, L. (2000). 'I'm working class and proud of it': Gendered experiences of non-traditional participants in higher education. *Gender and Education, 12*(2), 183–194.

The Education Committee. (2021). The forgotten: How white working-class pupils have been let down, and how to change it. Retrieved from https://committees. parliament.uk/committee/203/education-committee/news/156024/forgotten-white-workingclass-pupils-let-down-by-decades-of-neglect-mps-say/. Accessed on April 2, 2022.

Treloar, N. (2021). The weaponisation of the 'left-behind white working class'. Runnymede Trust. Retrieved from https://www.runnymedetrust.org/blog/the-weaponisation-of-the-left-behind-white-working-class-harms-us-all. Accessed on April 2, 2022.

Wilson, A., Reay, D., Morrin, K., & Abrahams, J. (2021). 'The still-moving position' of the 'working-class' feminist academic: Dealing with disloyalty, dislocation and discomfort. *Discourse: Studies in the Cultural Politics of Education, 42*(1), 30–44.

Yemini, M., & Maxwell, C. (2018). De-coupling or remaining closely coupled to 'home': Educational strategies around identity-making and advantage of Israeli global middle-class families in London. *British Journal of Sociology of Education, 39*(7), 1030–1044.

Chapter 5

Coming to Terms With the Academic Self: Place, Pedagogy and Teacher Education

M. L. White

Abstract

It is a rare challenge in academia to be asked to write about yourself, and rarer still to engage with the multiple (social, spatial, political, embodied and private) selves that impact on our practice. In this chapter I consider how who we are in academia is not simply a matter of adopting a professional role but rather involves identity management and negotiation practices to obscure, perform or disclose identities in professional contexts. This chapter is informed by my first ethnographic research project at a non-profit youth media centre in New York City; a study exploring innovative visual pedagogies for investigating how pre-service student-teachers articulate their views about the effects of poverty on educational attainment and my practices as a teacher educator on the MSc Transformative Learning and Teaching: a two-year, initial teacher education programme designed from a social justice perspective and working to produce graduates who position themselves as activist teachers. In this autoethnography I explore the complex temporalities of my academic identities, arguing the need for a critical spatial practice.

Keywords: Critical pedagogy; teacher education; identity; autoethnography; narrative research; space and place

Introduction

For more than 25 years I have identified as a teacher, first in secondary schools and now as a teacher educator and academic. I applied to university wanting to be a teacher, and looking back I now recognise that one of my aims was class mobility although I did not have the language to articulate this or the necessary knowledge of how to make my 'aspirations real and obtainable' (Treanor, 2017, p. 1). As, what we now refer to as, a first generation scholar (Thomas & Quinn, 2007) I did not know what was expected of me in higher education and without

The Lives of Working Class Academics, 57–72

Copyright © 2023 M. L. White

Published under exclusive licence by Emerald Publishing Limited

doi:10.1108/978-1-80117-057-420221005

the support of others – Sheila who bought all of my first-year books (I did not know that I would need my own copies); a sub-warden[1] in the halls of residence who helped me access and understand the classics that I had not read; and the students with whom I worked during summers and weekends at an outdoor centre (working as an assistant, cleaning, sorting and helping others and progressing over three years to the role of senior outdoor instructor) – I would not have survived the first term of university, never mind gone on to teach.

I grew up in a council house in a large Scottish town. My sister and I, and later our brother, received free school meals, commonly used as a policy tool and an indicator of poverty (Hobbs & Vignoles, 2010) and a proxy for socio-economic status (Jerrim, 2020).[2] As children, we understood that there were things that we could not afford and recognised the differences between ourselves and other families. In primary school I remember being asked why I did not have a dad and why my mum could not attend a school trip because she had to work. I remember feeling shame at those and other markers of difference. I am not sure when I first understood the impact of socio-economic status and its relationship to educational inequalities or when I became interested in 'a pedagogy of inquiry into personal positionality and into the social and economic roots of injustice' (Boyland & Woolsey, 2015, p. 5) but they both inform my academic practice.

Today in Scotland the poverty-related attainment gap is first identified in the early years and the gap grows wider throughout schooling (White, 2018). When I was growing up (long before devolution), the consequences of Thatcher's economic and education policies including section 28 of the Local Government Act (1986) were felt throughout the education system. Where we live, the places we grow up in and the spaces we inhabit impact on us. Then as now, education is spatial, because as Soja asserts

> ...human life is ... spatial, temporal, and social, simultaneously and interactively real and imagined. As intrinsically spatial beings ... we are at all times engaged and enmeshed in shaping our socialised spatialities and, simultaneously, being shaped by them.
>
> (2010, p. 18)

Our relationship to place is often understood and expressed as an aspect of identity – being *from* and *of* a place or not fitting *in* and feeling *out* of place. Who we are is associated with how we define ourselves, where we are geographically and socially (and metaphorically) and where we have come from. One of my secrets, kept hidden because of the shame I felt, is that I did not spend much time in school as a teenager and engage in the activities that help develop knowledge and skills and as Bourdieu (1990) writes in relation to habitus, a 'sense of one's place' (p. 131). I attended two high schools and yet did not complete a full school year in either. Appadurai (1996), writing about neighbourhoods, suggests that places, such as schools, are both context derived and generative, producing and affecting people and communities. My secret, hidden throughout college, an undergraduate degree, 12 years as a secondary school teacher, a part-time master's, a PhD studentship and more than 15 years as a teacher educator in higher education, has remained core to my identity and how I situate myself.

Space and Place

Much has been written about space and place in order to explore the genealogy of the terms and the many theoretical understandings and positions that exist. Space is an organising concept, an aspect of the ethnographic foundations of anthropology and sociology, and an understanding of space and place is one of many ways to understand our lives. In contrast to England and Wales, in Scotland most children attend their local school and the one geographically closest to them. This means that in spaces where people experience disadvantage, in for example, income, employment, education, health, access to services, and crime and housing as defined by the SIMD, there is a place-based disadvantage and a larger attainment gap (Sosu & Ellis, 2014). Places then are not equal and are differently positioned through what Massey calls a 'power geometry' (1994). Some places, some schools and communities are wealthier than others, have higher status and more resources confirming that 'inequality has always been at the centre of the education system' (Reay, 2017, p. 27). As Wilkinson and Pickett assert, the 'ways in which class and taste and snobbery work to constrain people's opportunities and well-being are, in reality, painful and pervasive' (2009, p. 165).

While I was able to acquire economic capital to attend university because I was eligible for a grant and was able to secure part-time employment, I lacked what Bourdieu (1986) calls cultural capital, later defined by Lamont and Lareau as, 'widely shared high status cultural signals (attitudes, preferences, formal knowledge, behaviors, goods, and credentials)' and a concept often 'used for social and cultural exclusion' (1988, p. 156). Throughout university I often felt out of place, and as noted by others (cf. Lawler, 1999; Reay, David, & Ball, 2005) anxious that my secrets – of health, economics, sexuality and class – would reveal themselves. In this chapter it is my contention that spatiality and identity are constructed, reviewed and remade throughout our experiences in education and in the academy. As Casey reminds us

> ...the relationship between self and place should point not just to reciprocal influence ... but, more radically, to constitutive coingredience; each is essential to the being of the other. In effect, there is *no place without self and no self without place.*
>
> (Casey, 2001, p. 406)

In considering the spatial, temporal, material and social practices of my academic life, I draw on the spatial theories of Lefebvre (1991) and Soja (2010) and of social geographers writing about space and place from sometimes contradictory and often intersecting positions. In this chapter space is socially constructed as well as material and embodied and thinking spatiality is a way to understand and experience education of being, researching, writing and retelling knowledge production (White, 2018). Writing about space and place is complicated by the familiarity and ubiquity of the terms which are used both literally and meta-phorically – *my place, your place, being in (or out) of place, knowing your place*. In popular discourse the terms define physical locations and social relations, struc-tured by and structuring social practice. As Tuan (1977) notes, both terms 'are familiar words denoting common experiences' yet when we seek to understand how these terms are used in research 'they may assume unexpected meanings and raise questions we had not thought to ask' (p. 3).

In this chapter I reflect on key experiences in my academic history: my first ethnographic research project at a non-profit youth media centre in New York City (NYC) (White, 2009); on a study exploring innovative visual pedagogies for investigating how pre-service student-teachers articulate their views about the effects of poverty on educational attainment and my practices as a teacher educator on the MSc Transformative Learning and Teaching – a two-year, initial teacher education (ITE) programme designed from a social justice perspective and working to produce graduates who position themselves as activist teachers (Sachs, 2003). In considering each of these experiences, in formal and informal educa-tional contexts and across geographical boundaries, I argue that our experiences in academia are spatial identity practices and rooted in our sense of place. Who we are in academia is not simply a matter of adopting a professional role but rather involves identity management and negotiation practices to obscure, perform or disclose identities in professional contexts.

The Ethnographic Self

After a number of years as a secondary school teacher I secured a PhD stu-dentship and left my job in high school to become a research-student-tutor and engage in a doctoral study. Over a period of 12 years, I had taught English, Media and Film Studies, been a form tutor, deputy and then head of year and led a department. I had worked in inner- and outer-city schools and had experienced first-hand the impact of policy reform on how society was organised, managed and experienced at the start of the 21st century. During my time in school (and in part-time jobs at a youth club and later a youth media organisation), I developed a growing awareness, what Freire (2000) refers to as a conscientisation, of the rise of social and economic inequality and its impacts, on the hopes and fears of digital, online and networked technologies and the changing role of education in late modernity.

Throughout my doctoral studies, I maintained my teacher education role at another university and, as is often the case in academia, worked across multiple boundaries and identifications. I had enjoyed teaching in high school and being recognised as a teacher was central to my identity (Gee, 2001) and a source of self-esteem and fulfilment (Nias, 1996). This made a return to study and the hybrid identity outlined by the university title (and represented by the hyphens) uncomfortable. As I worked to recognise my changed sense of self and develop my research focus, I introduced myself as someone who *used* to be a teacher. This historical placing of my identity articulates the centrality of the social and professional role I had worked hard to achieve. Yet over time and through study I realised that 'working the hyphens' (Fine, 1994, p. 70) and embracing a position of plurality represented the connection and interdependency of those hybrid and liminal identities and was an authentic articulation of who I was and wanted to be. In academic life we take on multifaceted professional roles and I am, among other identifications, a teacher educator, researcher, collaborator, facilitator, storyteller, administrator, manager, leader and writer.

In this section I reflect on my doctoral research project considering the importance of narrative and storytelling to ethnographic (and autoethnographic) practice. Drawing on fieldwork at a non-profit youth media education centre in NYC, I share stories from the research to argue that the experience of ethnographic research is a spatial identity practice. On the front page of my PhD thesis (and at home on the wall in the room where I work) I have a group picture, a visual reminder of the research project and the relationships developed with participants and collaborators. While the image represents an aspect of *my* story of the project, it is a collective artifact and a reminder there were many others involved and multiple stories that could be told.[3] Mitchell (2005) argues that the 'life of images is not a private or individual matter. It is a social life [of] ... the worlds they represent', (p. 93), and this image represents my developing research practice and exploration of the multiple identities and spaces I occupy in academic life.

> Although I had planned to arrive in the afternoon when it would still be light, at the airport I was offered a later flight in return for a flight voucher – to ease overbooking and when I arrived in NYC it was dark and cold. The five hour delay at Heathrow gave me more time than I needed to worry about what would happen when I arrived in NYC and I imagined a number of scenarios – all of which ended with me in danger and without a place to stay.
>
> At JFK I took a cab to the city and as I was driven through empty streets I looked out at buildings and signs that would become familiar to me, listening to the crunch of dirty snow outside. The cab driver let me out at Washington Square Park and I walked across the square to Waverly Place where the apartment I had leased a room in was. On the flight my concern was not for what would happen in the research, whether I had made a good decision temporally leaving my home or what would happen when I was in the classroom. My concern was that the room I had agreed to rent might not exist and I would be alone in NYC.
>
> Waverley Place runs across Washington Square and when I couldn't find 212 on the West side I went East assuming that I

had missed the building. When a doorman told me that there wasn't a number 212 and a girl in the coffee shop said she didn't know where it was it seemed that my worst fear was coming true. I phoned Amy (who I would be sharing the apartment with), and as she didn't answer the phone (did she exist?), left a message, I spoke to another doorman who said I could stay in his lobby until I 'worked it out' and later was invited to walk with a woman and her dog around the Square in order to look again.

Looking out into the darkness I refused more offers of help and phoned Amy one more time. I was relived [sic] to speak to her and find out that the number I should have been looking for was 123–212 is the area code for Manhattan and I had confused them. Why I didn't realize this when I looked in my book, I don't know. It was a stupid mistake (which I would laugh about later) but for now I had a place to stay and I was in NYC.

(Research journal extract)

The journey to begin fieldwork and my framing of an arrival scene (Weston, 1991) is a reminder of the anxiety I felt. When I arrived in NYC I was not concerned about the research process or what would happen the following day at the media centre. While the later flight paid for another journey, my focus was on the basic human need for safety and a place to stay. At the time I felt scared, inexperienced and alone, emotions that are identified in a number of ethnographic texts (cf. Coffey, 1999). Reading this account sometime after the event I wondered why I wrote it as a story to myself and I am struck by my use of colloquial language and the Americanisms I adopted. I described the 'cab' rather than the taxi, being 'let out' rather than dropped off, and 'an apartment' rather than a flat. The language forms we use provide some detail about our state of mind and here my casual description hides my not so casual fears. My choice of language also makes strange a difficult transition and might be an attempt to enact a new social identity in a new context.

Much of what is written about the process of ethnographic fieldwork refers to foreign countries and unknown cultures; however, this was not true in my research. The location for this research is important because the main fieldwork was carried out in NYC, a location regarded as *foreign* as I lived in London, but not exotic or unknown as has been the case historically with much ethnographic research.[4] For many ethnographers an understanding of and an engagement with the location of study is used to establish the authenticity of the project and the authority of the researcher. Like Pink (2001) who draws on the work of Massey (1994) and Ingold (2008), I am concerned with a different scale and am using spatiality as a framework for thinking about the research process and 'the situatedness of the ethnographer, as a multi-sensory concern' (Pink, 2001, p. 29).

Entering the building I was met by the school police officer who asked for photographic identification and telephoned reception before allowing me to enter the building (later after informal introductions and when I became a familiar face we would chat about the weather or our weekend plans). On that first day I entered the lift ('that's cute it's the elevator') and was confused to discover that there was not a button for the seventh floor where I had been told to go. On the sixth floor, classrooms and the noise of a school surrounded me, and I walked through the corridors concerned that I was missing an obvious sign before finding stairs that would take me to the seventh floor and begin the research.

(Research journal extract)

While this functions as the arrival story (and it does describe the moment I first entered the physical space of the research location), the confusion I felt represented an insecurity about my research role and might more accurately be described as part of my search for a border crossing (Giroux, 2005), and an eventual awareness and acceptance of multiple and hybrid identities: student, researcher, teacher and participant (Foucault, 1997). While Giroux (2005) uses the concept of a border crossing 'as a resource for theoretical competency and critical understanding' (2005, p. 6), borders and boundaries involve going into unfamiliar places and are often points of difficulty and a time to reassess and assert identity. My search for a border crossing was a search for a space where borders of place, disciplines (and their associated theories) and identities could coexist.

The research questions that form the basis of my PhD were focussed on young people and staff at the media education centre, but they also concern the identity of the researcher, my – self and the complex, multiple identities that affects the experience of research. Hall (1997) claims that 'identity' is formed in the 'interaction' between self and society (p. 276), and suggests that the inner core, the 'real me' is in continuous dialogue with the outside cultural world. While I struggled to acknowledge my multiple identities at the start of the research process (and believed that I successfully managed the identity I shared), I now recognise how much I did not share, the assumptions I did not challenge, the silences I held and the privileges of my white and, at the time young, female body. When I first arrived in NYC and couldn't find the (wrong) door, people wanted to help me, offering time, shelter and guidance. We experience the world through our bodies, and it acts as a boundary between self and other (Valentine, 2001). Our bodies and how we look have symbolic value and unlike the reprimand I received as a newly qualified teacher for not looking *like* a teacher in my first job, here my body provided privilege. In a context where race, poverty, geography and status impact on young peoples' educational experiences and outcomes (Kirkland & Sanzone, 2017) I wrote very little about the structural inequalities they faced and did not challenge many their assumptions about me.

For ethnographers the field, the research site or the spaces and places of research are central to our experiences and the relationships we develop. When we spend time in a research site, we deliberately and sometimes unconsciously work to create relationships with others as we try to develop and negotiate a place for ourselves. Describing the ethnographers' role Van Maanen (1988) suggests that we are 'part spy, part voyeur, part fan, part member' (p. 346).

In this research my previous experiences in education as a teacher and in ITE helped me to access and understand the actions, thoughts and feelings of other teachers and provided me with access to the site. Because of these experiences I was familiar with the physicalities of a school classroom and understood how important and value laden the space was. Further, my experiences in *informal* education, through youth work and extracurricular media arts practices, enabled me to have a 'deep familiarity' (Goffman, 1959) with the social processes I aimed to research. These experiences were important to the study because they were experiences that informed my educational beliefs and values. This did not mean that I was unable to make teaching and schooling 'anthropologically strange' (Becker, 1971), or that I took situations for granted but that my experience as a researcher (and the physical distance I travelled to the research) enabled analytical distance to be established and maintained, although this is an area I sometimes struggled with, falling into a teacher role in the classroom.

Davies (1999) notes that 'virtually all fieldworkers report experiencing emotional extremes, from great exaltation to serious feelings of inadequacy and self-doubt' (p. 83). Recognising that it is rare for ethnographers to leave fieldwork unaffected (Coffey, 1999), the research self and the relationships developed and maintained throughout the process becomes part of the research experience and of the academic self. However painful the process is, we must address our personal reasons for undertaking research and make clear 'that interpretations are produced in cultural, historical, and personal contexts and are always shaped by the interpreter's values' (Springer, 1991, p. 178). The more effectively readers can understand the account and its context (who produced it and why), the better they are able to anticipate the ways in which it may suffer from autobiographical influence and recognise the writers (or producers), point of view. On the first page of her doctoral thesis Vasudevan (2004) asks 'who am I to do this?', a question I continue to ask myself.

Seeing Disadvantage

More than a decade after my doctoral study and in my third academic role I worked with a colleague to explore pre-service, or student teachers' views of disadvantage and on an initiative to develop pedagogical frameworks for discussing issues around poverty and its effects on educational attainment (White & Murray, 2016). Following a BERA symposium (Thompson & Whitty et al., 2015) working with teacher education colleagues from around the United Kingdom, the project emerged in response to our context; a teaching-intensive post-92 university located in an area of disadvantage, and out of a concern to understand schools' and teachers' views on poverty and educational disadvantage and how these issues might be most effectively tackled in ITE.[5]

I was interested in this work in part because of my own school experiences but also because despite what might be considered a renewed interest in class (Lawler, 2005; Savage, Bagnall, & Longhurst, 2001, Skeggs, 2004; and more recently Friedman & Laurison, 2019; McEnaney, 2021) there is limited research about how student teachers, many of whom come from relatively privileged socio-economic backgrounds (Thompson, McNicholl, & Menter, 2016), understand structural inequalities and in particular how they conceptualise or *see* poverty and aim to address its effects on children's educational lives. Of particular concern is how best to prepare student teachers for the experiences they will have on the practicum, their school placements and in future employment both in schools in socially and economically deprived areas as well as in schools where poverty, though less prevalent, still has a significant detrimental effect on a minority of learners (Gorski, 2018; Treanor, 2017).

In this research we used a range of research methods to explore the attitudes and understandings that student teachers had in relation to and between these factors and educational outcomes and life chances. We surveyed student teachers at the beginning and at the end of their ITE programmes. We developed a series of workshops to gain insight from students and share our research findings, interviewed student teachers and other teacher educators and analysed the research materials produced by student teachers including photography and participatory maps.

In this project many of the student teachers reported that they had little personal experience of disadvantage, and for some of the students issues of poverty and disadvantage were to use their words *alien, unfamiliar* and *uncomfortable*. In the workshops it was clear that many student teachers viewed these issues through the lens of their own often self-identified class privilege and norm-referenced perspectives. In one workshop student teachers identified that they did not have the language to talk about class, the disadvantage some pupils experienced in their classrooms or its impact on schooling and education. This is significant because language is 'central not only in the production of meaning and social identities but also as a constitutive condition for human agency' (Giroux, 2005, p. 11). While our choice of language is complex and relational, we must consider the terms we use to describe ourselves and others in a way that recognises and dismantles structural inequalities.

We also found that some of the students shared limited aspirations of parents, schools and pupils as important factors in educational under-achievement. Stereotypical views of lack of parental aspirations, for example, were often explicitly or implicitly positioned as more influential on children's learning than the material and economic factors of poverty, and it was not unusual for students to report that they were informed by or sharing their mentor teachers' views. In one workshop when I asked students how poverty was defined, they briefly talked about finance and access to resources before moving from income to a deficit view and a lack of aspiration and access to culture, activities and community networks. As noted by Ladson-Billings (2006), the language of culture is often used by student teachers to talk about contexts and experiences including race, gender, sexuality and economics that do not match their own.

While this research was firmly located within our location, and its consequential geography (Soja, 2010), for student teachers their focus to 'pass the course' and 'start teaching' limited their engagement with and in the communities, the spaces they had been placed. Yet the discomfort student teachers experienced in talking about disadvantage, attainment and class and the silences we experienced in this project were important to disrupt student teachers' habits of *seeing* and the assumptions that they relied on (Brookfield, 2017). In one of the few studies on the social geography of teacher education, Hargreaves (1995, p. 32) argues that 'what it means to *be* in teacher education … can only properly be understood by firmly locating our studies of teacher education in space as well as in time' a position I agree with.

Transformative Learning and Teaching

At the end of 2019 and after more than two decades in London I returned to Scotland and to an academic role where I was appointed to lead one of the new and 'innovative' teacher education programmes in Scotland (Scottish Government Press Release, 2016). In this concluding section I consider my position as programme director of the MSc Transformative Learning and Teaching (TLT), a two-year ITE programme designed from a social justice perspective, and identify the tensions of space, place and identity that remain. Launched in 2017, the programme supports student teachers to engage in transformative teaching and to being committed members of an 'activist teaching profession' which Sachs describes as 'an educated and politically astute one' (Sachs, 2003, p. 154). Activist teachers are those for whom teaching is a critical and political endeavour (Apple, 2014; hooks, 1994), who seek to make education transparent and accessible and who engage productively and respectfully with the communities in which their learners live, acting as educators and advocates for their pupils (Kennedy, 2018). Since its inception there has been some resistance to a teacher education programme that qualifies graduate to teach across the transition, a boundary of disadvantage and a site of injustice where children from more affluent background fair better (Scottish Government, 2020).[6] This is challenging work for everyone involved because 'there is no one-shot inoculation for neutralizing the consequences of disadvantage' (Freeman, 2010, p. 693) and the programme was first described as an alternative route into teaching (Scottish Government, 2020). This marginal position highlights the implicit values and long-held assumptions and biases within ITE and reminds us that '*[t]here is no path to equity that does not include direct confrontation with inequity*' (Gorski, 2018, p. 102 original emphasis).

While I enjoyed my previous role and my values were aligned to a university committed to widening participation and rooted in its sense of place, my commitment to preparing beginner teachers to work in spaces of socio-economic disadvantage, reaching and teaching students in poverty and an explicit commitment to social justice motivated me to apply for the role. Yet, when friends and colleagues congratulated me on my appointment and a move to a Russell Group university, I considered that I was making the riskiest move of my career and my fears of being *out of place* resurfaced. But just as I benefitted from mentorship and support of those who understood what was expected at university at the start of my education, so I benefitted from colleagues and collaborators who included, encouraged and supported me as I crossed geographical and emotional boundaries.

The Need for Story

In one of the first TLT assignments, student teachers are asked to reflect on their identities and '[d]emonstrate and articulate critical awareness of their own professional values, identity and cultural self, and make informed judgements about how best to progress continued professional growth within a complex education environment'. Agar suggests that the process of writing adds 'critical reflection to our ongoing task of making sense out of who we are and what it is we do' (Agar, 1986, p. xi) and this task makes clear that:

> Teachers bring their entire autobiographies with them ... it is useless for them to deny this; the most they can do is acknowledge how these may either get in the way of, or enhance their work with students.
>
> (Nieto, 2003, p. 24)

Throughout this autoethnography I have worked to acknowledge my*self* and my relationships with others in order to develop a critical reflexive perspective and because others are implicated in what we write (Ellis, 2007). While writing the self can be a strategy for more reflexive practice, and is inextricably linked to theorising, it is through stories 'we constitute our very selves' (Charmaz & Mitchell, 1997, pp. 212–213).

So, what have I learned about myself through the process of writing this chapter, this story? In the academy our biographies, our bodies and the spaces and places we come from and inhabit, inform our practice. We are at all times spatial, temporal and social. And while I am hesitant to make any claims about my experience, not least because our stories are as unique as those they represent, there are a number of principles that I have strived for: to a transformative pedagogy and an understanding of who and *where* I am; to authenticity and an academic practice where I am actively and wholeheartedly engaged and to plurality and a recognition of the multiple identities, meanings and positions that we obscure, perform or disclose in professional contexts.

I used to believe that education could make up for social and economic inequality, that through education the experience of poverty, of class anxiety 'the feeling of vulnerability in contrasting oneself to others at a higher social level, the buried sense of inadequacy that one resents oneself for feeling' (Sennett & Cobb, 1972, p. 58) could be overcome. I now realise that self-awareness and reflection on one's own positionality and a pedagogy of discomfort (Boler, 1999), which can be painful and challenging, is important. In the academy we are in a unique and powerful position. Although it might look 'deceptively simple' (Grossman, Hammerness, & McDonald, 2009), the work of teacher educators is complex and multiple (Boyd & White, 2017), and we are not just teachers of teachers (Lunenburg et al., 2017). It is my view, we need to surface the fluidity and pluralities of the academy and of the sites, the spaces, the identities and relationships we engage.

As an undergraduate my main worry was about money and after that, that I doubted that I knew as much as everyone else, believing that it was luck that had enabled me to get *in* and that I would soon be found out (sometimes like many others I still feel that way). As a teacher I understood that material possessions did not indicate wealth and worked to reject a deficit discourse which blamed children and families for their socio-economic and class position (Crozier, Reay, & James, 2011). Now as a senior lecturer of teacher education when I recruit students to the programme and visit schools to coach and observe beginner teachers, I am working to support others to understand the impact of social, economic and political contexts. A critical spatial practice includes a community-engaged approach to teacher education (Zygmunt, Clark, Clausen, Mucherah, & Tancock, 2016) and is rooted in an understanding of space and place and the authentic experiences of the community the school serves.

In an autoethnography I am obligated to reveal both long-held and emerging tensions and questions about my academic identity – after all this is the challenge that was set. While much of this reflection and inward gaze feels uncomfortable (and perhaps indulgent), it has taken some courage to write and share this chapter. From the question who am I to do this? I also ask *where* am I and how has this changed my pedagogical practice, my view of education and of research. Like Ball (2003) I understand working class is a contested term and believe that there is no one way of being in the academy. Yet the experiences I describe in this chapter have enabled *my* 'transgressions – movements against and beyond boundaries' (hooks, 1994, p. 12), a practice I am committed to continue.

Notes

1. A sub-warden in a hall of residence works with the warden to manage the day-to-day running of the residence. This usually involves social, disciplinary, pastoral and administrative duties and the role often comes with free or reduced accommodation costs. In my third semester (in my second year of university), I became a sub-warden and benefitted from free accommodation.
2. The Scottish Index of Multiple Deprivation (SIMD), introduced in 2003, is the official measure of relative multiple deprivation in Scotland and used to identify the places where people are experiencing disadvantage across different aspects of their lives.
3. Here I use the term story as a way of bringing together context, information, knowledge and emotion, which Norman (1993) describes as the crucial elements of communication.

4. Here I am using foreign as an adjective to describe a country I do not live in and not to indicate *other*.
5. A London borough ranked 3rd highest on child poverty rates, and 13th in the United Kingdom overall, at 30%.
6. Research indicates that the transition between primary and secondary school adversely affects children's attainment and well-being (Scottish Government, 2019).

References

Agar, M. (1986). Foreword. In T. L. Whitehead & M. E. Conway (Eds.), *Self, sex and gender in cross cultural fieldwork*. Urbana, IL: University of Illinois Press.

Appadurai, A. (1996). *Modernity at large: Cultural dimensions of globalization*. Minneapolis, MN: University of Minnesota Press.

Apple, M. (2014). *Official knowledge: Democratic education in a conservative age* (3rd ed.). Abingdon: Routledge.

Ball, S. J. (2003). *Class strategies and the education market: The middle classes and social advantage*. London: Routledge Falmer.

Becker, H. (1971). Footnote. In M. Wax, S. Diamond, & F. Gearing (Eds.), *Anthropological perspectives on education* (pp. 3–27). New York: Basic Books.

Boler, M. (1999). A pedagogy of discomfort: Witnessing and the politics of anger and fear. In M. Boler (Ed.), *Feeling power* (pp. 175–202). Taylor & Francis.

Bourdieu, P. (1986). *Distinction* (Trans. R. Nice). London: Routledge and Kegan Paul.

Bourdieu, P. (1990). *The logic of practice*. Cambridge, MA: Polity Press.

Boyd, P., & White, E. (2017). Teacher educator professional inquiry in an age of accountability. In P. Boyd & A. Szplit (Eds.), *Teacher and teacher educator inquiry: International perspectives*. Attyka, IN: Kraków.

Boylan, M., & Woolsey, I. (2015). Teacher education for social justice: Mapping identityspaces. *Teaching and Teacher Education, 46*, 62–71. doi:10.1016/j.tate.2014.10.007

Brookfield, S. D. (2017). *Becoming a critically reflective teacher* (2nd ed.). Jossey-Bass.

Casey, E. S. (2001). Between geography and philosophy: What does it mean to be in the place-world? *Annals of the Association of American Geographers, 91*(4), 683–693. Retrieved from http://www.jstor.org/stable/3651229

Charmaz, K., & Mitchell, R. G., Jr. (1997). The myth of silent authorship: Self substance and style in ethnographic writing. In R. Hertz (Ed.), *Reflexivity and voice* (pp. 135–215). Thousand Oaks, CA: Sage.

Coffey, A. (1999). *The ethnographic self: Fieldwork and the representation of identity*. London, Thousand Oaks, CA: Sage Publications.

Crozier, G., Reay, D., & James, D. (2011). Making it work for their children: White middle-class parents and working-class schools. *International Studies in Sociology of Education, 21*(3), 199–216.

Davies, C. (1999). *Reflexive ethnography: Guide to researching selves and others*. New York: Routledge.

Ellis, C. (2007). Telling secrets, revealing lives: Relational ethics in research with intimate others. *Qualitative Inquiry, 13*(1), 3–29.

Fine, M. (1994). Dis-stance and other stances: Negotiations of power inside feminist research. In A. Gitlin (Ed.), *Power and method*. London: Routledge.

Freeman, E. (2010). The shifting geography of urban education. *Education and Urban Society*, *42*(6), 674–704.

Freire, P. (2000/1970). *Pedagogy of the oppressed*. New York, NY: Continuum.

Friedman, S., & Laurison, D. (2019). *The class ceiling: Why it pays to be privileged*. Bristol: Bristol University Press.

Foucault, M. (1997). What is critique?" translated into English by Lysa Hochroth. In S. Lotringer & L. Hochroth (Eds.), *The politics of truth*. New York: Semiotext(e).

Gee, J. P. (2001). Identity as an analytic lens for research in education. *Review of Research in Education*, *25*, 99–125.

Giroux, H. (2005). *Border crossings: Cultural workers and the politics of education* (2nd ed.). New York, NY: Routledge.

Goffman, E. (1959). *The presentation of self in everyday life*. New York: Doubleday Anchor.

Goodall, J. (2019). Parental engagement and deficit discourses: Absolving the system and solving parents. *Educational Review*, *73*(1), 98–110.

Gorski, P. (2018). *Reaching and teaching students in poverty: Strategies for erasing the opportunity gap* (2nd ed.). New York, NY: Teachers College Press.

Grossman, P., Hammerness, K., & McDonald, M. (2009). Redefining Teacher: Re-imagining Teacher Education. *Teachers and Teaching: Theory and Practice*, *15*(2), 273–290.

Hall, S. (1997). *Representation: Cultural representations and signifying practices*. London: Sage.

Hargreaves, A. (1995). Towards a social geography of teacher education. In N. Shimahara & i. Holowinsky (Eds.), *Teacher education in industrialised nations: Issues in changing social context* (pp. 87–124). New York, NY: Garland.

Hobbs, G., & Vignoles, A. (2010). Is children's free school meal 'eligibility' a good proxy for family income? *British Educational Research Journal*, *36*(4), 673–690.

hooks, b. (1994). *Teaching to transgress: Education as the practice of freedom*. New York, NY: Routledge.

Ingold, T. (2008). Bindings against boundaries: Entanglements of life in an open world. *Environment and Planning A: Economy and Space*, *40*(8), 1796–1810.

Jerrim, J. (2020). Measuring socio-economic background using administrative data. What is the best proxy available? Social Research Institute working paper. Retrieved from http://repec.ioe.ac.uk/REPEc/pdf/ qsswp2009.pdf

Kennedy, A. (2018). Developing a new ITE programme: A story of compliant and disruptive narratives across different cultural spaces. *European Journal of Teacher Education*, *41*(5), 638–653.

Kirkland, D. E., & Sanzone, J. L. (2017). *Separate and unequal: A comparison of student outcomes in New York City's most and least diverse schools*. New York, NY: Metropolitan Center for Research on Equity and the Transformation of Schools, New York University.

Ladson-Billings, G. (2006). It's not the culture of poverty, it's the poverty of culture: The problem with teacher education. *Anthropology & Education Quarterly*, *37*(2), 104–109.

Lamont, M., & Lareau, A. (1988). Cultural capital: Allusions, gaps and glissandos in recent theoretical developments. *Sociological Theory*, *6*, 153–168.

Lawler, S. (1999). "Getting out and getting away": Women's narratives of class mobility. *Feminist Review*, *63*, 3–24. Retrieved from http://www.jstor.org/stable/1395585

Lawler, S. (2005). Rules of engagement: Habitus, class and resistance. In L. Adkins & B. Skeggs (Eds.), *Feminism after Bourdieu*. Oxford: Blackwell.

Lefebvre, H. (1991). *The production of space*. Malden, MA: Blackwell. Original work published in 1974.

Lunenburg, M., Murray, J., Smith, K., & Vanderlinde, R. (2017). Collaborative teacher education development in Europe: Different voices, one goal. *Professional Development in Education*, *43*(4), 556–572.

Massey, D. (1994). A global sense of place. In D. Massey (Ed.), *Space, place and gender* (pp. 146–156). Oxford: Polity.

McEnaney, J. (2021). *Class rules the truth about Scotland's schools*. Edinburgh: Luath Press.

Mitchell, W. J. T. (2005). *What do pictures want? The lives and loves of images*. Chicago: University of Chicago Press.

Nias, J. (1996). Thinking about feeling: The emotions in teaching. *Cambridge Journal of Education*, *26*, 293–306.

Nieto, S. (2003). *What keeps teachers going?* New York: Teachers College Press.

Norman, D. A. (1993). *Things that make us smart – Defending human attributes in the age of the machine*. Reading, MA: Addison-Wesley.

Pink, S. (2001). *Doing visual ethnography: Images, media and representation in research*. London: Sage.

Reay, D., David, M. E., & Ball, S. (2005). *Degrees of choice: Social class, race and gender in higher education*. London: Institute of Education Press.

Reay, D. (2017). *Miseducation*. Bristol: Policy Press.

Sachs, J. (2003). *The activist teaching profession*. Buckingham: Open University Press.

Savage, M., Bagnall, G., & Longhurst, B. (2001). Ordinary, ambivalent and defensive: Class identities in the northwest of England. *Sociology*, *35*(4), 875–892.

Scottish Government Press Release. (2016, November 30). *New routes into teaching*. Edinburgh: Scottish Government. Retrieved from https://news.gov.scot/news/new-routes-into-teaching

Scottish Government Press Release. (2020, February). *Advice and guidance: Alternative routes into teaching*. Edinburgh: Scottish Government. Retrieved from https://www.gov.scot/binaries/content/documents/govscot/publications/advice-and-guidance/2020/02/alternative-routes-into-teaching-february-2020/documents/alternatives-routes-into-teaching-february-2020/alternatives-routes-into-teaching-february-2020/govscot%3Adocument/Alternative%252Broutes%252Binto%252Bteaching%252B-%252BFebruary%252B2020v3.pdf

Sennett, R., & Cobb, J. (1972). *The hidden injuries of class*. Cambridge: Cambridge University Press.

Skeggs, B. (2004). *Class, self, culture*. London, Routledge.

Soja, E. W. (2010). *Seeking spatial justice*. Minneapolis, MN: University of Minnesota Press.

Sosu, E., & Ellis, S. (2014). *Closing the attainment gap in Scottish education*. Joseph Rowntree Foundation.

Springer, C. (1991). Comprehension and crisis: Reporter films and the Third World. In L. D. Friedman (Ed.), *Unspeakable images: Ethnicity and the American cinema*. Urbana: Univ. of Illinois Press.

The Scottish Government. (2019). *Achievement of curriculum for excellence (Cfe) levels*. The Scottish Government. Retrieved from https://www.gov.scot/news/achievement-ofcurriculum-for-excellence-cfe-levels-1/. Accessed on August 20, 2022.

The Scottish Government. (2020). £50 million to improve attainment – Gov.Scot. [online]. Retrieved from https:/www.gov.scot/news/gbp-50-million-to-improve-attainment-1/. Accessed on February 22, 2022.

Thomas, L., & Quinn, J. (2007). *First generation entry into higher education*. Maidenhead: Open University Press.

Thompson, I., McNicholl, J., & Menter, I. (2016). Student teachers' perceptions of poverty and educational achievement. *Oxford Review of Education, 42*(2), 214–229. doi:10.1080/03054985.2016.1164130

Thompson, I., Whitty, G., White, M., Murray, J., Beckett, L., - Leeds Beckett University; Ellis, S., Burn, K., & Mutton, T. (2015, September). Perspectives on poverty and teacher education. In I. Thompson (Chair), *British educational research association conference*. Belfast.

Treanor, M. C. (2017). Can we put the poverty of aspirations myth to bed now?. In L. Kelly (Ed.), *Centre for research on families and relationships. CRFR Research briefing* (p. 91). Centre for Research on Families and Relationships. Retrieved from http://hdl.handle.net/1842/25787

Tuan, Y. F. (1977). *Space and place: The perspective of experience*. Minneapolis: University of Minnesota Press.

Valentine, G. (2001). *Social geographies: Space and society*. London: Routledge.

Van Maanen, J. (1988). *Tales of the field: On writing ethnography*. Chicago, IL: University of Chicago Press.

Vasudevan, L. (2004). *Telling different stories differently: The possibilities of multimodal (counter)storytelling with African American adolescent boys*. Unpublished doctoral dissertation, University of Pennsylvania, Pennsylvania.

Weston, K. (1991). *Families we choose: Lesbians, gays, kinship*. New York: Columbia University Press.

White, M. (2009). Ethnography 2.0: Writing with digital video. *Ethnography and Education, 4*(3), 389–414.

White, J. (2018). Children's social circumstances and educational outcomes. Retrieved from http://www.healthscotland.scot/media/2049/childrens-social-circumstances-and-educational-outcomes-briefing-paper.pdf. Accessed on March 18, 2022.

White, M., & Murray, J. (2016). Seeing disadvantage in schools: Exploring student teachers' perceptions of poverty and disadvantage using visual pedagogy. *Journal of Education for Teaching, 42*(4), 500–515.

Wilkinson, R., & Pickett, K. (2009). *The spirit level: Why more equal societies almost always do better*. London: Penguin.

Zygmunt, E., Clark, P., Clausen, J., Mucherah, W., & Tancock, S. (2016). *Transforming teacher education for social justice*. New York, NY: Teachers College Press.

Chapter 6

The Rubik's Cube of Identity

Khalil Akbar

Abstract

This chapter is an autoethnographic account of my working-class background into the lonely world of academia. It shares a small glimpse into my life journey from an intersectionality lens of being British born, of Pakistani heritage and a Muslim male. Thus, my working-class identity is one of several challenging identities amalgamated into one and silently interchangeable. This chapter is a rare occurrence to view my world from an introspective position. It shares the heavy constraints and challenges those of us who come from marginalised groups face daily. You will read how I cannot sever integral parts of myself which are deeply infused with the academic I am becoming. All of which I have struggled to maintain both personally and professionally. Subsequently, this chapter shares the complexity of these identities, my constant negotiation of them and my ongoing adaptation of now being uncomfortably viewed as middle-class.

Keywords: Dual identities; Islamophobia; microaggressions; role models; minoritised groups; othering

The Lives of Working Class Academics, 73–87
Copyright © 2023 Khalil Akbar
Published under exclusive licence by Emerald Publishing Limited
doi:10.1108/978-1-80117-057-420221006

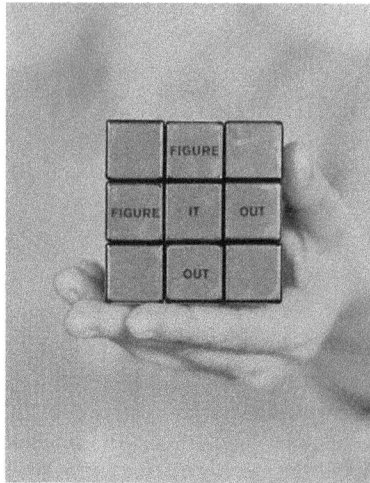

My story is not as simple as solely identifying from a working-class background. The latter is one of several complex layers of the dual identities amalgamated into one. Byrne (2019) argues that the categorisation of the working class is not homogenous; it is aligned with an intersectional approach related to race, gender, religion, etc. Thus, the negotiation of my identity has been fraught with many challenges from which I view the world through the lens of intersectionality; British born, Pakistani heritage and a Muslim male. Subsequently, to avoid concealing my true self, I write from the perspective of multiple social identities to delineate belonging, both in my personal and professional settings.

The start of this journey initiated well before my arrival into the world. My father certainly envisaged a utopia he had heard about from those who came before him. Amidst his intentions, my father envisaged a better life for himself, his nine children, a safer environment, security in freedom and, most importantly, the opportunity for a free and well-renowned education. Interestingly, the multitude of themes that arose with my father's arrival in the late 1960s in Britain are undoubtedly ones that have echoed throughout my own life, even in the modern day I write this.

My father's desire to better himself through education and the dream of a career was passionate and one he desperately wanted to pursue. The attempts for my father to enrol himself into education was short-lived and of disappointment. The language barrier was a significant hindrance due to not being a native speaker of the country he had just moved to. Thus, he felt he did not have time as a commodity since his allegiance lay with the financial care of his family back home and here. He also knew that he would not have the support of his family, who would question why he was pursuing several years in education in the Western world, where access to money was rife. Ironically, he escaped the clutches of a working-class background from Pakistan, straight into the same grasp in the western world. Therefore, in his life, this was the first face of immediate gratification that surfaced and would continue to do so for most of his life.

Unwelcome and Subliminal Messages

My father arrived in a country that was at times unwelcome to migrants and particularly those of colour. He was not oblivious of the systematic prejudice apparent in society. In particular, living in a town with a football stadium in the 1970s and 1980s brought numerous racial tensions. I was far too young then to understand that my skin colour was contentious to some people. I do recall clearly that we were never allowed out during a football match, lest we were embroiled in violence during those times. This caution was further perpetuated by mistrust of the police and their lack of training regarding community cohesion and issues of institutional racism, which was later exemplified through the McPherson report (1999).

Often enough, work demands were complex, with my father trying to fulfil his work duties amidst those who were unwelcome. He recognised that his job security often lay at the hands of such people, and thus, he realised that he was often expendable and was required to work hard. Admittedly, my father would agree that he could never speak out against unjust treatment due to the lack of support and an unawareness of how. Thus, how could he emancipate himself from a system he did not fully understand or was supported in (Freire, 2014). Interestingly, I have also felt this echo throughout my personal and professional life.

The Mcgregor-Smith Review (2017) stipulates that discrimination and bias arise throughout the careers of individuals and well before the start of it. I did not need this report to specify this because those around me were already highlighting the problematisation of my working-class, race and religious identity as I was growing up. Amidst a tight-knit South Asian community, I recall the subtle subliminal messages community elders were sending. All of which were in relation to the ugly face of systematic prejudice which I have viewed throughout most of my career; the lack of a diverse workforce (in particular, role models), micro-aggressions, the 'othering' and struggling to 'achieve the same progression opportunities as their White counterparts' (The Mcgregor-Smith Review, 2017, p. 9). Subsequently, I grew up aware of systematic oppression and later learnt how to deal with it accordingly.

My father was incredibly patient through the racial and working-class discrimination he often faced in the working world. It is disheartening for me to hear that he had become desensitised to this treatment and, in many ways, accepted his fate but was never defeated.

I now recognise that a small part of my father's high expectations of me doing well in education was to evoke what Freire (2014) refers to as the 'critical consciousness'. Both my parents understood that there was empowerment in being educated, ascertaining positions of power and having a professional career. Subsequently, my education has enabled a better critical consciousness, and thus I can engage with emancipation even if there are societal and institutional complexities.

The Move Towards Betterment

Ultimately, my parents envisaged manoeuvring me away from a working-class background and into a more privileged position even before the birth of their nine children. Having grown up in a predominantly South Asian area, undoubtedly also working class, my father recognised a high level of cultural and material deprivation. He noticed continuously; parents purposely advocated immediate gratification over a deferred one which temporarily increased their cultural capital. This subsequently devalued education's ideology, which did not sit comfortably with him.

Subsequently, my parents decided to leave a predominantly South Asian community early in my childhood and move into an all-white middle-class neighbourhood amidst affluent schools. It was evident to the surrounding neighbours that we were different; our ethnicity and working-class background were apparent in our external visage. Often enough, we were made to feel unwelcome, but my parents expected a high level of decorum in not responding to the racial and class negativity. Crew (2020) stipulates that classism is a bias that is hard to reverse. Amalgamate that with issues of race, and the complexity heightens. For this reason, it was often best not to engage in any negative dialogue lest the outcomes became worse.

To add further salt to injury, we were also often made to feel a sense of guilt at leaving the 'safety' of the South Asian community and often looked upon as those who had created some form of treason. Knott (2018) states that Muslim communities from Britain primarily identify themselves by their faith, ethnicity, language and kinship. I remember overhearing conversations with others in the South Asian community, that by moving to a predominantly white area, we would lose the characteristics stated by Knott. However, my parents were not overly concerned about spatial segregation but more focussed on our schooling and education. Without a shadow of a doubt, I had a disciplined upbringing which at times was constraining, but this was in line with my parents ensuring my 'roots' were not forgotten.

Language, Religion, Culture and Family

Both my parents had a high expectation that we learn our mother tongue and use it daily. Thus, my command of the English langue was not at a mastery level, and this was evident among my school peers due to being bilingual. For this reason, my language was undoubtedly in line with what Bernstein (2002) refers to as 'restricted codes.' Consequently, my English language was often a hindrance to my academic achievement and one that remained with me for a good part of my education. Moving to an all-white school was challenging and one where I had to make a conscious effort in altering the way I spoke and conducted myself. Thus, not only was I learning my parent's native tongue but also the English language simultaneously.

I certainly resonate with Matthys (2012), who states that when you move away from class cultures regarding speech, writing and thinking, there are risks of alienation from that culture. Ironically, from being advised by community elders not to leave, it was this same South Asian community where the 'othering' became apparent. Moving to a middle-class area and a well-established school did not come without its problems when I mixed with peers from my South Asian community. My use of the English language drastically differed from theirs, and my ideology regarding numerous topics was also varied. I was often 'othered' by exercising my agency, and derogatory comments were usually made about me not being 'fully Pakistani' and racial slurs with my association with 'sounding and acting white'.

For this reason, there are still times when I am conscious of the way I converse with others. Often enough, trying not to use overly academic jargon and revert to adopting slang and colloquialism that is now alien to me. Subsequently, this repeatedly thrusts me back to my working-class roots, giving me a more welcoming approach from specific audiences. However, this negotiation of my identity is not necessarily a choice but one of necessity. One that I found I could not escape, no matter where I have lived and who I associate myself with.

Crew (2020) states that accents and social class in Britain have a long history. I have never made any pretence about not being from a working-class background within my professional context. I am often reminded of that social class and my heritage by professionals making comments such as, 'you are very well spoken' throughout my career. Often enough, I have felt that this is alluding to a particular stereotype and even profiling that has been both overt and covert in nature. However, my ability to code-switch my language has been beneficial in accessing various audiences of people. I now feel it is of great advantage, particularly when engaging my students in Higher Education.

My cultural and religious upbringing resonates with what Scourfield, Gilliat-Ray, Khan, and Otri (2013) discuss regarding issues of embodiment and habitus; I unconsciously amassed habits and moral behaviours regarding my Muslim identity. These echoed a 'hidden curriculum' in that my norms, values and beliefs were achieved through observations and imitations. These were not just enacted values but also the espoused ones regarding my Muslim identity and how I was expected to foster those ideologies daily.

Adding further complexity to this was my Pakistani heritage and abiding by those separate norms that were not in line with religiosity. This often created confusion; on one side, I was expected to adhere to scripture, and on the other side, cultural norms which were opposite to each other. The additional layer of being British, and identifying with that more than my Pakistani heritage, certainly evoked an identity crisis; who am I? Where do I belong? How should I behave?

Subsequently, not only was I from a working-class background but then torn between a traditional Islamic upbringing and Pakistani culture. All of which I was navigating through a secularised multicultural society. Consequently, living as a minority within a minority, I had to deal with an increased level of cognitive dissonance whilst trying to develop a more cohesive and personal identity (Suleiman, 2016).

In the outside world, I often felt a sense of betrayal to both my religious and cultural identity by engaging with things that I knew would be displeasing.

Subsequently, in the latter environments, I also felt a sense of guilt at wanting to be my authentic self (away from both religion and culture) but not having the confidence to do that. This was one of my earliest recollections about the complexity of negotiating my identity depending on my social positioning.

University, the Silent Departure and Ineffective Role Models

There was no presupposed notion of not attending university; it was an expectation set by my parents from a young age. There was never any dialogue about the choice of this – only the anticipation of where and what academic discipline I would forge for my future career. In fact, even the field required dialogue and approval from my parents. Subsequently, the academic rigour expected from this was challenging at times. There was intense pressure to secure high grades, complete additional work, read vast amounts of books for pleasure and ensure that our focus was solely on schooling. The work ethic they instilled in me certainly comes from my working-class roots and remains with me to this very day.

Yes, both my parents remain uneducated, but I resonate entirely with Goodall and Montgomery's (2013) literature, which states that parents from ethnic minorities find engagement with schools challenging but desire to take an active involvement with their children's education. Both my parents were incredibly active in supporting me in my education; it was important for my working-class parents to ensure that my siblings and I had better lives than they did. Their ideology of this was synonymous with education and success.

For me, the opportunity to attend university was dual in nature. I was already prepped to participate, so the decision was not negotiable. But more significantly, the intention of going to university also concerned my complex identity. I resonate with Knott (2018), who states that university offers young Muslims the opportunity to forge their own identities, away from what they have been initially exposed to.

Whilst negotiating my identity, a lot of what I was navigating through did not always sit comfortably with me. I had become constrained, and a part of me felt shackled by expectations and adherence to norms that were not befitting of my nature and ideology of life. My inquisitive mind searched for the world's mysteries outside religious, cultural and family boundaries. Thus, I saw university as a form of escapism that I grasped, and subsequently, it was the first time in my life where I felt free to explore, seek and trial and error.

Amidst my short time at university, it felt like a great adventure and a new sense of freedom. Admittedly, my focus shifted away from university, and I lost both focus and passion for it. An integral element of this was the consequence of my identity crisis and searching for the 'self', which was still unknown to me at that time. If I did not 'know thyself', how could I ever understand my life, the journey ahead and what my ultimate destination was. So, staying at university at that time was not part of my identity journey.

My decision to leave university, after the first year, was one that I look back in slight bewilderment; what was I thinking, and why was there no support from the university? However, these fleeting thoughts are now from someone who is somewhat wiser and looks back with reflectivity. I resonate with Malik and Wykes (2018), who argue that Muslim students are a particular group most likely to leave Higher Education with no award. Unbeknown to me, I had become part of the statistics immersed in widening participation issues in Higher Education sectors.

Sharing my decision with my parents was one of the most challenging conversations I had with them. They tried to convince me to stay and continue, but my decision had been made at heart, and there was no changing that. Reflecting on this time, I remember the complete devastation my parents experienced. I now realise that leaving education was a sense of betrayal of their hard work, inability to pursue education themselves and the impression of not wanting more from life as they had once dreamt for themselves and their children.

At that age, the problem with my own experience was the lack of role models in line with my lived experience. I resonate with Bhopal and Jackson (2013), who state that universities lack the representation of BAME staff. The DfE (2021) states that BAME teachers and leaders are under-represented within the teaching workforce; statistics show that in 2019, 85.7% of all teachers in state-funded schools in England were white British, and 92.7% of head teachers were white British. Yes, there seems to be a call for male role models, but Tembo (2020) states that no such call is made for those under-represented in the profession. I look back and realise how alien I was in a system dominated by white academics. Thus, how could I ever explain the complexities of my identity crisis and a new sense of freedom to those unfamiliar with me and my background?

Boliver and Powell (2021) state that the Office for Students now expect a strategic and systematic plan to encounter those issues related to ethnic inequalities and deploy initiatives to support those from minoritised backgrounds. This was not the case with my sudden decision to leave university at a different time. There were no meetings, suggestions for an alternative plan or my voice being heard. Subsequently, my departure from university was relatively silent, which most likely went unnoticed at the time.

The Return to University and a Career Was Born

I had numerous jobs in London that I feel did not involve any career potential. However, at that time, the concept of deferred gratification was not something I understood. Having spent years refining my spoken language, this often alluded to others that I was highly educated. Once again, the presumption that those who speak well are more likely educated. Confusingly, it constantly surprised people that I had left university. Over time, there were a number of these conversations, and I started to develop a sense of regret that I had the potential for betterment but seemingly threw away that opportunity. UCAS (2021) states that in 2019, British South Asians Higher Education participation was a mere 50%. Looking at these statistics, I realise that I possibly perpetuated people's negative impressions of working-class and ethnic backgrounds by leaving education.

During my time working in London, it was not surprising that I naturally drew closer to those from a working-class background. There was familiarity with them, a sense of belonging, understanding and no judgement. I now thank these people because their encouragement and advice enabled me to want more. They reignited my passion and focus for betterment, and subsequently, I chose to return to university. Even now, many years on, I am still drawn to minoritised groups for these very reasons.

Going back to university was not an easy venture for me. Boliver (2016) states that students from ethnic minority groups are considerably under-represented in elite universities. I was not confident to apply to more reputable Russell Group universities because I was unsure about my academic abilities. It was unfortunate that I did not understand the concept of impostorism back then because that is what it was. I was fighting the internal battle that I had marginalised myself, by perpetuating the claim that working-class boys are least likely to attend university. Ardy, Branchu, and Boliver (2021) state that those from ethnic minorities have a higher risk of not completing their degree programmes. I was weary about not further contributing to more statistics if I did not complete it.

Also, the university I attended seemed unimportant because I needed to stay in my locality due to ease of travel and convenience. Donnelly and Gamsu (2018) state that studying locally is often situated by those from disadvantaged backgrounds. I indeed related to this because the affordability of working full time and completing studies in the evenings was financially more manageable. I was fortunate to have this flexibility; otherwise, I would not be where I am today.

Leaving employment for full-time education was not an option, and thus, I had to do both. Working full time and completing my studies in the evenings was incredibly challenging. I did not have a laptop, so I had a reliance on the on-campus facilities. Eventually, I purchased an archaic desktop computer which was often more problematic than good. I also did not possess a car and needed to get to the other side of town, so I was always late. Comments were often made about this, but no one ever sat me down for me to explain my circumstances. It was an incredibly stressful time, and if it had not been for a key few people in my life, I most likely would have left.

Completing my degree did not feel as liberating as others around me might have wanted. I thought I was incredibly behind both in academia and my career and thus, needed to catch up with others. After a few very challenging years of studying and working simultaneously, I was undoubtedly exhausted, but my drive to betterment was strong. I completed my teacher training qualification and had a very successful career as a Primary school practitioner, where I held a number of strategic and transformational roles.

I felt this achievement was a turning point in my life where even though I still felt working class, I was now treated by others as someone who had manoeuvred into a different realm that was alien to me. It was a surreal experience to suddenly be viewed as middle class due to my education and career. However, I took no benefit from that due to still feeling working class. Ultimately, I thought I existed in two different worlds, further exasperating my identity crisis.

During my time working in Primary schools, I decided to complete my Master's degree and continue my pursuit of knowledge and education. Again, I finished this over some years whilst working full time amidst some senior roles. Completion of my Master's degree was undoubtedly my first monumental feeling of success. Until then, any achievements felt like a catch-up programme, and thus, the intrinsic rewards were nothing compared to achieving a postgraduate degree.

My graduation was incredibly memorable because both my parents were present. This was very symbolic because even though I had dropped out of university, I had managed to acquire the highest qualification in my family. For me, the Master's degree had repaired the internal damage of disappointing my parents many years before. Subsequently, my venture into a postgraduate qualification gave birth to my passion for research, writing and making a difference in a different capacity than I was used to.

An Outsider Amidst the Insiders

There has been a counterapproach to the issue of gender diversity in schools, with a call to ensure more male role models are recruited (DfE, 2017). Subsequently, I was very much valued in Primary schools due to being a South Asian male. All the head teachers I encountered encouraged me to be a positive role model for ethnic minority communities. Even though this experience was somewhat optimistic, a diverse workforce in related educational sectors has not been similar. Bhopal and Jackson (2013) state that universities lack the representation of BAME staff and are also under-represented within senior levels. I have earlier stated the significate disparity between ethnic monitory groups in education compared to white colleagues, which became even more apparent in Higher Education.

Consequently, I have sometimes felt like an outsider trying to establish positionality and creditability in an environment where I am aesthetically different. Thus, it surfaces the question of what institutional aims and objectives set regarding race equality show? Subsequently, I have often wondered if education establishments are even aware that they might be viewed as perpetuating overt and covert discriminatory practices, by not evidencing a diverse workforce. In particular, I resonate with Vieler-Porter (2021), who states that the problematisation of educational outcomes cannot be fully addressed when there is an under-representation of BAME educators. Thus, it is safe to say that people like myself bring value to organisations from which the better ones will harness.

Islamophobia, the Power of Language and Microaggressions

Bush, Glover, and Sood (2006) argue that BAME educators and leaders are prone to barriers through covert and overt forms of discrimination. Ipsos MORI (2018) found that Muslim graduates and younger Muslims felt that prejudice increased and thought they lacked opportunity. I must admit that there are truths in this matter, as uncomfortable as this might be to read. The impact of fundamentalist Islam has sadly impacted many Muslims who are in line with British life, both personally and professionally. Consequently, the birth of Islamophobia has undoubtedly cast a dark shadow over me throughout most of my career. Islamophobia has enabled the rhetoric that Muslims, such as myself, are a monolithic group different from those in the West.

Further adding to the complexity is what Farrell (2016) argues regarding policy and political rhetoric surrounding the notion of Muslims being a suspect community. Consequently, anti-terrorism strategies such as British values have reinforced Muslims 'othering' and marginalisation (Bamber, Bullivant, Clark & Lundie, 2018). However, Muslims like myself do not feel their faith conflicts with Britishness; I have a strong sense of belonging with our nationality and have commonality with other British and ethnic groups (Ipsos MORI, 2018). I further resonate with The Runnymede Trust (1997), which found that Muslims are routinely challenged regarding their values, loyalties and commitments. Subsequently, I have often kept my religiosity intensely private throughout my career, lest I create the impression of orthodoxy and conservatism, which is not my reality.

There have been numerous times when I have had to renegotiate my faith by modifying my exterior, such as trimming down my beard to secure a job position, ensuring I pray in places that are not visible and never discussing issues of faith in a professional setting. I will undoubtedly avoid political dialogues where faith is the centre of the topic lest there are repercussions. Thus, my voice and agency are constrained, even with freedom of speech and individual liberty in the free world I reside in.

Du Bois (1903 cited in Holloway, 2015) talks of 'double consciousness' and how it depicts the feeling of having more than one identity and how this complexity makes it challenging to develop the self. Thus, for me, it has become second nature to look at myself as a Muslim academic through the eyes of others. This has engaged me with a sense of self-criticality and constant reflexivity in how my behaviour might be perceived. Me adopting a liberal stance with my faith is a personal choice. However, I must advocate liberalism to those around me, which I feel is not a choice.

I resonate with Said (1997), who maintains that 'Islam is synonymous with terrorism and religious hysteria'. Islam is synonymous with terminologies such as terrorism, radicalisation, extremism, etc. Subsequently, I often wonder, now that these terms are associated with Islam, is it possible for people to divorce those connotations from me as a Muslim? If we think about something long enough, does that not then form our ideologies and thus, impact the way we behave?

Subsequently, when I am new to an establishment where no one knows me, I am often left internally dejected by my thoughts that people are consciously and inadvertently profiling me. This has been evidenced by comments such as, 'you're not how I thought you might be'. Maybe part of the problem is that I am yet to challenge these assumptions, but that is not so easy when new to an establishment and trying to forge positionality.

A problem often not spoken about, most likely due to the challenge of evidence, is that of microaggressive behaviours that I have experienced and viewed within professional settings. At times, comments have been made regarding my various identities, be it working class, ethnicity, faith or even sexuality. Subsequently, focussing on those areas where there is an awareness of discriminatory attitudes has made me feel the subject of stereotypes. The more covert experiences of microaggressions certainly resonate with Rollock (2012), who states that such behaviours can be subtle such as being interrupted, spoken over and even having the legitimacy of contributions questioned. All of which I have unfortunately experienced throughout my career.

Yes, I am protected by law – the Equality Act (2010) and the Protected Characteristics (2010), etc. However, I am not protected against covert discrimination with classism, race, faith, etc. I have found that they are all incredibly challenging to evidence. Thus, even within the charted waters of law, I have often felt I am navigating through such storms by myself. In saying this, such oppressive behaviours have only made me a better person and a more effective academic.

Meritocracy Challenged and Imposter Syndrome

Numerous times, my meritocracy has been challenged within a professional setting. The commitment to diversifying establishments is not necessarily a new phenomenon but has undoubtedly evoked challenges for me. When I have secured a new job, a promotion, recognition of my hard work etc. there have been open reminders of my marginalised identities through comments such as, 'you secured that due to being male, due to being Pakistani, the establishment diversifying etc'. Consequently, at times I have felt that my meritocracy is negated, and the self-feeling I have been reduced to a 'poster boy' to fill the 'status quo' regarding diversity.

Wilson, Reay, Morrin, and Abrahams (2020) make a pertinent point regarding how we counteract the tokenistic use of bodies through familiar networking, spaces where we can engage in open dialogues and create support structures. My minoritised identities, which include that of being working class, naturally flock to others like me who identify as coming from marginalised groups. Even within professional settings, I now can decipher who is inherently part of my 'tribe' and theirs with little effort.

The complexities of these dual identities have been fraught with issues of accepting myself as an academic and novice researcher. If one looks at the amalgamation of my intersectionality and marginalisation issues, the concept of failure has undoubtedly contributed to imposter syndrome (Sakulku & Alexander, 2011). The 'othering' that I have experienced has made me question myself as a professional and thus, at times, shadowed my true potential. For this reason, I have had to try to ensure that the stains of impostorism did not become yet another face of my day-to-day identity.

Subsequently, I have grown much more confident with accepting that my agency has a voice, credibility and respect from experienced academics and other professionals alike. I have learnt that reminding myself of my meritocracy is not self-indulgent. I am still navigating my self-confidence as an academic and reminding myself of my hard work and value. This slowly removes my notions that I cannot work at elite universities, even though my working-class background is sometimes reluctant to accept this (Binns, 2019).

My Identity, My Students and Our Familiarity

I have come to understand that class can be invisible at times, and thus the exterior can often be deceptive in who comes from what background. Due to the way I articulate myself and often enough, the way I dress smartly, I feel there is a misconception about my class background. Amidst conversations with both students and peers, I have always made an effort to ensure that my true self is brought to the surface with no pretence about being someone I am not.

Crew (2020) states that staff in new universities were more likely to identify as working class. This aligns with my identity and the positive change the universities are now adopting in recruitment. I come from a working-class background, and I proudly hold onto that identity. For this reason, I feel my class disclosure has enabled a whole perspective and ideology on how academia is and should be viewed; academics come from varied backgrounds.

My working class background and coming from an ethnic minority group have been beneficial in the establishments I have worked in. It has enabled me to have lived experiences that are often alien to those in other classes but familiar to those from similar backgrounds. Joseph-Salisbury (2020) argues that a diverse teaching force could assist with raising positive academic outcomes for students due to them feeling represented. These experiences have helped me create an effective rapport with students and colleagues.

What is significant to appreciate is that students from minority backgrounds will be drawn to institutions where there are BAME staff (Bhopal & Jackson, 2013). I have found that those from marginalised groups will often rely on me for support, guidance and encouragement due to our familiarity and accessibility. Even though Bhopal and Jackson further argue that this is burdensome due to working over and above, I feel it is a service to all the students under my care.

Subsequently, it is vital for me as a practitioner, with a lived experience of being marginalised, to ensure that my students have a good understanding of issues of race, class and identity formation. I envisage that this will enable them to think critically and establish a firm acceptance of their belonging and own acceptance as British citizens, regardless of their backgrounds (Habib, 2018).

The Face of Oppression, My Agency and Structure and Who Am I?

Young (2011) stipulates there are five faces of oppression, and one in particular, 'powerlessness', is essential for me to recognise. Undoubtedly, there is a division between the working and middle classes. Thus, the labour division also exists – professional and non-professionals. The latter are classed as powerless; they 'lack the authority, status, and sense of self that professionals tend to have' (Young, 2011, p. 76).

I have had the privilege of a high education, professional development, authority, influence, a rise in status and recognition, which Young (2011) refers to as 'respectability'. This is all well and good, but what has been essential to me is not forgetting that I come from a working-class background. Thus, I was undoubtedly from the powerless, a place where I lacked authority, presence and autonomy and often felt expendable. Now having manoeuvred into being categorised as middle class, I am in this constant state of reflexivity, lest I inadvertently become one of the oppressors.

Manoeuvring away from a working-class identity echoes a sense of guilt. Not because of any conscious abandonment of that identity but merely because others see the illusion of middle-classness, which I feel is not befitting how I view myself. To many, my background may seem irrelevant whilst considering my current position. Some may even say that I need to describe myself as middle class and move on actively. However, I have not been able to adhere to this class adaptation, and there has been no metamorphosis for me to transcend into another being of some sort.

This chapter was never going to be merely about me being a working-class academic. It would have been impossible for me to have written this 'story' without it intersecting with my gender, race and faith. Giddens (1976 cited in Best, 2003) states that both human agency and structure are intertwined. Altering the structures around me is not plausible because each of these social systems I belong to is deeply rooted in their ideologies and practice. Thus, my agency is often interchangeable depending on the various environments I belong. Therefore, the academic you meet will depend on who you are, where you meet me, in what context and why. Subsequently, I often see my multiple identities as that of a Rubik's cube; each identity face revolving depending on where I am and whom I need to be within that context.

I am working class at my core and always will be. Amidst that identity, I am also British, South Asian, Muslim and male. I cannot let go of my history to date; I cannot forget my parents' sacrifices and challenging lives; I cannot let go of my work ethic; I cannot compromise on the relationships I have forged with working-class friends, peers and students. To commit to anything else would be inauthentic, disingenuous and an abandonment of myself. Even if I make attempts to alter myself, I always feel displaced. Thus, to ignore any one of my multiple identities would consequently negate an integral part of who I am.

References

Arday, J., Branchu, C., & Boliver, V. (2021). What do we know about black and minority ethnic (BAME) participation in UK higher education? *Social Policy and Society, 21*(1), 1–14.

Bamber, P., Bullivant, A., Clark, A., & Lundie, D. (2018). Educating global Britain: Perils and possibilities promoting "national" values through critical global citizenship education. *British Journal of Educational Studies, 66*(4), 433–453.

Bernstein, B. (2002). Theory of social class, educational codes and social control. *British Journal of Sociology of Education, 23*(4), 525–526.

Best, S. (2003). *A beginner's guide to social theory.* London: Sage.

Bhopal, K., & Jackson, J. (2013). The experiences of black and minority ethnic academics: Multiple identities and career progression. Retrieved from https://scholar. google.co.uk/scholar?q=The+Experiences+of+Black+and+Minority+Ethnic+ Academics:+Multiple+Identities+and+Career+Progression&hl=en&as_sdt=0 &as_vis=1&oi=scholart. Accessed on March 2, 2022.

Binns, C. (2019). *Experiences of academics from a working-class heritage: Ghosts of childhood habitus.* Newcastle upon Tyne: Cambridge Scholars Publishing.

Boliver, V. (2016). Exploring ethnic inequalities in admission to Russell group universities. *Sociology, 50*(2), 247–266.

Boliver, V., & Powell, M. (2021). Fair admission to UK universities: Improving policy and practice. Retrieved from https://www.nuffieldfoundation.org/wp-content/uploads/2021/01/Fair-admission-to-universities-in-England.pdf. Accessed on March 2, 2022.

Bush, T., Glover, D., & Sood, K. (2006). Black and minority ethnic leaders in England: A portrait. *School Leadership & Management, 26*(3), 289–305.

Byrne, G. (2019). Individual weakness to collective strength: (Re)creating the self as a 'working-class academic'. *Journal of Writing in Creative Practice, 12*(1–2), 131–150.

Crew, T. (2020). *Higher education and working-class Academics: Precarity and diversity in academia.* London: Palgrave Pivot.

Department for Education. (2017). Early years workforce strategy. Retrieved from https://www.gov.uk/government/publications/early-years-workforce-strategy. Accessed on March 2, 2022.

Department for Education. (2021). Ethnicity facts and figures: School teacher workforce. Retrieved from https://www.ethnicity-facts-figures.service.gov.uk/workforce-and-business/workforce-diversity/school-teacher-workforce/latest. Accessed on March 2, 2022.

Donnelly, M., & Gamsu, S. (2018). Regional structures of feeling? A spatially and socially differentiated analysis of UK student im/mobility. *British Journal of Sociology of Education, 39*(7), 961–981.

Farrell, F. (2016). 'Why all of a sudden do we need to teach fundamental British values?' A critical investigation of religious education student teacher positioning within a policy discourse of discipline and control. *Journal of Education for Teaching, 42*(3), 280–297.

Freire, P. (2014). *Pedagogy of the oppressed.* London: Bloomsbury Academic.

Goodall, J., & Montgomery, C. (2013). Parental involvement to parental engagement: A continuum. *Educational Review, 66*(4), 399–410.

Habib, S. (2018). *Learning and teaching British values.* Manchester: Cham Springer International Publishing.

Holloway, J. S. (2015). *The souls of black folk.* New Haven, CT: Yale University Press.

Ipsos MORI Social Research Institute. (2018). *A review of survey research on Muslims in Britain.* Retrieved from https://www.ipsos.com/en-uk/review-survey-research-muslims-britain-0. Accessed on March 2, 2022.

Joseph-Salisbury, R. (2020). *Runnymede perspectives: Race and racism in English secondary schools*. London: Runnymede Trust.

Knott, K. (2018). *Muslims and Islam in the UK: A research synthesis*. CREST (Centre for Research and Evidence on Security Threats. Retrieved from https://www.research.lancs.ac.uk/portal/en/publications/muslims-and-islam-in-the-uk(672ce62b-46ee-488c-8041-7aa7e15e962b).html. Accessed on March 2, 2022.

Malik, A., & Wykes, E. (2018). *British Muslims in UK higher education: Socio-political, religious and policy considerations*. London: Bridge Institute.

Matthys, M. (2012). *Cultural capital, identity and social mobility: The life course of working-class university graduates*. London: Routledge.

Rollock, N. (2012). Unspoken rules of engagement: Navigating racial micro-aggressions in the academic terrain. *International Journal of Qualitative Studies in Education, 25*(5), 517–532.

Said, E. W. (1997). *Covering Islam*. London: Vintage.

Sakulku, J., & Alexander, J. (2011). The impostor phenomenon. *International Journal of Behavioral Science, 6*(1), 75–97.

Scourfield, J., Gilliat-Ray, S., Khan, A., & Otri, S. (2013). *Muslim childhood: Religious nurture in a European context*. Oxford: Oxford University Press.

Suleiman, O. (2016). Internalized islamophobia: Exploring the faith and identity crisis of American Muslim youth. *Islamophobia Studies Journal, 4*, 1–12.

Tembo, S. (2020). Black educators in (white) settings: Making racial identity visible in early childhood education and care in England UK. *Journal of Early Childhood Research, 19*(1), 70–83.

The Equality Act. (2010). Retrieved from https://www.legislation.gov.uk/ukpga/2010/15/contents. Accessed on March 2, 2022.

The Protected Characteristics. (2010). Retrieved from https://www.equalityhumanrights.com/en/equality-act/protected-characteristics

The Runnymede Trust. (1997). Islamophobia: A challenge for us all. Retrieved from https://www.runnymedetrust.org/publications/islamophobia-a-challenge-for-us-all. Accessed on March 2, 2022.

The Mcgregor-Smith Review. (2017). Retrieved from https://assets.publishing.service.gov.uk/government/uploads/system/uploads/attachment_data/file/594336/race-in-workplace-mcgregor-smith-review.pdf. Accessed on March 2, 2022.

Universities and Colleges Admissions Service. (2021). *2020 entry UCAS undergraduate reports by sex, area background, and ethnic group*. Cheltenham: UCAS.

Vieler-Porter, C. G. (2021). *The under-representation of black and minority ethnic educators in education: Chance, coincidence or design?* London: Routledge.

Wilson, A., Reay, D., Morrin, K., & Abrahams, J. (2020). 'The still-moving position' of the 'working-class' feminist academic: Dealing with disloyalty, dislocation and discomfort discourse. *Studies in the Cultural Politics of Education, 42*(1), 30–44.

Young, M. I. (2011). *Justice and the politics of difference*. Oxford: Princeton University Press.

Chapter 7

Uptown Top Ranking: From a Council Estate to the Academy

Marcia A. Wilson

Abstract

This chapter will examine the intersectionality of race, class and gender as defining my experience of being a Black, working-class woman in academia over a 30-year period in the United States and United Kingdom. Drawing on Critical Race Theory (Delgado & Stefancic, 2013) as the framework for positionality, early childhood experiences will be discussed along with my entry and journey in academia. My early experiences are important to document as they are influential in defining my working-class heritage. I will also discuss the importance of intersecting issues related to being a Black working-class woman such as my accent and the politics of my hair in the academy. There are unique challenges faced by Black working-class women, so I conclude with some personal tips for staying in academia.

Keywords: Working class; racism; Black women; academy; hair; accent

Advisory: This chapter contains a racially offensive term.

Introduction

When I was initially asked to write this chapter, I had to think twice about accepting the offer. One issue was the tension in my mind about claiming a working-class identity given my current career position. I am a Professor and a Dean at a university. However, I would argue that being working class is much more than one's job and financial standing. It is borne out of one's values and the way the world is experienced. It is 'a way of being, relating, and thinking that culminates in a shared cultural experience often invisible to the privileged...' (Case, 2017, p. 17). I work in a sector that was not established for people who look like me or have my background, and I have always felt a lack of belonging

The Lives of Working Class Academics, 89–100

Copyright © 2023 Marcia A. Wilson

Published under exclusive licence by Emerald Publishing Limited

doi:10.1108/978-1-80117-057-420221007

and connection in the academy despite having a successful career. However, my key motivation for staying in academia is to positively contribute to the equity, diversity and inclusion agenda. My mission is a social justice one, and it is to leave higher education better than I found it. It is also important to me that Black, working-class women see academics who are like them and are appropriately represented at all levels across the sector. I hope that others find this chapter useful as I discuss the challenges of staying in academia, trying to reach one's potential and in that process – work towards change that would be beneficial for everyone.

Humble Beginnings

As stated earlier, I tussled with my claim to be a working-class academic. My roots are working class but I now have a senior management position, and over the past couple of years have sat on the executive committee of two universities. To understand why I position myself as a working-class person, it is important to share some information about growing up in the East End of London in the late 1960s to the early 1980s.

Historically, to be born within the sound of Bow Bells denotes being an authentic Cockney. I'd like to say that I was born within the sound of the Bow Bells but in my heart, I know that's not strictly true. I was born a few miles from Bow in Forest Gate, East London, but I remember seeing the Pearly Kings and Queens on parade and they even visited my primary and secondary school. I also remember people using Cockney rhyming slang in everyday conversations and going to the market stalls every Saturday morning to buy fresh food. Our shopping was always a combination of fruit and vegetables bought from the market and non-perishables from a supermarket. My mum and I would pull our shopping in a small food trolley and take the underground tube home. We did not own a car. If my local football team, West Ham United, was playing at their home ground (the Boleyn), we had to do our shopping extra early because the streets would be lined with police from Upton Park station to the market and down to the Boleyn because some of the supporters were notorious for violence and racism.

My parents were of the Windrush Generation and came to England from Jamaica in the early 1960s. Both came in search of a better life and were invited over as British citizens because Jamaica was a colony until 1962 and Queen Elizabeth II was the Head of State. On arrival, both lived in London and experienced daily overt racism that made life in the 'Motherland' very difficult. Securing accommodation was challenging as white landlords often had signs in their windows saying 'No Blacks, No Irish, No Dogs'. My parents were reliant on friends and family who were already settled to give a helping hand so that they had basic amenities. My father worked for British Rail and my mother worked as a care home assistant looking after elderly people. Both worked shifts and had the strongest work ethic I have ever seen.

We were the first Black family on our street in a new Council home in West Ham, East London, in 1976. Prior to that, we lived a short distance away in an area called Plaistow on a council estate in a small two-bedroom maisonette. I was pleased that we were moving to a house where I could have my own bedroom. All the other families on our new street were white. Some spoke to us and some ignored us, but I do have mostly good memories of playing outside with the neighbourhood children. The racism was evident among some neighbours to the extent that one of them had a black cat and decided to call it 'Nigger'. That was my first introduction to the word. The news that our new neighbours called their cat a racial slur quickly reverberated down our street, but no one said anything to them. It was just accepted as the way it was.

I attended the local primary and then the secondary comprehensive school, and this was during the reign of the Conservative government with Margaret Thatcher as Prime Minister. During this era, unemployment steadily rose and state-owned enterprises were privatised. I saw the poor getting poorer and the rise of the right-wing. Thatcher was very vocal about immigration by stating on TV that (white) people in Britain were afraid that the country will be swamped by people of a different culture. It was during the 1980s that Black people experienced increasing racist hostility and police brutality which culminated in riots in Bristol, London and Liverpool. The hostility was evident in the daily walk to my secondary school. Racist slogans and logos were spray-painted everywhere by the National Front and the British Movement which were far-right organisations. Although everyone in the neighbourhood was working-class, white people had the privilege of not dealing with racism and the hostile environment that was directed at racially minoritised people.

My parents worked hard in manual labour jobs where we had the essentials but could not afford luxuries. I count myself fortunate that I always had a roof over my head, have always known where my next meal is coming from and we could always afford heating. From a young age, I remember my father emphasising the importance of education as the way out of poverty, and in particular, urging me to be a doctor as he believed that I would always be employed if I was a medic.

I left school with a few 'O' Levels and went to work in a shop in Central London. It was the norm for working-class children to leave school at 16 years old and go to work. After four days in my new job, I decided to leave because I was constantly bullied and shouted at by my line manager. I did not want another job so decided to return to school and study 'A' Levels. I did not have a plan. The other children in the sixth form were talking about which university they would apply to and what they were going to study. I was silent as I did not think I was smart enough to go to university and the truth was that I was doing 'A' Levels because I didn't know what else to do. During that time, only 2% of students went to university and I didn't know anyone who had studied beyond secondary school. The Head of the Sixth Form called me into her office and told me to apply to university. I went to Open Days at a few universities and loved visiting Bangor, North Wales. I could see the snow on the peaks of Snowdon from the campus and fell in love with the beauty of the city.

Gaining entry to university was not straightforward. I received a conditional offer and but did not achieve the grades required, so I decided to visit the

Department Head. I did not realise that university was unlike school and that it was very possible that the Head of Department might not be in his office. I travelled from London to Bangor on the off chance that I could just speak to a member of staff. He was not in his office when I arrived so I sat outside his office and waited for a couple of hours. When it became obvious that I needed to travel back to London before it got too dark, I wrote the department head a note and slipped it under his office door and then went home. A couple of weeks later, I was offered an unconditional place to study sport and education. Perhaps my main motivation for attending university was to avoid working in a job where I was constantly disrespected. Although the four days of bullying by my line manager in the shop was horrendous, I actually have a lot to be grateful for because if I enjoyed the shop work, I might have never left! Being in an environment where there was a mix of different social classes was a new experience to me. I had not met anyone from a private school before or students whose parents bought them a house to live in or people who came from such wealth that they had all of their needs catered to. University broadened my horizons beyond East London and enabled me to think about endless possibilities in relation to a career.

My secondary school experience was very different to most of my Black friends in East London. I do not know of any other Black children from my school who went to university the same year as me. In general, teacher expectations were low for working-class children and even more so if you were Black (Gershenson & Papageorge, 2018). The impact of teacher expectations and student attainment has been well documented (Brophy, 1983; Dusek, 1985; Jussim, 1989) since the seminal study entitled 'Pygmalion in the Classroom' by Rosenthal and Jacobson (1968). The body of research on teacher expectations influenced my decision to learn more about how people in positions of power can negatively or positively impact others depending on whether they hold high or low expectations of those people. I decided to study this topic for my PhD and apply the framework to sport, so I examined how coach expectations influence athletes' cognitive process, behaviour and outcomes. My research interests have developed further as I continue to examine power dynamics in relation to racism and racial trauma. I completed my postgraduate studies in the United States and worked over there for a 10-year period. I did not plan to study in the United States. I applied for PG positions in the United Kingdom but was not successful. It was my undergraduate lecturer who encouraged me to study in the United States because he had a very positive experience during his sabbatical in Eugene, Oregon.

I define my entry to the academy as 'accidental', very similar to Kwhali (2017). I did not know what career I wanted, and I did not know enough about different viable options. After my early experiences when I left school, I just knew that I wanted a secure job where I was respected. I did not know where that was or what it looked like. As Pulley (2019) argues, Black working-class women academics are generally raised in families that do not have the economic, social and cultural capital power typically rooted in being racialised as white, middle-class and male. I was the first person in my family to attend university and achieve postgraduate qualifications. I just kept going with no real thought as to what career I would have when I eventually finished. As I was studying for my PhD, I was also teaching and found that I could relate to students and they were receptive to me, so I started applying for Assistant Professor positions as I was still living in the United States. Having secured a position at a small Liberal Arts College in South Carolina, I did not feel as though my class status was an issue for colleagues or students. I was living in the deep south where the locals have a distinctive southern drawl and were probably unaware of the roots of my accent. Being a Black woman, on the other hand, was the dominant factor related to experiences of racism and sexism.

'You Wot?': The Problem with My Accent Is Yours, Not Mine

I moved back to the United Kingdom in 2001 to spend time with my aging parents. I secured a lecturing position in a university that was in the South West of England and that was my first experience of my accent being commented on by a student. A young white male was sitting in the lecture towards the front saying loud enough for me to hear that he couldn't understand what I was saying. His friend was smiling but hushing him at the same time. Although this experience was new to me as a lecturer, it is not uncommon for working-class academics to experience frustration regarding their accent as being perceived as incompatible with their job (Larcombe, 2016). Accent Prestige Theory posits that a person who speaks with the accent of the dominant group in society will be perceived more positively compared to people with regional or foreign accents (Fuertes, Potere & Ramirez, 2002). Furthermore, in their meta-analysis, Fuertes, Gottdiener, Martin, Gilbert, and Giles (2012) indicated that the standard accent as spoken by the dominant group within society was more strongly associated with higher intellectual and social class status; solidarity and trustworthiness; and dynamism.

I have spent the majority of my academic career working in a post-92 university in the East End of London. My accent was accepted by the majority of colleagues as most of us sounded very similar. In fact, 'standard accents' were more out of place in that particular environment. My accent also helped to forge a connection between me and my students. I was able to identify with them because I was from the local area and had an upbringing similar to many of them. A working-class accent can be a positive attribute for connecting with poorer students (Coogan, 2019). Although some people choose to tone down their accent or modify it to gain greater perceived acceptability and respectability in the academy, I think there is something lost when this happens. All students, especially those who are marginalised, need to see and hear people who look like them in positions of power. Authentic representation is crucial if we are to resist and challenge the status quo.

Black Hair: The Personal Is Political

In addition to accents that maybe seen as problematic by some in the academy, Black people's hair has long been perceived as contentious in various domains. This has been dominant in the education sector where Black children have been excluded from school for wearing their natural hair (such as afro, braids and locs) with schools contending those styles are against school uniform policy (Dabiri, 2020). Black women's hair is personal but also political and is intimately associated with our historical and social heritage. In some quarters of our communities, it is not uncommon to hear Black people talk about 'good' and 'bad' hair. Good hair is that which is closely connected to European hair texture which tends to be long and straight. Bad hair is typically short with tight curls (Lester, 2000). As can be deduced by this 'good' and 'bad' hair situation, 'good' hair is closely aligned with whiteness (Brown, 2014). bell hooks encapsulates why the personal choice of hair style is political in her essay 'Straightening my hair'.

> There are times when I think of straightening my hair just to change my style... Then I remind myself that even though such a gesture could be simply playful on my part... I know that such a gesture would carry other implications beyond my control. The reality is: straightened hair is linked historically and currently to a system of racial domination that impresses upon black women, that we are not acceptable as we are, that we are not beautiful. To make such a gesture...would make me complicit with a politic of domination that hurts us.
>
> (hooks, 2007, p. 6)

While studying for my PhD, I decided that I would have a hairstyle that reflects who I am and who I want to be in the academy. I have had locs for over 20 years and my feelings about my hair are reflected in my resistance to conform with social norms and expectations about Black hair. hooks argues that locs can be seen as the 'total antithesis of straightening one's hair, as a political statement' (hooks, 2007, p. 5). It is important to note that I am not anti-straightening of one's hair as I see it as a personal choice. However, it is frustrating and concerning that some Black women feel pressure to ensure their appearance is closely aligned to what would be deemed professional, and therefore acceptable. In the same way that working-class accents are sometimes regarded as a problem, Black natural hair is rarely accepted as an appropriate way to be in the academy.

My only memorable experience of my hair being an issue for someone was many years ago when I was invited to join a team of managers to host a delegation of academics from China. My boss had arranged to take them for dinner and before we left, he asked me to put my hair up. I was taken aback by his comments and replied that I would not be doing that. He looked at me for a moment as if to think about what to say but then said nothing. We did not discuss this incident because I knew that he did not have the level of racial literacy required to understand the implications of his request. I think with locs, it is easier to disguise them if they are pulled up and tucked away rather than having them down, which relates to what is deemed as potentially an unprofessional look for the workplace.

If I had acquiesced to the request to change my hairstyle, I might have found myself on the road to code-switching. Code-switching is when people interact and behave in different ways depending on the context they are in (Case, 2017), and when this occurs within the workplace, they embrace the dominant culture. There is a body of literature that focuses on code-switching among professional Black women who work in predominantly white spaces (Cheeks, 2018). Although code-switching has garnered more attention in the United States, it also occurs in the United Kingdom where in relation to class and code-switching, changes in accent and language may occur. In relation to race, there have been accounts of Black women being pressured to change their authentic selves in the workplace. The most common issue is non-acceptance of natural hair as a professional style (Sini, 2016). Code-switching and requests to change hairstyle is based on little or no value given to cultural and racial capital that Black people bring to the workplace. The expectation is that we fit into and embrace the existing culture and leave ours at the door and collect it as we leave the workplace at the end of the day. There is no thought that we might add value to what is already present and it does not need to be in conflict with existing cultural norm.

A Round Peg in a Square Hole: Being in the Academy

Over the years, I have often pondered whether my gender, race or class is the defining characteristic that shapes my experiences in the academy. It is perhaps an impossible question to answer because the intersectionality of those characteristics provide different experiences and meanings in life at different times depending on the situation. Kimberlé Crenshaw's work on the experiences of African-American women has been hailed as the work that typifies intersectionality. It is important that an intersectional framework is used as a way of understanding Black working-class women's experiences in the academy as this provides a more nuanced understanding from a feminist and multicultural perspective (Showunmi, Atewologun, & Bebbington, 2016). Race and racism cannot be denied as having a central feature in the experiences of Black people in the academy. Regardless of class, Black people still experience racism as highlighted by Showunmi and Maylor (2013).

All three of my degree experiences (Bachelor's, Master's and Doctorate) were steeped in middle-class whiteness. The academics were white and middle-class, the curriculum was unapologetically largely white and male by way of content, books and journal articles, and the environment was white (portraits on walls and statues on the campuses). At undergraduate level, I gravitated to working-class students of all ethnicities for friendship. At postgraduate level in the United States, I still gravitated to working-class peers for friendship but class seemed to matter less to them. Throughout my studies, I did not question out loud the Eurocentricity and middle-classness of my experience. I was often the only Black person in my class, on my degree programme and in my department as an academic. As Delgado and Stefancic (2013) argue, one of the theoretical tenets of Critical Race Theory is that race and racism are endemic, normalised and central to the functioning of our society. It became normal to be the only Black person in the academic space. Roxanne Gay encapsulates my feelings in her reflective account as a Professor:

I am the only child of immigrants. Many of my students have never had a Black teacher before. I can't help them with that. I am the only Black professor in my department. This will probably never change for the whole of my career, no matter where I teach. I am used to it. I wish I weren't. There seems to be some unspoken rule about the number of academic spaces people of color can occupy at the same time. I have grown weary of being the only one.

(Gay, 2014, p. 22)

Almost 40 years ago, Carroll (1982) expressed a similar sentiment:

There is no one with whom to share experiences and gain support, no one with whom to identify, no one on whom a Black woman can model herself. It takes a great deal of psychological strength 'just to get through a day', the endless lunches, and meetings in which one is always 'different'. The feeling is much like the exhaustion a foreigner speaking an alien tongue feels at the end of the day. (p. 120).

It was not until I studied for my PhD that I experienced being taught by a Black woman academic – Professor Audrey Qualls who was one of my mentors. There is a dearth of Black professors in the United Kingdom, and it has become somewhat normalised. There are no data on the number of working-class professors across the sector, but I would hazard a guess that the numbers are shockingly low as well. As an example of the scarcity of Black people in senior positions, across the UK higher education sector, there has only been one Black woman who has led a Higher Education Institution (HEI). Baroness Valerie Amos was appointed Director of School of Oriental and African Studies (SOAS) in 2015. There are only 45 Black women professors out of approximately 23,000 full professors in the United Kingdom. The Higher Education Statistics Agency (HESA) data indicate that 0.6% of professors in the United Kingdom are Black (2019–2020). The paucity of Black women senior staff is directly related to systemic failures across the sector from undergraduate student to professor in academia.

Although compared to the national population, Black, Asian and Ethnic Minority students are over-represented in higher education. They account of 26.7% of students, whereas they make up 14% of the UK population. However, the percentages decline at postgraduate level (18.6%) and again for academic staff (11.2%) and professors (9.3%). It is important to disaggregate the data as they mask the percentages for each racialised minoritised group. For example, Black people are under-represented and comprise 2.8% of staff in the higher education sector, whereas Black people make up 3.3% of the UK population. To date, there has only been two Black leaders of a higher education institution in the United Kingdom, with the most recent appointment being made in 2020 when Professor Charles Egbu was appointed Vice Chancellor of Leeds Trinity University. The under-representation of Black staff, in general and working-class Black staff in particular, has an impact on the student experience for all regardless of their race and class. Under-representation reinforces white middle-class supremacy as the natural and unwavering order of the structures within our institutions. The lack of Black people working within higher education is problematic because the absence at all levels is normalised. This is particularly an issue at senior management levels because there is a lack of attention to address one of the most persistent and concerning issues in the sector which is the degree awarding gap. This is the percentage points difference in good degrees (a 1st or 2:1) between different ethnic groups. The degree awarding gap across the sector is currently 19.7% between white and Black students. This translates into 86% of white students are awarded a 1st or 2:1 degree, whereas 66.3% of Black students are awarded the same. There has been much discussion about the causes of the degree awarding gap and specific interventions that are needed to address it. Although it is a complex issue, attention to closing the gap is urgent as it has been estimated that if the sector continues at the same rate, the gap will not close until 2085/86 (Loke, 2020).

In the summer of 2020, one could be forgiven for thinking that there were changes ahead in the higher education sector. The murder of George Floyd shone a light on racial injustice. Coupled with COVID-19 and the impact that the virus had on people racialised as minority in the United Kingdom, it was evident that there were two pandemics – the virus and racism. Many higher education institutions posted statements of solidarity with Black Lives Matter as there were global protests highlighting police brutality and racial inequities. For the first time, the people who took to the streets were from all ethnicities. Promises were made about changes that would be implemented to create opportunities but 18 months on, there has been little sustainable change. Dismantling a racist, classist system requires allies who are part of the change for the long term. It is not enough to protest against the system then return to business as usual the next day.

Although having worked in academia for 30 years, I feel largely accepted by most colleagues, but I do not feel as though I fit in as expressed by Crew (2021). If invited to social engagements, I now know which knife and fork to use for each food course and I know how to pronounce words that were not part of my vocabulary when I first entered academia. I have been fortunate to meet interesting people from across the globe and all walks of life. However, most of my experiences have been where I have been the only Black women in the room which has often been an overwhelmingly lonely and, sometimes, hostile place. The academy continues to be a white middle-class space where racism and classism can thrive, and although both are a constant, they have been a changing and evolving feature throughout my career.

In May 2019, I was promoted to the Professoriate. Unfortunately, this a rarity for Black women regardless of their socio-economic status. In 2020, there was a celebration of Black women professors in Central London after the University and College Union (UCU) commissioned a report about the career experiences of Black women professors (Rollock, 2019). A portrait of each professor was displayed in one room for all to see. In other words, it was possible to fit a portrait of *every* Black woman professor in the United Kingdom in one room.

Final Thoughts…

Regardless of who you are, the academy can be a challenging place to carve out a career, so self-care is essential. Audre Lorde asserted that self-care was an act of self-preservation and an act of political warfare. Self-care is undeniably important especially given the trends documented by Black women regarding higher workloads compared to their white counterparts as well as the additional emotional labour involved in simply existing in a space that was not designed for you.

People create the culture within the institution so we can choose how we are going to behave and interact with each other. I would advocate for a kinder, more compassionate culture where collaboration and support are rewarded. True allyship, where we see people using their privilege for change is needed in the academy. Being in a space where colleagues feel supported and valued for who they are and what they bring to the table is critical if we are to engage in the culture change. Many of the academics that I have met on my journey, especially those starting out in their career, give me hope that we can change the culture and have a different vision of what success looks like in the academy. However, this will not happen unless the gatekeepers are also on the journey – meaning those who have the power to reward aspects of work that are not currently valued or prized in the promotion process. Mentoring and sponsorship of others is crucial, especially those who are under-represented in the academy. Helping colleagues navigate the system and championing them can be the difference between that person staying and thriving or deciding to leave. Finally, I would like to stress the importance of authenticity and link this to the title of my chapter. 'Uptown Top Ranking' was a hit reggae song for Althea and Donna in 1977. I clearly remember seeing both Black women singing their song on the television at a time when it was a rarity to see Black women on TV. A line in their song is 'Nah pop no style, I strictly roots' which I interpret loosely as not following others, be it in fashion or other areas of life and 'strictly roots', is remaining true and proud of your heritage or origins. It is important to succeed as you are rather than be an imitation of who you would like to be (Anthony, 2012). There are small steps that we can all take on this journey of change, and I urge courage and bravery to embrace your authentic self. It is important to stand in our truth and create opportunities to speak it. If we can engage in small changes, we are committing to leaving academia in a better state than when we found it.

References

Anthony, C. G. (2012). The Port Hueneme of my mind: The geography of working-class consciousness in one's academic career. In G. Gutierrez y Muhs, Y. F. Niemann, C. G. Gonzalez, & A. P. Harris (Eds.), *Presumed incompetent: The intersections of race and class for women in academia* (pp. 300–312). Boulder, CO: University Press of Colorado.

Brophy, J. E. (1983). Research on the self-fulfilling prophecy and teacher expectations. *Journal of Educational Psychology, 75*, 631–661.

Brown, N. (2014). "It's more than hair...that's why you should care": The politics of appearance for Black women state legislators. *Politics, Groups, and Identities, 2,* 295–312.

Carroll, C. M. (1982). Three's a crowd: The dilemma of the Black woman in higher education. In G. T. Hull, P. Bell Scott, & B. Smith (Eds.), *All the women are white, all the blacks are men, but some of us are brave.* New York, NY: The Feminist Press.

Case, K. A. (2017). Insider without: Journey across the working-class academic arc. *Journal of Working-Class Studies, 2,* 16–35.

Cheeks, M. (2018). How Black women describe navigating race and gender in the workplace. *Harvard Business Review.* Retrieved from https://hbr.org/2018/03/how-black-women-describe-navigating-race-and-gender-in-the-workplace

Coogan, R. (2019). A working-class accent in academia is a blessing and a curse. *Times Higher Education.* Retrieved from https://www.timeshighereducation.com/opinion/working-class-accent-academia-blessing-and-curse

Crew, T. (2021). Navigating academia as a working-class academic. *Journal of Working-Class Studies, 6,* 50–64.

Dabiri, E. (2020). Black pupils are wrongly being excluded over their hair. I'm trying to end this discrimination. *Guardian.* 25 February 2020. Black pupils are being wrongly excluded over their hair. I'm trying to end this discrimination | Emma Dabiri | The Guardian.

Delgado, R., & Stefancic, J. (2013). *Critical race theory: The cutting edge.* Philadelphia, PA: Temple University Press.

Dusek, J. B. (1985). *Teacher expectancies.* Hillsdale, NJ: Lawrence Erlbaum Associates.

Fuertes, J. N., Gottdiener, W. H., Martin, H., Gilbert, T. C., & Giles, H. (2012). A meta-analysis of the effects of speakers' accents on interpersonal evaluations. *European Journal of Social Psychology, 42,* 120–133.

Fuertes, J. N., Potere, J. C., & Rameriez, K. Y. (2002). Effects of speech accents on interpersonal evaluations: Implications for counselling practice and research. *Cultural Diversity and Ethnic Minority Psychology, 8,* 346–356.

Gay, R. (2014). *Bad feminist: Essays.* London: Corsair.

Gershenson, S., & Papageorge, N. (2018). The power of teacher expectations: How racial bias hinders student attainment. *Education Next, 18,* 64–70.

hooks, b. (2007). Straightening our hair. In *Z Magazine: The spirit of resistance lives.* Woods Hole, MA: Z Communications. Originally published in September 1998 by Sargent, L, & Albert, M.

Jussim, L. (1989). Teacher expectations: Self-fulfilling prophecies, perceptual bias, and accuracy. *Journal of Personality and Social Psychology, 57,* 469–480.

Kwhali, J. (2017). The accidental Academic. In D. Gabriel & S. A. Tate (Eds.), *Inside the Ivory Tower: Narratives of women of colour surviving and thriving in British Academia* (pp. 5–24). Stoke-on-Trent: Trentham.

Larcombe, P. (2016). I'm a professor with a working-class accent – Get over it. *Times Higher Education.* Retrieved from https://www.timeshighereducation.com/blog/im-professor-working-class-accent-get-over-it

Lester, N. A. (2000). Nappy edges and Goldy Locks: African American daughters and the politics of hair. *The Lion and the Unicorn, 24,* 201–224.

Loke, G. (2020). Time's up for the awarding gap. *WONKHE*. Retrieved from https://wonkhe.com/blogs/times-up-for-the-awarding-gap/

Pulley, T. W. (2019). *An intersectional analysis of Black working-class women becoming members of the academy.* LSU doctoral dissertations (p. 4805). Retrieved from https://digitalcommons.lsu.edu/gradschool_dissertations/4805

Rollock, N. (2019). *Staying power: The career experiences and strategies of UK Black female professors.* London: University and College Union (UCU).

Rosenthal, R., & Jacobson, L. (1968). *Pygmalion in the classroom: Teacher expectations and pupils' intellectual development.* New York, NY: Holt Rinehart & Winston.

Showunmi, V., Atewologun, D., & Bebbington, D. (2016). Ethnic, gender and class intersections in British women's leadership experiences. *Educational Management Administration & Leadership, 44,* 917–935.

Showunmi, V., & Maylor, U. (2013). Black women reflecting on being Black in the academy. Retrieved from https://discovery.ucl.ac.uk/id/eprint/10012147/

Sini, R. (2016). Wear a weave at work – Your afro hair is unprofessional. Retrieved from https://www.bbc.co.uk/news/uk-36279845

Chapter 8

One's Place and the Right to Belong

Iona Burnell Reilly

Abstract

Higher education (HE) in England and other parts of the United Kingdom (UK), traditionally and historically, has been dominated by privileged and powerful social groups. In recent decades, universities have opened their doors and encouraged participation by a diversity of learners including women, working class, minority ethnic groups and many others that might be deemed historically under-represented in HE. This movement came to be known as 'widening participation'. I consider myself to be a product of the widening participation movement having returned to learn in 1994 after a 10-year break in education. However, providing access to participate is only the first step. For many HE students from under-represented groups, like the working class, the journey through the academy, while earning their degree, can be fraught with profound and difficult experiences. This chapter charts my own journey into HE as a student, and back into HE as an academic, with some equally fraught and profound experiences.

Keywords: Widening participation; working class; habitus; imposterism; academia; social structures

> There is risk and truth to yourselves and the world before you.
>
> —Seamus Heaney[1]

How Did I Get Here?

Bimrose and Barnes pose a question: 'Are individuals actually able to navigate their way effectively and "choose" their career biographies or do the social structures within which they make decisions constrain freedom to determine their own destiny'? (2011, p. 2). For a long time I presupposed that I would not go to university, that it was not a place for me; not because anybody had told me that, but because there were never any conversations about university,

The Lives of Working Class Academics, 101–121

Copyright © 2023 Iona Burnell Reilly

Published under exclusive licence by Emerald Publishing Limited

doi:10.1108/978-1-80117-057-420221008

careers and professions amongst the working class people and the family that I grew up with. Therefore, my assumption was 'it is not for the likes of us'. Bowl notes this when she states 'working class people may not think they are eligible for opportunities to achieve because of their internalised assumptions that certain opportunities are "not for the likes of them"' (2003, p. 129). Another reason that further perpetuated the idea that university was not for the likes of us was that the working class, historically, had very little history or presence in higher education (HE). For a long time, HE had been dominated by middle/upper class participation. 'Universities traditionally have not been places for the working class', according to Crozier, Reay and Clayton (cited in David, 2010, p. 74). We did not see people like us entering the doors of universities, unless it was via the back tradesman's door. Yates has discussed the factors that influence people's career paths and questions whether they are 'a product of their circumstances and to a degree, pre-destined by factors such as geography and social class' (2014, p. 25).

Given my early circumstances, the area that I grew up in, the failing school that I attended, and the values and practices of my family, I would have to agree that, to an extent, my path was pre-destined. Ryan and Sackrey might also agree as they assert that 'We do not get to choose a class to be born into – and since significant mobility is blocked to most people – our life experiences are importantly the outcome of a spin on the wheel of fortune' (1984, p. 3). Ryan and Sackrey also discuss the myth of social mobility and how it 'functions to make it appear as though one's position in life were a consequence of a fair game with all participants playing by the same rules, all with the same starting points – hence it is the individuals' efforts and talent that are determinative, not the class into which one is born' (1984, p. 2).

When my father arrived in England from Ireland in the 1960s looking for work, he was greeted by signs up in windows which said 'no Irish, no blacks, no dogs'; this was his starting point. He had just turned 16 and had left Ireland during what was the country's period of economic stagnation and emigration. He settled in East London, married, my brother and me arrived and my parents started a haulage business. As I was growing up in a traditionally working-class and culturally diverse community, which included an Irish migrant diaspora, I was well aware that we were all working-class – everyone was – we didn't know any different because we didn't see anyone different from us. Everyone worked, we possessed a strong work ethic and, growing up, I saw work as the route to freedom, to independence and having control over your own life. My father was the family role model and demonstrated to us that hard work meant not having to rely on anyone – including the state. He, most likely, inherited this mindset from his family – a long line of Irish farmers, some of whom survived the 'famine'.[2] Both of my grandmothers were also incredibly hard-working women and given that this was in a period when women were yet to be deemed equal, they were also juggling child-rearing and the domestic chores. Thankfully, I inherited this ethos and grew up knowing that I need not be afraid of hard work.

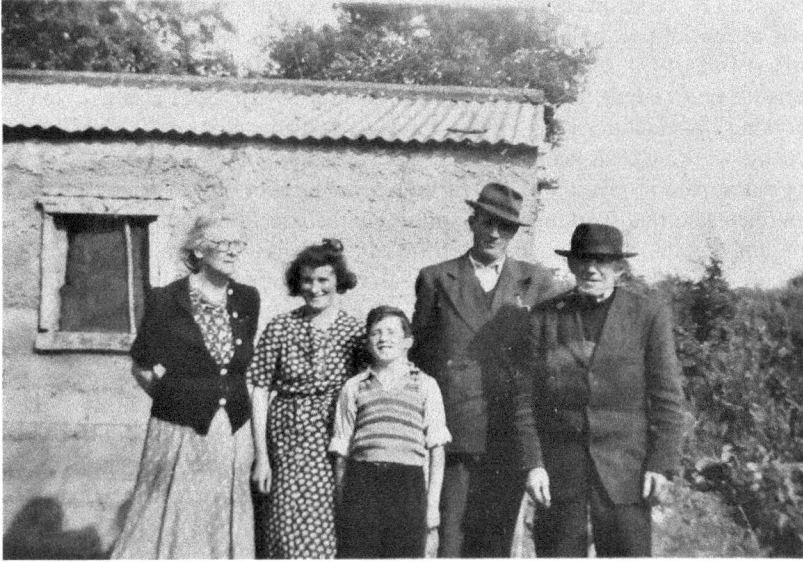

The Irish farmers: my father, my grandparents and my great-grandparents.

When I left school, the only expectation of me was to get a job; any job would do. As long as I was earning enough to keep myself, nobody minded what I did. Typical of most working-class families in this period of the 1980s and 1990s, education was not valued or held in high regard. Families had to work to keep themselves, and people of my background rarely had the privilege of staying on in education, even if they wanted to. Because of my lack of formal qualifications, I spent most of my young adult life bouncing from one meaningless job to another. That is, they were low-paid, unskilled positions that anybody could do. They did not feel like careers or vocations; they were not professions, or skilled work. Some jobs I really enjoyed, like delivery driver – driving a van around central London every day was a lot of fun. However, I knew that if I wanted a skilled profession, a career, I would need to return to education and acquire some qualifications. An additional reason for wanting a career was that I felt under-used and unfulfilled by the jobs that I was doing prior to going to university. I felt as though I was not fulfilling my potential. Reay reminds us that there are 'very many different ways of being working-class' (2017, p. 5), and this was certainly evident in the area that I grew up in. My parents ran their own business and this was our source of income; other families relied on other means, sometimes through illicit activities. Some families had very limited opportunities and were extremely poor.

Class is a social structure and social structures shape and socialise us into adult members of society. My working-class culture, values and practices socialised me into believing that education was not important – but working was. Bourdieu, the great French sociologist, asserted that some people will succeed in education, and some will not, and this is largely down to which social class they belong to

(Bourdieu & Passeron, 1977). Bourdieu explained that, through no fault of their own, aspirations of the working-class culture do not include education (Bourdieu & Passeron, 1977). Therefore, coming from the working class can have implications on one's educational achievement. Reay (1997, p. 552) also asserted that 'working class identities are not associated with academic success'; quite possibly because working-class people tended to leave school and go to work. If they did not participate in HE it was out of the economic necessity to find a job. When Bourdieu said that working-class culture limited educational aspirations, he was not implying that excluding oneself from education is a deliberate decision on the part of somebody from the working class, but rather it is a situation that is created and reproduced unconsciously and 'without any conscious concertation' (1984, p. 173). In addition, Bourdieu noted, the exclusion is 'internalised as a second nature' (Bourdieu, 1990, p. 56) and becomes what he called 'habitus'. As well as my working-class habitus, I lived in what the Higher Education Statistics Agency (HESA) (2021) calls a 'low participation neighbourhood'.[3] In fact, nobody that I knew when I was growing up went to university. The notable lack of visible role models further strengthened the notion that university was not for the likes of us. However, in a previous publication I claim that:

> Bourdieu's theory of habitus is compelling. He asserted that one's habitus is deeply engendered within individuals and that this creates a disposition below the level of consciousness which determines how we act or think …However, Bourdieu did not account for individual differences within the working class, and that some people may aspire to different goals.
>
> (Burnell, 2015, p. 106)

Evidence from my previous research strongly implies that 'habitus is not as enduring as the theory suggests' (Burnell, 2015). As I approached my mid-twenties, I had an epiphanic moment and decided to enrol myself into college. Initially, I was aiming for a vocational qualification in sport and fitness; I was a sport and fitness enthusiast and had an idea that I could work at my local leisure centre. While on this course, a chance remark from the tutor about my academic ability led me to enquire about an Access to Higher Education course. This was to be the beginning of my journey into HE, and not via the tradesman's door. According to Bourdieu and Wacquant (1992) 'One of the great achievements of the English HE widening participation policy and strategies is that it has helped working-class students to overcome that sense of place that leads to self-exclusion from places that they do not feel that are rightly theirs' (cited in Crozier, Reay, & Clayton, 2010, p. 68). This was an opportunity for me to work hard, not in the traditional working-class sense of getting your hands dirty, but working in the academic arena to achieve and succeed educationally, and start to build a career – a profession. At this point I didn't have a plan, I just knew it was the right path to pursue.

Strangers in Paradise: Academics from the Working Class (Ryan & Sackrey, 1984) is one book that has influenced my motivation to produce this one.

Strangers is concerned with the issue of social class mobility and, in particular, what happens to people from the working class who choose academia as their path to a 'higher social station' (Ryan & Sackrey, 1984, p. 1). *Strangers in Paradise* was published in 1984 when I was 15 years old. I had already left school – a year before the legal leaving age. It was a sub-standard failing secondary comprehensive – what would now be called a 'sink school' (Reay, 2017). I was a bored, disruptive and disillusioned pupil who could not see the point of going to school. There were far more interesting things to spend my time on. Interestingly though, there was a university campus about 1.5 miles from where I lived; it was, until 1992, a polytechnic. However, I did not 'see' this building; I had no con-ceptualisation of what it was. I was aware of a building – bricks and cement – but had no understanding of what it contained, that it was an institution of education, that people went there to obtain degrees; I had no understanding of what a degree was. This was because, as a value, education was not part of my habitus. Bourdieu used his theory of habitus to explain how working-class culture limits educational aspirations and that, consequently, being from the working class is like a barrier to educational success (Bourdieu & Passeron, 1977). According to Webb, Schirato and Danaher, habitus can be understood as the 'values and dispositions gained from our cultural history that generally stay with us across contexts' (2002, p. 36–37). In other words, if education is not valued in your family as you are growing up, and its success is not celebrated, then it is unlikely to be something that you aspire to. However, Leathwood and O'Connell explain that 'poor self-esteem or lack of confidence are not individual traits or personality failings but the product of social relations' (2003, p. 609). In a previous publi-cation, I argued that:

> ...the relation is one built on history – of the middle/upper class being in a dominant position, and the working class being in a subordinate position. Leathwood and O'Connell (2003) explain that it is this social relation between the two classes that has manifested feelings of self-doubt and caused people to question their position as they move into middle-class territory and experience feelings of not belonging.
>
> (Burnell, 2015, pp. 100–101)

Given that habitus is operating below the level of consciousness, with habits 'internalised as a second nature' (Bourdieu, 1990, p. 56), it might seem that changing one's habitus to include educational aspirations would be too difficult. However, Reay, Crozier, and Clayton (2009, p. 1104) suggest that habitus is 'permeable', and can be adapted and modified as one's circumstances change. One of the most significant changes in circumstances for many working-class people was the widening of participation into HE. This was one of the major educational reforms that was to take place in England and other parts of the United Kingdom. It was decided by the then government that HE was too exclusive, that too many social groups were under-represented in it, and one of those was the working class. Zinciewicz and Trapp (2004) define under-represented groups as 'those with no family history of HE experience, from low participation neighbourhoods, socio-economically disadvantaged students, students from ethnic minorities, and students with disabilities' (cited in Taylor & House, 2010, p. 46). Widening participation aimed to redress the balance and enable these under-represented groups to benefit from accessing HE and achieving degree success. However, this change in circumstances meant that our habitus would be changed too and would now include HE as a new practice. The result was that the habitus we had been socialised into, and could identify with, would be altered and adapted, as a result of participating in HE.

After a dismal start in education, I resigned myself to thinking that I would never be academically successful or gain a professional position in employment. However, the New Labour government of the 1990s changed people's perception of HE by opening up possibilities for participation in HE that had not been explored before. In addition, the access course movement had created an alternative route into HE that meant people like me, without formal or traditional qualifications, could apply for places on undergraduate degree courses. Learners who entered HE this way came to be known as non-traditional students, and I became one such person. I returned to education after a 10-year period of absence, completed an access course and progressed to university. I could be deemed a widening participation success story, or, in Bourdieusian terms, 'un miraculés' (1988). A miracle, according to Bourdieu, is somebody who survives through unfortunate circumstances; in this context, a member of the working class who becomes educationally successful. Similarly, Ryan and Sackrey state that they 'considered ourselves to be exceptionally lucky to have risen from non-professional families to middle-class careers. We are the "exceptions" upon which the American social mobility myth was based' (1984, p. 4). In Britain, we too have the social mobility myth; however, Bourdieu would argue that because the culture of the dominant classes continues to be held in the highest esteem, they use their power to maintain their advantages. In this way, class inequalities are normalised and perpetuated. Jones calls this a 'rigged society' and explains that 'the demonization of working-class people is a grimly rational way to justify an irrational system. Demonize them, ignore their concerns – and rationalize a grossly unequal distribution of wealth and power as a fair reflection of people's worth and abilities' (2020, pp. 182–183).

Accessing Higher Education

Access to Higher Education courses became the popular route for non-traditional students who wanted to return to learn and enter HE but lacked formal qualifications. By the late 1980s, a wide range of subject areas were on offer. Students could gain entry to a range of degree courses from physical sciences to philosophy by progression from the access course route. Burke refers to this as the 'access movement' (2002, p. 7) and she explains the phenomenon as 'education that explicitly aims to widen access to groups who have been socially and culturally excluded from educational participation' (Burke, 2002). This also meant that non-traditional learners, such as the working class and minority ethnic groups who may not have considered entering the historically white middle/upper class elitist institution of HE, could now aspire to pursue a degree course. Burke asserts that these courses were begun in order to widen the participation to marginalised groups: 'The access movement was initially driven by a commitment to redress the balance set by the legacy of institutional classism, racism and sexism' (2002, p. 64). Thompson, interestingly, notes that 'It was largely women who had been denied education earlier in their lives who took up the opportunities offered by Access' (2000, p. 25). Many working-class students are also women, and, historically, women were excluded from HE. Arnot notes that 'it was not until 1948 that the last bastions of male privilege fell and women were allowed to take the same degrees as men in Cambridge University...this battle for equal rights and equal treatment of men and women still has resonance today' (2002, p. 188).

Access courses have, therefore, become the popular choice for people like me – mature working-class students returning to learn after a break in education. Burke argues that a lack of confidence in this type of learner is not as a result of being out of education for a long period. She explains that western binary thinking reinforces the notion that '...middle-class culture is superior and working-class culture deficient...' (2002, p. 86), implying that working-class students have internalised feelings of failure. I certainly had internalised feelings of failure, having left school early with no formal qualifications. Reay points out that 'The university sector, more than any other sector, epitomizes middle classness ... How then can the mature working-class student maintain a sense of authenticity and still hope to fit in?' (2002, p. 338). Access courses were designed to accommodate a new type of learner, one that was, historically, excluded from education and unlike those students who progressed from the earlier and traditional A-levels. Access courses, therefore, have evolved out of the widening participation drive, and educational reform, based on raising HE participation rates of learners who were non-traditional and/or returning to learn. This was a significant and lasting social change.

Having completed the access course, I went to my local university to embark on a degree in Linguistics. There were opportunities for careers in teaching and, although I was not inspired to teach children, I was interested in teaching adults so, after leaving university, I trained to teach English to Speakers of Other Languages (ESOL) and began working at the local college. Whilst there, an opportunity to teach academic skills on the access course came my way. I ended up teaching on this course for eight years. I felt very passionate about the access course and the students on it. I could empathise with how they were feeling, having felt the very same myself when I was an access student. Preparing and sending cohort after cohort off to university every year, seeing people transform their lives, realise their potential and fulfil their dreams was, for me, extremely satisfying and rewarding, and I thoroughly enjoyed my job. Being an access course tutor in a college of further education (FE), often referred to as the 'second-chance nature of FE provision' (Green & Lucas, 2000, p. 172), certainly fitted with my personal values, given my class, background and non-traditional route into HE. However, I also felt that my job was part of my identity; I had been an access student, gone to university as a mature student, completed teacher training and returned to teach students like myself, about whom I felt passionately. Yates discusses the concepts of 'career identities' and 'professional identities' (2014, p. 30). She quotes Schein (1978) who defined the professional identity as a 'relatively stable and enduring constellation of attributes, beliefs, values, motives and experiences in terms of which people define themselves in a professional role' (Yates, 2014, p. 30). I felt as though my job was a part of my identity as a working-class, non-traditional student, who had returned to learn after failing in education first time round. These circumstances were what brought me to the job, which actually felt more like a calling.

After 13 years of working in a college of FE, I decided it was time for a change. Two changes in government had meant that the political landscape of the sector had shifted; I felt that the job no longer fitted with my personal values and I began to feel discontented. The FE sector had begun to be run like a business, with a profit margin, and the ethos of learning and education seemed to be mislaid. However, I had not lost my passion for students, teaching, and enabling learners to reach their potential, so I wanted to remain in the industry of education. While in FE, I had completed further degrees at master's and doctoral levels, so I was now qualified to teach in HE. It was a hard decision to make, given all that I have discussed around values, identity, a calling, etc. but I had an instinct that I could continue my good work in the HE sector, making just as much difference there, and although my identity would shift a little, I could still 'pay forward' by enabling learners to believe in themselves and reach their potential. My doctoral thesis was on the topic of widening participation into HE, and the experiences of working-class students, so I felt something of an authority on this subject, which further strengthened my professional identity.

Fish Out of Water

While I was extremely grateful for being given the opportunity to study in HE, given my dismal educational background and lack of formal qualifications, I was also aware that learners like me had no history and very little to identify with within this historically and traditionally middle/upper class institution. Until World War II, university education was the preserve of a small elite, less than 2% of the relevant age cohort were attending university, and among women, the percentage was less than 0.5 (Blackburn & Jarman, 1993). Moreover, the concept of mature students at this time did not exist. Even though the Robbins Report (1963) endorsed the principle that a HE should be available to all those who had the ability and qualifications to benefit, it was not until the government Department for Education and Science (1987) white paper *HE: meeting the challenge*, that alternative routes to HE started to become popular and non-traditional and mature learners like myself were really able to participate in HE. Even then, it would take another 10 years and a new government's educational reform for the widening participation movement to get into full swing. I entered university to complete my first degree in 1997 at the height of the widening participation movement.

Widening a traditionally narrow arena to include learners from under-represented groups is a major step towards social inclusion. However, if this new type of learner does not feel comfortable, included, or does not have any history in that arena, then the effects will be felt. In a previous publication (Burnell, 2015) I addressed the question posed by Bourdieu and Passeron (1977) – of why people from middle-class backgrounds are more likely, and those from working-class backgrounds less likely, to attend university. Maton (cited in Grenfell, 2008) explains how habitus works in practise, and in relation to the social field, or social setting, in which we find ourselves:

> Imagine, for example, a social situation in which you feel or anticipate feeling awkward, out of your element, like a "fish out of water". You may decide not to go, to declare it as "not for the likes of me", or (if there already) to make your excuses and leave. In this case the structuring of your habitus does not match that of the social field... Social agents thereby come to gravitate towards those social fields (and positions within those fields) that best match their dispositions and try to avoid those fields that involve a field-habitus clash.
>
> (cited in Grenfell, 2008, pp. 57–59)

For me, the effects of field–habitus clash were minimal. I attended the local university where many learners were from similar backgrounds. This university had taken full advantage of widening participation policies and strategies by encouraging large numbers from the local working-class community to participate in what the university had to offer. This meant that I studied alongside people from my own social class who were also enjoying the benefits of widening participation. I did not consider applying to an elite university, or even an institution outside of my local vicinity. In fact, while at the local college of FE, completing my access course, I was encouraged by my tutors to apply to universities that had a large proportion of mature and working-class students. It was felt that widening participation students should apply to universities who were engaged in the widening participation movement; they felt that otherwise we would feel out of place and experience the 'fish out of water' phenomenon, as described by Maton (cited in Grenfell, 2008). Interestingly, Crew notes that 'Research on students by Donnelly and Gamsu (2018) found "staying at home and studying locally" is something that tends to be found in disadvantaged communities' (2020, p. 27). Maybe the safety net of remaining close to home is what minimises the effects of field–habitus clash?

Reay, Miriam, and Ball (2005) write about how education amongst the working class is far from straightforward; '...the link between class and education, in which failure is emblematic of the working class relationship to schooling, frequently makes working class transitions to higher education complex and difficult' (p. 84). Another contested area is the question of what type of HE we are preparing learners for. Reay has also examined the stratified system of HE in terms of the elite and mass institutions (1997). In more recent work, she comments that the 'majority of working-class students end up in universities seen to be "second class" by both themselves and others' (2017, p. 121). The statistics for the two types of universities indicate that non-traditional mature learners are also severely under-represented within the elite universities. Northedge argues that widening participation has meant that 'non-traditional students have been treated as "charity" cases to be rescued from ignorance. The stately home of elite education is simply extended by adding a large paupers' wing. "Proper" students continue to define the norms, whilst the rest tag along behind as best they can' (2003, p. 17). If this is an accurate interpretation of the situation, then the purpose of widening participation to give people fair and equal access to a once elite education system is undermined. Nevertheless, for me, going to a 'working class university' in my local area and studying alongside people like myself was a transformative experience and one that I benefited from, both personally and professionally, as it set me on the path that I am on now.

During Reay et al.'s (2005) research into the overlapping effects of social class in the process of applying to HE, and especially on the issue of which HE institution to apply to, they used Bourdieu's (1984) theory of 'objective limits'. Placing objective limits on oneself means to avoid places where we have no history or sense of identity: a 'sense of one's place which leads one to exclude oneself from the goods, persons, places and so forth from which one is excluded' (p. 471). More recently, Reay notes that 'children from working-class backgrounds account for just 1 in 20 enrolments into the elite Russell Group of universities' (2017, p. 118); although the number increases as those working-class students pursue postgraduate degrees. As my academic journey progressed, and my confidence grew, I found that applying to more elite universities in order to complete higher degrees, did not seem so unusual, and many of my peers were also applying. I went on to complete a master's degree, and then a doctorate at a Russell Group university; and although elite, I did not experience it as elitist. Crew notes that:

> Classism has been the hardest bias to reverse as it requires the redistribution of wealth, and opportunity and 'class' is not a protected characteristic under the equalities legislation. One could argue that by virtue of having a PhD or being employed as a lecturer or researcher in the academy, this redistribution has been successful (2020, p. 82).

Introjected Values

Introjected values, according to counselling psychology, are messages absorbed in childhood, from, for example, family and education. Carl Rogers, a prominent psychotherapist, believed that introjected values get in the way of people being their true selves (Rogers, 1951). We become conditioned to believe a myth about ourselves and the myth becomes our internalised core belief; this is a similar concept to Bourdieu's habitus theory. Wakeling comments on 'what Bourdieu calls *hysteresis:* the habitus of their family and community of origin is ingrained and will not easily go away, leading to the reported (and very real) feelings of guilt, inadequacy, alienation but also anger' (cited in Taylor, 2010, p. 43). As we grow into adults, these messages from childhood that have formed our beliefs about ourselves become our script and we live our lives according to this script. In my case, as a child I left school early, before the legal leaving age, before sitting any exams, and in the belief that, educationally, I was a failure. This was the message that I received from the education system, backed up by some of the adults in my life. I had swallowed the message from school and others around me that I would 'never amount to anything', that I had failed in education and therefore in life. I felt written off by the system. Not only that, according to my experience, I was a failure. This, then, became my script, and for many years during my teens and early twenties, I lived my life according to this belief, backed up by my experience. I had internalised these ideas and didn't attempt to do anything professionally or educationally for many years.

Wakeling notes that 'many traditional working-class occupations are literally dead end jobs' (cited in Taylor, 2010, p. 38), meaning that they do not lead to increased social status, promotions or higher salaries. For 10 years I drifted from one dead-end job to another, believing that was my lot, that I was not capable of, nor deserved, anything more. Then, I discovered what was inside that building one and a half miles from my home. I hadn't 'seen' the building, despite travelling past it a million times. What came into my awareness, what I had not been conscious of, was that it was a university, a place of education, a place where people like me, working-class educational failures, would be welcomed through its doors in order to get a second chance at education. However, that also brought other kinds of feelings, such as imposterism, and a constant questioning of one's place and the right to belong. Wilson, Reay, Morrin and Abraham note that 'There probably aren't too many individuals who feel at ease with every aspect of the academy and that never encounter some form of imposter syndrome' (2020, p. 6). Wilson et al. go on to argue that 'there are powerful and affective class-based experiences, particularly when you have been and become upwardly socially mobile. This is particularly acute for those who occupy positions of intersecting marginalisation. . .' (Taylor, 2010). Although I have only alluded to it briefly here, my gender, as well as my social class, undoubtedly had an impact on the ways in which I experienced the world.

The problem, according to Rogers (1951), is that often, our experience cannot be relied upon and the messages we have internalised, that become our core beliefs, are not true. My perception gave me a way of seeing the world, a 'truth'. However, the ways of the world can contaminate who we really are and lead us to hide our true selves. Therefore, our 'way of knowing' is not a reliable source and often these 'truths' can be challenged and changed. If, like me, you grew up in a working-class family, in a working-class community, and attended a failing school, and were consistently made to believe that you were 'not going to amount to anything', that becomes your truth. I now know that wasn't true, I was not a failure, the system was – the education system and the social class system was fraught with systemic failures, and to an extent still is. Introjected values are little more than assumptions and, like habitus, when the illusion is shattered, anything is possible. A chance opportunity can often be the key to breaking down the barrier of a lack of self-belief, leading one to fulfilling one's potential.

Widening participation into HE opens doors that might have remained forever closed. However, entering these doors may have certain profound effects on people's personal lives. The phenomenon of 'imposter syndrome' has been written about extensively (Leary, Patton, Orlando, & Funk, 2000; Sakulku & Alexander, 2011; Slank, 2019; Wilkinson, 2020) since Clance and Imes (1978), two American psychologists, noted that 'despite outstanding academic and professional accomplishments, women who experience the imposter phenomenon persist in believing that they really are not bright and have fooled anyone who thinks otherwise' (p. 241). Breeze suggests 'that we cannot understand feelings of imposterism as an individual problem or private issue, isolated from the social contexts in which they are felt' (cited in Taylor & Lahad, 2018, p. 195). Imposterism is the effect of deep-rooted social, historical and political structures of the institution; these structures contain oppressive forces such as neoliberalism, class stratification, class privilege, racism and other inequalities. It is these social structures that emanate the absorbed messages which condition us to believe a myth about ourselves – that then becomes our limiting core beliefs. My own experiences of imposterism are entrenched within my social class, my gender and my cultural heritage. These characteristics and their intersections heightened my sense of risk, the fear of being found out. Breeze explores imposter syndrome as a 'potential source of action and agency, in relation to the feminist ambivalences of being "within and against" university institutions, as feminist academics are both complicit with and struggle against the neoliberal university' (cited in Taylor & Lahad, 2018, p. 193).

'You're getting ideas above your station, Iona', one family member told me when I announced my intention of returning to education and enrolling into the university. I almost choked on my introjected value but decided to dismiss it and push on; after all – what was the worst that could happen? Actually, although I didn't realise it then, this was to become an example what Reay termed 'class-lessness' (1997). In other words, you would now be deemed middle-class, according to your education and qualifications, but you weren't born there, so you're not really middle-class. Issues of identity and social class, and their personal struggles to fit into a social class, may not be issues that, generally, traditional students who are progressing to HE straight from school, would have to deal with. One such issue, for example, and one that I can empathise with, is re-negotiating one's identity within the social class into which one is born, after having been re-educated into a different social class. Freeborn asserts that 'Educating yourself out of your own class, but doing it at an age where assimilating into the educated class is not realistic, not even entirely desirable, means that you become, forever, neither fish nor fowl' (2000, p. 10). The metaphorical concept of 'neither fish nor fowl' is one I can intensely identify with. 'We are often told that a working-class scholar is a contradictory notion' (Crew, 2020, p. 24); that the term 'working class academic' is a contradiction in terms – an oxymoron. I may feel working-class, possess working-class values, and come from a family/background who all very much identify as working-class, but I am perceived as middle-class. People often look at me and assume I am middle-class. My students often say that because of my job, my salary, my qualifications and education, that I am middle-class – and they don't know where I live! (I live in a middle-class postcode). However, maybe these are now the yardsticks with which to measure one's social class; it seems to be less about perception and more about conceptualisation. Wakeling, in his article 'Is There such a Thing as a Working-Class Academic?', argues:

> ...there is no 'going back' to working class origins because university education and upward mobility change the individual psychologically and set them apart in the eyes of those 'left behind'. At the same time, coming from a different class background to that dominant within the academy means one is similarly marked out and never quite able to gain full acceptance (or self-acceptance).
>
> (cited in Taylor, 2010, p. 41)

These are the after-effects of widening participation into HE.

Speaking the Wrong Language

When I got to university, as a student of Linguistics, I realised that my cockney accent, with its glottal stops, and *th*-fronting, was going to be a hindrance to me. I was already alive to the impact that my regional accent could have because I had experienced a very embarrassing moment while at the second high school that I had been sent to for a brief period at aged 14, before making the decision that school was definitely not for me and left for good. It was a drama lesson. The school was three miles from where I lived – in the wrong direction. It was in a posh middle-class area that is now considered to be part of East London due to expansion of the Greater London area. I had managed to stay silent for most of the time in the new temporary school but when I entered the drama lesson, we were required to speak. 'You're new' the teacher said, 'do you like drama?' 'Not really' I said. 'Not really? alright mate, alright mate' the teacher mimicked. Everyone laughed. My face turned beetroot red. The teacher had mimicked my cockney accent because nobody else in the school spoke like that. Crew discusses the concept of 'microaggressions' (2020, p. 81):

> Bourdieu (1990) would describe this as symbolic violence, a "soft" violence that includes actions that have discriminatory or injurious meaning such as racism, sexism or classism... Microaggressions appear to be a common ingredient of professional life both for women and for people of colour, but they are also found to be present in the experiences of professionals from disadvantaged social backgrounds.
>
> (Bourdieu, 1990)

Moving socially means moving your language and the way you speak. Accentism is a prejudice – people make social judgements when we speak, it's a subtle and covert type of discrimination, making connections and assumptions between speech styles and stereotypes. This is also a type of classism; one of the assumptions made about you if you have a regional accent is that you are from the working class. Crew comments that 'the association between accent and social class in Britain has a long history. Hiraga (2005) found speakers of urban accents like Birmingham were perceived to be the lowest in status measures such as wealth and intelligence, whereas speakers with received pronunciation (RP) were classified highest' (2020, p. 72).

I hadn't spent much time outside of the East End of London, so I had no awareness of there being regional varieties of English. Apart from my neighbours' non-native English speakers' accents, the only other accent I was aware of was Irish. Cockney is one variety of English, a dialect found in the region of London where I grew up. Standard English is also a dialect, not a regional one but one associated with the middle class. Standard English is also used as the medium for education – it is the language of the classroom, lecture theatres and academics. Returning to learn and entering HE, particularly as a student of Linguistics, meant that I became conscious of my language, and the features of my regional dialect. During my final year of the degree in Linguistics I decided that I wanted to become an English language teacher; this was the real test of my language mettle. Learners of English as an additional language will model your pronunciation so if you say 'erf' instead of 'earth', they will say that too. The importance of modelling accurate language for students learning English was drummed into me during teacher training and I became adept at switching between dialects – Standard English for the workplace and my regional variety for home. However, language, and one's dialect, is very much a part of identity, especially class identity. Previously, I quoted Freeborn, who alludes to the idea of 'Educating yourself out of your own class... assimilating into the educated class is not realistic' (2000, p. 10). For me, this became part of that re-negotiating one's identity that I have previously discussed – in fact, what I developed was a dual identity; some aspects of myself were retained and some were changed. I can relate to one of Skeggs' research participants when she said: 'what I was is not what I am now' (Skeggs, 1997, p. 97).

Lynch and O'Neill note how working-class identities are changed by HE: 'no other group finds that school is about learning to be the opposite to what one is' (1994, p. 322). This strongly suggests that pursuing a HE means you can no longer occupy a working-class identity. This is a frustrating situation to be in for people who have constructed their identity, especially while growing up, around being working-class. Experiencing this shift in class identity put me into a complex subject position where I had a foot in both worlds. Previous relationships were forged within the constraints of working-class values, and those values did not include education. Becoming an academic, with an emerging sense of identity set within the boundaries of the dominant class, meant the need to negotiate both worlds simultaneously. Byrne, in his own autoethnography, reflects that, 'Existing, now, as a working-class academic, I realize that I am neither entirely working-class, nor entirely academic. Being among academic people, who act, speak and think in unfamiliar ways, has meant building a new identity that has become simultaneously less and more working-class' (2019, p. 145).

Byrne's experience heavily resonates with me when he reveals 'I have all but lost my regional accent: when with my family, I sound different to them, and yet the occasional rhotic "r" still betrays me, revealing my West Country origins to my colleagues. ... when the accent creeps in unexpectedly, there is a risk of being caught trying to "pass" as something you are not' (2019, p. 143). By the time I started work as an academic in HE I was a confident Standard English speaker, and reserved my native dialect for informal occasions, where I felt it was more acceptable, and where I felt more comfortable with it. This could be an example of what Abrahams and Ingram (2013) term the 'chameleon habitus' – the ability to adapt to both environments, 'Despite being immersed within two somewhat contradictory fields they can sometimes develop various strategies to enable them to overcome any internal conflict' (p. 213). Although I wasn't aware of any internal conflict, and I felt fairly well equipped when I entered HE as an academic, Coogan points out that 'Prolonged exposure to the academic environment can affect the way we dress, the way we behave – both in public and online – and even the way that we articulate our thoughts in everyday conversation. Over time, we might find ourselves passing as academics so naturally that we don't even realise that we have changed' (Coogan, 2019).

Changing the way one speaks is often seen as pretentious. Addison and Mountford (2015) conducted research into features of classed identities in HE. They describe one of their research participants who:

> ...sees herself as being part of a respectable working class and emphasizes her difference to those she sees as being part of a more devalued working class in her discussion. She does this by working on her accent to converge with what she views to be a more middle class version of her own. She is conscious of slippages and how this might be read negatively by others, signifying a lack of fit... (p. 8).

For me, it's less about pretending and more about developing and evolving into a comfortable and confident version of myself. I have evolved with my job role into a member of the *neo* working class, one that has adapted her working-class habitus to include HE, both as a practice and a value. Although my cockney dialect is not quite as strong as it used to be, I'm definitely comfortable with dropping the odd 'h', or slipping in a glottal stop, and although I don't *th*-front very often, when I do, it is done to assert my working-class identity – which I don't attempt to hide.

Who Am I Now?

Previously, I cited Maton (Grenfell, 2008) who explains the 'fish out of water' phenomenon and how that leads to a field–habitus clash. For me, the effects of field–habitus clash were minimal as I learnt to re-negotiate my identity within my professional position. Looking back, I can say that the transitional journey – from access student to widening participation undergraduate, then into the teaching profession, completing doctorate and becoming a HE lecturer – was fairly seamless and integrative. Hodkinson (cited in Grenfell & James, 1998) discusses how people find 'turning points' in their lives, which means that they change course and, in turn, alter their habitus; 'As a person lives through a turning point the habitus of the person is changed' (p. 101). Hodkinson also explain that 'At a turning point a person goes through a significant transformation of identity' (Grenfell & James, 1998). My transformation began as soon as I enrolled at university as an undergraduate student. Nevertheless, Crozier et al. (cited in David, 2010) assert that 'Universities traditionally have not been places for the working class' (p. 74), and they, therefore, have no history and nothing to identify with in the academic arena. The uneducated working class were traditionally excluded from HE, the educated middle and upper class were included. This was our starting point – striving for a place and an identity within the academy, a place where we can feel that we belong. The widening participation movement enabled that to happen and several decades later, working-class academics are firmly established within HE.

There have been many debates and discussions about people from the working class entering HE and what that experience is like for them. Reay (2002), for example, and her 'imposters', so called because they felt that they did not belong in the world of HE. Askham discusses the anxieties and identity conflicts of 'the adult who chooses to leave one world to enter the intellectual world of learning' (2008, p. 89). Askham cites Elliott (1999) as calling this 'inhabiting two discourses at once' (Askham, 2008). Reay also uses a case study to highlight issues of 'classlessness' (1997), and recounts how Christine, a working-class woman with a degree deems herself 'classless' because she is now not working-class, but nor is she middle-class:

> Christine told me later in the interview that she "came from a very working-class background". To claim middle-class status for Christine would constitute a denial of her past, while to continue to call herself working-class could be construed as a denial of her educational achievements. For Christine, classlessness is the consequence of compromise (1997, p. 228).

However, the research at this time was implying that there were two polarised positions – the uneducated working class and the educated middle class – and that learners inhabited one or the other. What seems to be the case now is that we have a foot in both worlds, with a requirement to negotiate both worlds simultaneously. Baxter and Britton comment that 'The process of moving between classes has very strong emotional and affective aspects which colour the lives of those who experience it' (2001, p. 95). For me, the negotiation has been an interesting experience; I started working as an academic in the university where I had been a student – a post-92, ex polytechnic, with a strong tradition of educating the working class. Although it now has university status, it has not lost its ethos, and remains committed to widening participation. For a while, I felt like an imposter in the academy, a trespasser even, not because of my class but because of my job role. Binns, interestingly, cites Warnock as asserting that 'Behaviours that appear to the working-class academic to signal arrogance are viewed by the middle-class as markers of confidence and self-assuredness ... Because self-promotion and networking are necessary to professional class success, the working-class academic is once again at a disadvantage' (Warnock, cited in Binns, 2019, p. 94). After a couple of years, I settled into the role, grew in confidence, started to use own my voice, and my views, and was not afraid to express them in the company of other experienced academics, some middle class, who also became my network of colleagues. Crew notes that her 'respondents from "new universities" were the most likely to describe themselves as being working-class' (2020, p. 22) and this might be because the new universities employ the most number of lecturers who identify as working-class. I don't describe myself as being anything else.

Crew quotes one of the participants from her own research whose words are reminiscent of Reay's participant, Christine, who she interviewed 23 years previously:

> I look around at my life and I think I have no right to call myself working class at all because me and my partner have more money...we live in a very sort of proper kind of middle-class area and we do very middle-class things... But then I can't describe myself as being middle class because I always feel like I have one foot in the working-class world (2020, p. 23).

However, Crew goes on to explain that the phenomena are not always as straightforward or easily explained:

> We already see a fetishization of working-class culture in fashion, music and in the street food revolution, while in academia, inequalities experienced by working class people are colonised by middle class academics for publications. There are examples of white elite academics, oozing with privilege, who desire that attractive working-class status, until it's not inconvenient, and then they shed it like a second skin.
>
> (Crew, 2020, p. 23)

Byrne's experience doesn't concur with Reay's 'imposters' (2002), or Askham's 'identity conflict' (2008), but rather he cites Tapp's (2013) 'hybrid identity' and describes his experience as conforming to an 'internal duality' (Byrne, 2019, p. 139). Having a dual identity is certainly a concept that I can identify with; although I don't hide my working-classness, there are aspects of the working-class culture that I leave at the door as I enter HE because they don't fit with what the expectations of being an academic are. As I previously stated, I have evolved with my job role into what might now be deemed a member of the *neo* working class, one who has adapted and changed her habitus to include working in HE, a job not traditionally associated with being working-class. I have learnt to re-negotiate my identity from where I was to where I am now, and that re-negotiation includes inhabiting two worlds simultaneously, something that very many working-class academics do. Wakeling (2010, p. 38) argues that an occupation as an academic cannot be compared with 'solidly' working-class occupations 'such as bus driver, cleaner, supermarket checkout assistant or lathe operator' (I confess I had to look up *lathe operator*, never having come across that job); maybe not, but that is not to say that, given the right opportunity, that bus driver or cleaner could not become an academic. Crew makes reference to the 'organic intellectuals who, on the other hand, emerged from their own culture and could act as change agents' (2020, p. 112). I have used the phrase here '*neo* working class' to describe my adapted working-class habitus, with added practices and values to the existing traditional practices and values of my social class, and to indicate that working-class habitus has changed in many respects, as well as acting as an agent of change.

Nevertheless, HE is still shrouded in elitism and snobbery does exist in many institutions, albeit more so in one type of institution than another. I have experienced some uncomfortable exchanges with academics at elite institutions that I would attribute to snobbery. Despite these challenges, more and more of the working class are finding their way into academic roles in HE and this is partly due to the widening participation drive: HE widened its participation to allow under-represented groups to take part, 20+ years on and many of those students are now academics; not only did we take advantage of that opportunity educationally, we also benefitted vocationally. To use Wakeling's phrase: 'there is no going back' (cited in Taylor, 2010, p. 41).

Notes

1. Seamus Heaney (1939–2013), my favourite Irish poet, made this comment as he addressed the graduating class of The University of North Carolina, 1996: '...the true and durable path into and through experience involves being true to the actual givens of your lives. True to your own solitude, true to your own secret knowledge. Because oddly enough, it is that intimate, deeply personal knowledge that links us most vitally and keeps us most reliably connected to one another' (The Marginalian).
2. The 'famine' in Ireland was a period of great hunger and starvation while the country was under British rule. 'Ireland was part of the United Kingdom, which was the richest and most powerful nation in the world. Ireland was producing a surplus of food. However, between 1845 and 1852, more than 1.5 million Irish people starved to death, while massive quantities of food were being exported from their country to Britain. A half million people were evicted from their homes, often illegally and violently, during the potato blight. Another 1.5 million had no choice but to emigrate to foreign lands aboard rotting, overcrowded "coffin ships". The famine left a scar so deep within the Irish people, that it set in motion a war that would finally gain Ireland its independence from Britain in 1922' (Mulvihill, 2017).
3. HESA, the Higher Education Statistics Agency, collects, processes and publishes data about HE in the United Kingdom.

References

Abrahams, J., & Ingram, N. (2013). The chameleon habitus: Exploring local students' negotiations of multiple fields. *Sociological Research Online, 18*(4), 213–226.

Addison, M., & Mountford, V. G. (2015). Talking the talk and fitting in: Troubling the practices of speaking 'what you are worth' in higher education in the UK. *Sociological Research Online, 20*(2), 4.

Arnot, M. (2002). *Reproducing gender: Essays on educational theory and feminist politics.* London: Routledge Falmer Press.

Askham, P. (2008). Context and identity: Exploring adult learners' experiences of higher education. *Journal of Further and Higher Education, 32*(1), 85–97.

Baxter, A., & Britton, C. (2001). Risk, identity and change: Becoming a mature student. *International Studies in Sociology of Education, 11*(1), 87–102.

Bimrose, J., & Barnes, S. A. (2011). Adult career progression and advancement: A five year study of the effectiveness of career guidance. Retrieved from [PDF] Adultcareerprogression&advancement:Afiveyearstudyoftheeffectivenessofcareer guidance|SemanticScholar

Binns, C. (2019). *Experiences of academics from a working-class heritage: Ghosts of childhood habitus.* Cambridge: Cambridge Scholars Publishing.

Blackburn, R. M., & Jarman, J. (1993). Changing inequalities in access to British universities. *Oxford Review of Education, 19*(2), 197–215. doi:10.1080/0305498930190206

Bourdieu, P. (1984). *Distinction.* London: Routledge and Kegan Paul.

Bourdieu, P. (1988). *Homo academicus* [Trans. by Collier, P.]. Cambridge: Polity, Press.

Bourdieu, P. (1990). *The logic of practice.* Cambridge: Polity Press.

Bourdieu, P., & Passeron, J. C. (1977). *Reproduction in education, society and culture.* London: Sage Publications.

Bourdieu, P., & Wacquant, L. (1992). *An invitation to reflexive sociology.* Cambridge: Polity Press.

Bowl, M. (2003). *Non-traditional entrants to higher education.* Stoke on Trent: Trentham Books.

Burke, P. (2002). *Accessing education: Effectively widening participation.* Stoke on Trent: Trentham Books.

Burnell, I. (2015, Autumn). Widening the participation into higher education: Examining Bourdieusian theory in relation to HE in the UK. *Journal of Adult and Continuing Education, 21*(2). doi:10.7227/JACE.21.2.7

Byrne, G. (2019). Individual weakness to collective strength: (Re)creating the self as a 'working-class academic'. *Journal of Writing in Creative Practice, 12*(1 & 2), 131–150.

Clance, P. R., & Imes, S. (1978). The impostor phenomenon in high achieving women: Dynamics and therapeutic intervention. *Psychotherapy Theory Research and Practice, 15*, 241–247.

Coogan, R. (2019). A working-class accent in academia is a blessing and a curse. *Times Higher Education (THE).*

Crew, T. (2020). *Higher education and working-class academics precarity and diversity in academia.* London: Palgrave.

Crozier, G., Reay, D., & Clayton, J. (2010). The socio-cultural and learning experiences of working-class students in higher education. In M. David (Ed.), *Improving learning by widening participation in higher education* (pp. 62–74). London: Routledge Falmer Press.

David, M. (2010). *Improving learning by widening participation in higher education.* London: Routledge Falmer Press.

Department of Education and Science (DES). (1987). *Higher education: Meeting the challenge.* London: HMSO.

Freeborn, C. (2000, October). Now or never. *Guardian Education, 3,* 10–11.

Green, A., & Lucas, N. (2000). *FE and lifelong learning: Realigning the sector for the twenty-first century.* London: Institute of Education.

Grenfell, M. (2008). *Pierre Bourdieu key concepts.* Durham: Acumen Publishing.

Grenfell, M., & James, D. (1998). *Bourdieu and education.* Oxon: Routledge Falmer Press.

HESA. (2021). Widening participation summary: UK performance indicators. Widening participation summary: UK Performance Indicators | HESA.

Jones, O. (2020). *Chavs: The demonization of the working class.* London: Verso.

Leary, M. R., Patton, K. M., Orlando, E., & Funk, W. W. (2000). The impostor phenomenon; self-perceptions, reflected appraisals and interpersonal strategies. *Journal of Personality, 68,* 725–726.

Leathwood, C., & O'Connell, P. (2003). 'It's a struggle': The construction of the 'new student' in higher education. *Journal of Educational Policy, 18*(6), 597–615.

Lynch, K., & O'Neill, C. (1994). The colonisation of social class in education. *British Journal of Sociology of Education, 15*(3), 307–324.

Mulvihill, J. (2017). *The truth behind the Irish famine.* Jerry Mulvihill.

Northedge, A. (2003). Rethinking teaching in the context of diversity. *Teaching in Higher Education, 8*(1), 17–32.

Reay, D. (1997). Feminist theory, habitus, and social class: Disrupting notions of classlessness. *Women's Studies International Forum, 20*(2), 225–233.

Reay, D. (2002). Class, authenticity and the transition to higher education for mature students. *Sociological Review, 50*(3), 398–418.

Reay, D. (2017). *Miseducation inequality, education and the working classes.* Bristol: Policy Press.

Reay, D., Crozier, G., & Clayton, J. (2009). 'Strangers in Paradise'?: Working-class students in elite universities. *Sociology, 43*(6), 1103–1121.

Reay, D., Miriam, E., & Ball, S. (2005). *Degrees of choice: Social class, race and gender in higher education.* Stoke on Trent: Trentham Books.

Robbins, L. (1963). *Higher education, report and appendices* Cmnd 2154. London: HMSO.

Rogers, C. (1951). *Client-centered therapy.* London: Constable Publishing.

Ryan, J., & Sackrey, C. (1984). *Strangers in paradise.* Boston, MA: South End Press.

Sakulku, J., & Alexander, A. (2011). The impostor phenomenon. *International Journal of Behavioural Science, 6*(1), 75–97.

Skeggs, B. (1997). *Formations of class and gender.* London: Sage Publications.

Slank, S. (2019). Rethinking the imposter phenomenon. *Ethical Theory & Moral Practice, 22,* 205–218. doi:10.1007/s10677-019-09984-8

Taylor, Y. (2010). *Classed intersections: Spaces, selves, knowledges.* Farnham: Ashgate Publishing.

Taylor, J., & House, B. (2010). An exploration of identity, motivations and concerns of non-traditional students at different stages of higher education. *Psychology Teaching Review, 16*(1), 46–57.

Taylor, Y., & Lahad, K. (2018). *Feeling academic in the neoliberal university: Feminist flights, fights and failures*. Cham: Springer International Publishing AG.

Thompson, J. (2000). *Stretching the academy: The politics and practice of widening participation in higher education*. Leicester: NIACE.

Webb, J., Schirato, J. T., & Danaher, G. (2002). *Understanding Bourdieu*. London: Sage Publications.

Wilkinson, C. (2020). Imposter syndrome and the accidental academic: An autoethnographic account. *International Journal for Academic Development, 25*(4), 363–374. doi:10.1080/1360144X.2020.1762087

Yates, J. (2014). *The career coaching handbook*. Oxon: Routledge.

Chapter 9

Who Do You Think You Are? The Influence of Working-Class Experience on an Educator in a Process of Becoming

Peter Shukie

Abstract

What does it 'feel like' to be working class and an academic? This chapter explores the significance of working-classness both from influences in childhood, and experiences as an adult, when entering academia. Asking what feelings are involved makes autoethnography the perfect lens for analysis, while immediately challenging the objectivity of a distanced neutrality preferred by much academic process. A provocation comes from the question, 'who do you think you are?' that reverberates through my life and reinforces that as autoethnographers, we become both subject and analysts; as such working-class subject analysts, the reflections amplify the importance of experiences lived and offer more than mere diversity in research methodologies. This is an account of what it feels like, and how these feeling have altered what my work in the academy looks like, how theory, pedagogy and practice have changed and how a working-class praxis emerged.

Keywords: Gonzo pedagogy; toxic narratives; media representation; new academy; haunted nostalgia; shame

Introduction

There have been points writing this chapter when I have found myself thinking 'what is the point?'. Class, being working class, is something I have held close and struggled to understand, over five decades. I have been warmed by it and tired of it, and I know that very often the sensation that comes with any identification with working-classness is one of futility, frustration, depression and competition. Competition to 'prove myself', a process so worthless that involvement in such

The Lives of Working Class Academics, 123–134

Copyright © 2023 Peter Shukie

Published under exclusive licence by Emerald Publishing Limited

doi:10.1108/978-1-80117-057-420221009

proving grounds makes us self-loathe, shuddering with the ugly clumsiness of having to define our families, communities, histories and backgrounds for the edification of others. It makes writing this chapter difficult, a lifetime of 'chip on your shoulder' reproaches that silence any reflections of what has shaped me. There is also the sense of betrayal, of discussing what we did not have that denies the struggles of parents also living with five children in a two-bedroomed terrace. Remaining working class as an adult seemed an additional badge of dishonour, as if a salvation narrative was necessary to talk about class from higher peaks. There is the ultimate purpose here too, the point that drove me to write, that working class, experiencing poverty, is important in shaping what education looks like. I realised, as the writing emerged, how owning my working-classness is absolutely necessary in facing the power of an academy that seeks to nullify it.

How to write this was the ensuing challenge. A question surfaced, something that echoed across my early life and into Higher Education, 'who do you think you are?'. Not a question in any authentic sense, operating as an admonishment, a check, a dark shadow stepping in front of fledgling steps on newly dreamed pathways. Neither does it need to be articulated every time, it can appear in a sneer or belittling comment. Over decades I have heard from others of their experiences of this form of blockage. Some successfully overcoming it, others not, all of us aware of how much harder it makes movement. Many face this on some level, but there is an insidious presence of this within class. Ingrained in the ways we see ourselves and are taught by institutions to see ourselves, there is the familiarity of Plato's call for us to 'know your place'. This is destructive, not only to the individuals bound by rigid structures, the whole communities confined by low expectations and thwarted ambition, but for the whole of society. Like some monstrous panopticon, our lives are made hideous by media representations of working-class incompetence and reinforced by fear and loathing of our ambition that threatens the stability of other classes. Lisa McKenzie (2015a) described a feeling of being in university spaces as one in which,

> My gender, my class and my background is exposed: the way I speak, the way I use words, my research respondents, their stories, their lives and mine are no longer reduced to flat words on a page hidden in a ream of impenetrable panegyric fence-sitting. We become animated, in hyper colour, with hyper sound; we are multi-dimensional and consequently easy to see, and easy to target.
>
> (McKenzie, 2015a, np)

The sense of exposure McKenzie describes is significant, in seeking out work on class experiential accounts are essential. Writing around class has had to change to reflect what it means to be working class operating within dominant/ dominating middle-class narrative space.

In later years, I worked to create a working-class academic conference, and it happened because there were many of us out there, many more than I imagined. I started to reflect on the extent to which class had influenced everything I had done. Without the gagging of 'chip on shoulder' rebukes, it was apparent that working-classness had not been a barrier to what I had achieved, it had been the source of power that allowed me to achieve anything at all. This chapter is no celebration of education and transformation to a more palpable ideal state, rescued from poverty. Todd (2017) warns of the 'myths of social mobility' and it is important to recognise the ways in which education can be used to further promote a narrative that celebrates education as an individualist escape route. My experiences were not that. My initial forays into Higher Education were accompanied by my becoming homeless, much of the work since has been precarious. What has stuck has been a drive to realise the need for fairness and equality that are absent in many educational structures.

Inspiration comes too from others writing about their experiences. Tanya Shadrick (2022), on deciding whether to write, what to write, says 'it's not much, but neither is it nothing' (p. 302). The courage required is likely to go unnoticed, but through telling our stories we can become 'calling cards and quiet invitations' (Shadrick, 2022) that encourage others to step from the silence and reveal hidden lives. That we often feel small, insignificant and unworthy is part of being us, and the cruelty of our confinement being that we are encouraged never to tell our stories. Academic distance insists these experiences remain only ours, a secret to hide and to see as dysfunctional, broken and in need of fixing. I have for almost all of my life answered, 'who do you think you are?' with some form of outward bravado, some cockiness and noisy demonstration when I was at my strongest. 'Not much' is what I thought mostly, and even in strong moments, self-denigration lay inches below the surface ready to wash over the temporary islands of confidence. It is other working-class writers and speakers that allowed me to think, 'neither is it nothing'. This chapter, that I have worried over, lay down and left, returned to and seen as a gnawing but troublesome necessity, is important because it is part of my own 'not nothing'.

This has to be bound to the future, not the past. Recollection involves looking backwards but it is the influences and practices of a working-class approach to education that I believe are helping shape new thinking and action. My work is infused with a necessity to include class, make it manifest as a formative power in our lives in the face of it being eradicated, replaced with 'toxic poverty narratives' (O'Hara, 2020) that depicts the poor as the architects of our own despair. I also had to create alternate pedagogies in how class was introduced, of a gonzo pedagogy that prioritised the lives we lived as a form of analysis and creativity. This was important in seeking to evade the mega-theories built around us, populated with increasing verbosity, built almost entirely on misrepresented concepts of our wretchedness. This continued pressure to have who we think we are controlled by others is insidious and destructive, it is happening around us. I speak with students encouraged to deny class exists in the UK, seeing their own struggles as part of personal failings for having a family, not achieving school, arriving late to education, not being confident enough. I am continually faced with the realities and contradictions of the academic and the lived world. 'It's all academic anyway' is a hackneyed response to something that is of limited or no relevance. It can well be applied to much academic discussion around class, where the lives involved are seen as generalisable and thus made invisible by massifi-cation of argument and alienating theory. Mirlees (2015) writes on how the millennial generation is manipulated to see themselves outside class, as individuals within generalisable narratives of youth, consumer, worker-to-be-managed and victim of hard times (p. 298). We are encouraged to silence experience and talk of education only in terms of attainment, progress and economic achievement. Class may be a painful but necessary basis from which to begin societal change, to have it eradicated is to lose any possibility of a collective and shared experienced that recognise the necessity for such change. Mirlees suggests the optimum approach to change narratives that erase class awareness is to 'speak with' (p. 298) people rather than dictate to. It is different talking about poverty and education when your own home has no heating, when you are hungry, when you are frightened of a future you feel is out of your control. Our gonzo pedagogy approaches use projects and community-inspired activism, art that reflects on lived experience, psycho-geography that has students walk their towns and feel the society as they experience it. Dialogue was the first instinct that came to me as an educator, in my thirties after returning to study and having to work several jobs and attend the local college to gain the degree begun a decade earlier. I was given my first job in a group of excluded young people, with the interviewing manager saying that, 'you live on the same estate as most of them, so you might find a link'. I, like them, was defined as 'being given a chance', the largesse of an Other that we should be grateful for and welcome this opportunity. It was natural to me to begin with dialogue, we walked canals, read to each other, made films, watched films, wrote songs, poetry, painted and had discussions. We gradually got rid of reams of supplied resources based on writing CVs and cover letters. Attendance was high, and that meant I was 'safe' as a risk that had paid off, the funding metrics ach-ieved. The organisation found this 'a miracle', but nothing miraculous happened here, just a recognition of how we were all people and could treat each other with love and respect. When I asked for a library, a corner with book shelves and books, the managers collectively burst out laughing. It was a laugh I recognised throughout every encounter I had with education, from school, college, poly-technic and university. Anything good we had achieved was lost, what that laugh forced into us was a reminder of who we were and how fixed our identities were in these spaces.

When reflecting on this two decades later, I was struck by the words of one of O'Hara's (2020) interviewees when writing about the power of shame, Reverend Barber, who said, 'We have to shift the narrative. But you can't do that without shifting the narrators' (p. 82). It is absolutely the case that the narrators around class cannot be solely from privileged middle- or upper-class background. Of course, they almost always are. The shift toward first-person experience makes all the difference to what we read around class, it is the way we avoid faux objec-tivity, as if it is possible to consider class from a position of neutrality. McKenzie (2015a, 2015b), Reay (2018), de Waal (2019), Hudson (2019), O'Hara (2020), and Shadrick (2022) all write powerfully about class not only through statistical data and theory, but through experience and 'what it feels like' to be to be oppressed, demeaned and ignored (O'Hara, 2020, p. 114). As educator, researcher, activist and academic the significance of voice has been paramount in my work, but recognising this is far from the end of the problem. Grossman (2005) was one of the first researchers I encountered that recognised that voicelessness was never the issue. Our communities may well be noisy, verbose, opinionated and loud but that counts for little in an academy that '*cannot or will not hear* [those that do not] *echo with their own assumptions and beliefs*' (p. 79). Reverend Barber is right to identify the need for new narrators, but we also need much work to create spaces in which their narration can be heard. The 'presumption of ignorance' (Grossman, 2005, p. 79) that comes from dominant narrators is purposeful in silencing the diversity of working classes, especially those from poverty. Not because we are incapable of noise but what we have to say often challenges the neatness of theoretical concerns with who we are. It is important we hear each other and demolish mediation between the branches of working-class communities, between regions, races and cultural backgrounds. It is important to recognise ongoing evidence-based reflection, such as the Alston Report (2020) on poverty in the United Kingdom and the United States. While Alston makes clear that, 'poverty is a political choice and will be with us until its elimination is reconceived as a matter of social justice' (Alston, 2020, p. 19) it is *what this feels like* that can galvanise our responses.

Like the ironic title of Valerie Walkerdine's (1991) film *Didn't She Do Well*, the power of our existence in the academy comes from the way *we* change *it* – not how successfully *it* has changed *us*. My background makes me powerful in my teaching approaches and the ways I come to see learning. There is celebration here, as Kit de Waal (2019) advocated in her working-class writers' anthology, but not of social mobility; a celebration of working-class craft, creativity and strength is what characterises those that have influenced my work and that I will show as a pulse through this auto-ethnographic account of a working-class experience of the academy. Who I think I am, how I manage to establish this within academia, *is* the point of this chapter. By writing ourselves into the narrative of Higher Education, we broaden perceptions of academia and who it includes. By forming new narratives we continue the push away of dominating toxicity that destroys and replace these with our own voices, cultures, knowledges and ways of seeing.

The Search for Who I Thought I Was/Might Be

My experiences of childhood are not entirely negative, yet there is a gnawing residue that comes from poverty, of overcrowded housing, hunger and growing awareness of being somehow less than others. Bullying in free school meal queues ultimately makes up less than a few days of a lifetime, and regardless of later reflection and contextualisation that it was not our fault, these memories come mixed with anger, shame and bitterness. What becomes apparent is that you only start to feel shame in the presence of others, from elsewhere, from the middle-class gaze. It grows across life and the ironic recognition is that education, that route of transformation, becomes also the site of greatest exposure and judgement.

I am, like all of us, partly defined by my time too, an era in which we grew awareness of who we were. The fact that working-classness is continually represented as a negative space means we are often left desperate for images of ourselves that are not already overlaid with caricatures formed by a toxic narrative (McKenzie, 2015b; O'Hara, 2020) or part of a grand silencing of our own cultures in place of a bestowed, sanitised and sterile national culture (Sczezelkun, 2020).

There was a feature of The Smiths and the period of the 1980s that used images from two decades earlier, of images on record sleeves from black and white filmic depictions from *A Taste of Honey*, of film noir depictions from a British New Wave. I recognised this then, not as a nod to art, or a recognition of a style or cultural movement. Shelagh Delaney, the film of her work, among others like *Saturday Night Sunday Morning, This Sporting Life, Spring and Port Wine, Billy Liar* remained the only depictions of working class as heroes, of agents of change, of accent and poverty with a voice, no matter how dark. We were desperate for representation, for cultural depictions we could relate to, for signs of our existence outside our own immediate experience. The sense of inclusion, of being part of a wider network is what culture brings, a sense of belonging denied us apart from fragments collected over decades. Seeking out positive representations of ourselves is crucial to allow us to see what we might do, how we might become different versions of ourselves. It is an absence of representation that has long enraged communities and people around race (Coard, 1971), gender, cultural diversity, *of us*, that is *by us*. Entering the academy is to recognise the extent to which those of us outside must abandon our own cultures, linguistics richness, spaces and histories to fit into the accepted normative processes of a middle-class academy. To do this we are encouraged to adopt new accents, values, ways of seeing that further impoverish our own working-class cultures by shadowing them in this other light, as if we must learn to despise ourselves before we are improved. Without the opportunity to write our own representations, we become reliant on those given us of ourselves by others. I look back on those images and cultural artefacts and see how my desperate need for recognition, to see others living a life like mine. Those Sunday night films from decades earlier provided something, library shelves a little more, seeking out those stories of outsiders, of triumph over adversity. In literature and film, this search often had to go back decades, to the haunting brass jazz in *A Taste of Honey* contrasted with the jaunty brightness of a Terry Thomas world of tennis and travel. Decades old by my viewing of these in the early 1980s, the mono-chromed worlds of Arthur Seaton (*Saturday Night Sunday Morning*), Frank Machin (*This Sporting Life*) and the failed escape bids found in *Spring and Port Wine* and *Billy Liar* became rare beacons of places in which we could see ourselves. In each of these films and others like them, there came the aching presence of dysfunction, of broken spirit and adversity. Billy Fisher (*Billy Liar*) was a lower-middle class character but one written and played by working-class talent. His condition affected me most, the trapped animal, living schizo-delusional existence and unable to breaks his chains, to join Julie Christie and take a London-bound train and start a new life. In the humdrummery of such a life, the necessary pretend world of Ambrosia, where Billy Fisher was king/emperor/dictator, drew him closer than any real-world opportunity could. The working-class backgrounds of the author (Keith Waterhouse) and star (Tom Courtenay) offered inspiration while also familiar as they bound aspiration to a trope, of angry young men, in black and white, distanced already from our lives of miners' strikes, overcrowded housing and industrial decay. Theirs was the world of our fathers, mothers, the adults beyond us that lived a life of possibility so long as the gritty anger came with talent and courage. *Billy Liar* affected me because he highlighted the ways we were encouraged to see the weakness of existence as our own fault; it was my failure to live in poverty. O'Hara (2020) argues that poverty is not an illness (p. 89) but there is a sense of it making us ill. Not the many illnesses that hunger and poor housing can bring, but that anxiety and gut-wrenching inadequacy we have foisted upon us and that can last a lifetime. The development of my identity from this background required therapy, not theory.

My own story is not one of triumph, but it is one of survival. I am working class, from poverty and surprised that I am looking at my experiences for the first time as ones of class and not of my own failings. I was not just in poverty as a child, but also as an adult, working in temporary jobs, often in precarity, in squats, in houses without heating, working but in emergency accommodation. I do not have that schizophrenic inbetweenness, of the tension between being working class and academic, as I have never had long away from actual struggle. Perhaps it is because although with a PhD from Lancaster University, with 20 plus years as a lecturer, these are in working-class spaces, in College Based Higher Education (CBHE).

Crew (2020) opens her work on working-class academics with a range of the measures and stratifications that are applied, societally and more academically, such as Bourdieu's concepts of cultural and social capital. These seem important in allowing for authenticity, of seeking interlopers claiming poverty for kudos or credibility. What this continued emphasis on authenticity does do is muddy the waters and start the process of defining class to the extent that often we get no further. What it means to be working class in the academy is immediately turned into an objectification of class, a pressing call to remove experience and replace it with distanced and clear-cut definitions. The fact that attending university in my late teens effectively made me homeless in my early twenties is not simply a tale of adversity, a *prolier-than-thou* account that raises my own flag of authenticity. It was a part of a crushing of self and a flailing impotent anger that manifested in a decade of struggle and survival that was forged in those periods of fear and outsider status. I learned in a polytechnic in London that I was not part of this system, that my experiences were detrimental to study and almost entirely my own fault. When I left home, thinking I was bound to be something other than I was despite nobody else thinking that, I left a room shared with my three brothers and sister. The day I left, a shoving up of a bed and the replacing of a couple of posters meant I was gone. The space was no longer available. I had all the fears and anxieties of anyone travelling to a new city, to a new experience, but added to that was the knowledge that the road behind me had been washed away.

It might be that free school meals through all stages of education made a difference, I do not know. It led to bullying, to fights, to a character shaped by often being a clown, distracting from my lack of designer brands or cash in any form. I read nightly in the town library, voraciously, but I did not achieve well in school, I was caned a lot and on detention weekly. Education was something I did for myself, in secret and for free, and schooling was system of oppression delivered to me without any visible benefit other than making me frightened and rebellious. Education of the self and the education system were not the same thing. Only reflecting from a parallax view some decades later can I consider that social conditions massively impacted what study means and what chances of success I had. As I decided that Higher Education allowed something of the self-study benefits of growth and personal development, I decided on the escape route to polytechnic. Nobody at home saw me as vanguard, or pioneer. This was not the act of bravery or courage that I might have hoped. I was more viewed as an idiot walking a path that was beyond me. On the Friday before I left for London on the Sunday night 'milk train' my dad took me to a wholesale warehouse that he got his ice cream van stock from, introducing me to Margaret with the intention that I would 'get on'. I said again, 'I am going to university in London, on Sunday'. The look on both their faces, Margaret who I had met just minutes before, was one of incongruity, of mocking smiles, the faces of 'who do you think you are?'. 'Don't be so bloody stupid' was enough of a paternal push and slap on the back that I could have expected, so it was with that I left with rucksack and bin bag for East London. Who we think we are comes in all sizes and acts of bravado, delusion, vision, drive and hope, but the extent to which we follow these is also shaped by those around us. While Bourdieu's concepts of capital have some use (Crew, 2020), they are not the only factor. Rage and dreams, delusion and obstinacy are equally significant. It was not just that I was the first person in the family to go to university (or polytechnic, nobody knew the difference); I was the first person in the entire street, the streets around our street, my wider family and relations, to have even attended sixth form. Presumably the teachers at my school had been to universities, but these were not people I could claim any link or relation to. Certainly, the children of teachers at our school were going. They always had been and we all knew it. It was spoken about in public, their celebrations held aloft at assemblies as regularly as mine was included in the detention list of shame that closed proceedings. We all knew the word university, even had some vague idea about what it was and where they were located. That others would be going, that they spoke about it, was still no revelation, no clarification. All it did was affirm the difference between the teachers and us. They were largely the angry, violent distributors of verbal coshes and wooden strikes. I was naughty, it seemed, before I even arrived. All the children waiting to be caned, or in detention, were similar to me; we walked from the free school meal queues to the waiting lines for canings, admonishments, detentions and suspensions. All of this was in-house as we all were the ones without home phones, no parents called to attend, just a silent and hidden group of those who could be blamed, and so were. The violence seemed never-ending, our communities 'the enemy within' according to Margaret Thatcher, and the teachers responding as if they believed every word of it. That anyone from this line-up would go to university was simply not a consideration. Not for us, not for anyone that was involved with us. We were also the first generation to enter a world of no-work, of mass unemployment, closed factories and mills, a mining industry in a final death thrall. Not that any of these options appealed, I saw myself as a poet without recognition, a wandering philosopher, a social justice warrior who was fighting a cause of eternal inequality. I would be freed from my current terrors and trauma, I was sure, although never certain how that might happen.

Entering the Academy

Morrisey had said, around the time I left for London in 1986, that 'If Prince came from Wigan he would have been slaughtered by now' (Coupland, 2006). A rare mention of the town outside the sports pages, and while dismissive, I knew what he meant. London allowed for play and reinvention, fashion and experimenta-tion. For the first time, a room of my own with a metal camp bed and four walls. But just for me. Back home, these discoveries of a new self often meant being swift of tongue and feet to avoid Morrisey's predicted slaughter. But by then I *had* London, it was education that had took me there, and allowed these growing spaces. For those denied that, like forced rhubarb, crowded in the dark and grown in uniform space, there was a resistance to difference and often violent retribution. What Morrisey said of Prince seemed clear to me then, there was no communal growing grounds, no romantic free space of free expression and growth. When I see back those brilliant minds and creators that came out of our spaces, it is always with respect for the intensity of effort that forces poetry, song, art, liter-ature from hard soil. In those urban clubs, terraces and repurposed warehouses, the intense and furious brilliance of music, fashion, art, writing was forged from working-class energy. The collectives of those nomads and creatives were devel-oped through necessity, of the impulse to make/build/generate despite the lack of support. The ambition and the permission had to come from within, and it made newness, originality and brilliance possible. Such creation reached out and trig-gered engagement from others, and it was only ever possible from working-class space, from seeing the struggle against 'go to work and shut your mouth' men-talities that proliferated. While it is possible to look at working-class spaces and say all is well, the artists and the successful can emerge, such an approach ignores the many who are never able to make their mark. Education remained the accessible space for all but was not the place shaped by these thinkers and cre-ators. It was cold, harsh and often brutal in assessing who would be included. I could name artists, writers, musicians and sports people from my communities, and those like it – but not a single academic.

In London, the interview had included a meeting with a Literature lecturer. Part of the well-worn outline was around Shakespeare re-imagined, 'right here, in Stratford East, the irony is not lost on us!' he chortled. It was lost on me. It was probably three years before I worked out this allusion to Stratford upon Avon, the cultural differences, the separation of class and geography. They were both in the south after all, which seemed to me populated by posh people with a singular world view and calling that I had no part in. We are all bound by class perceptions, but access and belonging accompany middle-class understandings of academia as much as they were absent in mine. Although new to me then, the prevalence of imposter syndrome is established and something I am conscious of. What these reflections remind me is that we are not the only ones to award ourselves the identity of imposter and while I recognise this syndrome, I did not create my experiences of it alone.

It took little time for me to see there is a chasm between the educational purpose and power of Higher Education, and the cultural and value practices they have become wrapped up and entangled in. The purpose/power, of knowledge, sharing, creating, development of an understanding, collaboration, exposure to others and other ideas is strangled by the weeds of aspirational, me-first, prestige riddled concepts of education as status. It was a chasm that had a profound impact on me. I studied Cultural Studies, and the new books and ideas, alternate thinkers and ways of seeing were exciting and illuminating. A module in socio-linguistics brought new ways of seeing language, English embedded in life and actively shaping who we were, who we thought we were. I loved these ideas but found myself struggling to stay afloat. In the first few weeks in a socio-linguistics lecture, the excitement I felt (and still feel) when encountering new knowledge raged through me. I almost levitated upwards as I saw the knowledge discussed resonated in my world, feeling I just might make this whole academic thing work, bursting with enthusiasm. I raised my hand and stood, making an impassioned outline of the importance of accent in my home town, of identity, of conflict and shifting language patterns. Our lives, my reflections, this lecture, all coming together. Then, the students in front giggling, their accent familiar from the television but never from conversation, of their whispered 'listen to his voice', more giggling, of my shame and the reddening, burning and forcing me down deeper into my chair. Of later loathing of my own weakness, of not spouting something back, but knowing I would not, even if it happened again. Many more of these little acts happened, amplifying my cultural alienation, my cultural insignificance. Shame, as O'Hara (2020) writes, is an inevitable conclusion of a toxic poverty narrative; it is systematic intention that we carry this hot rock burning in our bellies and behind the eyes. Along with this was the sense of my feeling I was getting above myself, a 'chip on my shoulder' pretentiousness, inability masquerading as exclusion. On many occasions I got as far as the lecture theatre, having read what was needed, but looked in and fear made me walk off, wandering alone and drenched in self-loathing. I cannot know this was all rooted in class. I do know there was nobody I could talk about this to, not a soul I knew who had experienced this. I knew if I said a single word about this at home, it would have confirmed the stupidity of the move and the unpalatable *told you so* inevitability of another failed dream. Education did not feel as if it was a gateway out, a rising platform of social mobility, if anything it felt as if it was intensifying my sense of being outside, unworthy and ridiculous.

I left after two years, unhappy, homeless and a failure. My return a decade later was in desperation but in the North, in a college, with others like me. The learning became powerful and valid and started me toward post-graduate qualifications, research roles, educator status, writing degrees and designing projects. I am now an External Examiner at the London University I left in a state; the courses are brilliant and show working-class students making impassioned presentations and lecturers praising their insight, their brilliance. My experiences have not gone away, my work is all about class not as homogenous groups to be analysed. Instead, working-classness is the basis of projects that matter, of art and psycho-geography, of new pedagogies that we write papers on and share with our communities. Class always remains, still gnawing and painful as well as bringing solidarity and the rage to make other dreams possible. Working as an adult, I felt angst, not irony, in a PhD world in which I was told I needed to 'find my voice' in a system that had taken such efforts in ensuring I lost it. I get excited now by seeing others have lived this and are 'out there' and making claims for change. Maria Fusco (2020) talks of 'working-classness as method' (p. 13) and leaves spaces of fluidity, for ever-changing worlds, a method that is not numbered, flow charted, torturous in detail. Instead, a question, 'what does working classness as method actually mean?' (Fusco, 2020, p. 13), and a wondering response, 'how you go about things; how you imagine something will turn out; the juicy combinatorial possibilities; how it actually turns out; wanting but never sure' (Fusco, 2020). Valerie Walkerdine (2020) calls for a 'working class mode of research' (p. 11) that can counter 'pathologising assumptions' and allow us to read 'research and policy in a different way' (Walkerdine, 2020). Both are energising, both show a change is possible and response is forcing its way to the surface. *Who do you think you are?* remains a pertinent question; one we can infuse with that sense of this being reflective, encouraging and powerful. A question we see anew when encountered through a working-class praxis, a working-class pedagogy and a recognition of the necessity of ourselves to reimagine a new academy.

References

Alston, P. (2020). *Report of the special rapporteur on extreme poverty and human rights*. New York: United Nations.

Coard, B. (1971). *How the West Indian child is made educationally sub-normal in the British school system: The scandal of the black child in schools in Britain*. London: New Beacon Books.

Coupland, D. (2006). Papal attraction. *The Guardian*. Retrieved from https://www.theguardian.com/music/2006/mar/19/popandrock.morrissey

Crew, T. (2020). *Higher education and working-class academics: Precarity and diversity in academia*. Cham: Palgrave Pivot. doi:10.1007/978-3-030-58352-1_1

Fusco, M. (2020). *A belly of irreversibles*. Chapter in Edwards, Sean (2020), *Undo Things Done*. Liverpool: Bluecoat.

Grossman, J. (2005). Workers, their knowledge and the university. In J. Crowther, V. Galloway, & I. Martin (Eds.), *Popular education: Engaging the academy*. Leicester: NIACE.

Hudson, K. (2019). *Lowborn: Growing up, getting away and returning to Britain's poorest towns*. London: Vintage Publishing.

McKenzie, L. (2015a). Who would be a working-class woman in academia? *Higher Education*. Retrieved from https://www.timeshighereducation.com/lisa-mckenzie-who-would-be-working-class-woman-academia

McKenzie, L. (2015b). *Getting by: Estates, class and culture in Austerity Britain*. Bristol: Policy Press. doi:10.1177/0261018315600836b

Mirlees, T. (2015). A critique of the millennial: A retreat from and return to class. *Alternate Routes: A Journal of Critical Social Research, 26*. Retrieved from http://www.alternateroutes.ca/index.php/ar/article/view/22321

O'Hara, M. (2020). *The shame game: Overturning the toxic poverty narrative*. Bristol: Policy Press.

Reay, D. (2018). A life lived in class: The legacy of resistance and the enduring power of reproduction. *Prism Journal, 2*(1). doi:10.24377/LJMU.prism.vol2iss1article287

Shadrick, T. (2022). *The cure for sleep*. London: Weidenfeld & Nicolson.

Szczelkun, S. (2020). *Silence: The great silencing of British working class culture*. London: Routine Art.

Todd, S. (2017). The six myths of social mobility. In Social History Society's 2017 conference at the UCL Institute of Education. Retrieved from https://socialhistory.org.uk/shs_exchange/myths-of-social-mobility/

de Waal, K. (2019). *Common people: An anthology of working class writers*. London: Unbound.

Walkerdine, V. (1991). Didn't she do well. Retrieved from https://www.youtube.com/watch?v=uHxwTYZX2P4

Walkerdine, V. (2020). What's class got to do with it? *Discourse: Studies in the Cultural Politics of Education, 42*(1), 60–74. doi:10.1080/01596306.2020.1767939

Chapter 10

John Constable Was My First Art Teacher: Construction of Desire in a Working-Class Artist/Academic

Samantha Broadhead

Abstract

The development of 'desire' in a working-class artist/academic is explored through an analysis of the reminiscences between the author and her mother. It is argued that the notion of cultural capital implies a deficit in working-class subjects that is deterministic and does not fully explain those who are successful in the art world and/or academia. Rather than thinking about works of art and art practice in terms of cultural capital, they are conceptualised as resources that can have existential significance for some people. This is because early interactions with the arts enable people to connect with the world and at the same time enable them to recognise their own desires and talents while learning to think critically about their lives. The findings of this study suggest a nuanced approach based on cultural assets and resources rather than cultural capital should be considered in educational policy and practice.

Keywords: Working class; desire; artist; academic; cultural capital; cultural assets

Introduction

This chapter explores the initial critical incident that ignited my desire to become an artist and academic. First, I establish that I was raised in a working-class environment and subject to many of the indicators of disadvantage such as low income, eligibility for free school meals and being the first-in-the-family to attend higher education. I consider how Bourdieu's notion of cultural capital provides an account of why social inequalities are resistant to change, and on the other hand that it does not fully explain the experiences of working-class artist/academics. I

The Lives of Working Class Academics, 135–153
Copyright © 2023 Samantha Broadhead
Published under exclusive licence by Emerald Publishing Limited
doi:10.1108/978-1-80117-057-420221010

draw upon a critical incident from my childhood that helped provoke the desire in me to be an artist. The analysis of this incident is informed by the writings of Biesta (2017, 2020) where he considers the intersection between the arts and education and how these two disciplines enable us to 'be in dialogue with the world'.

The autoethnographic approach that underpins this chapter was based on reminiscences exchanged between me and my mother whilst looking at the family photograph album from the early 1970s when she would have been in her early 20s and a 'stay-at-home' mother. She was meticulous in describing the contents on the back of the photographs. We also looked at the remnants of my art work done in my childhood that my mother had kept.

Rather than adopting the language associated with widening participation, referring to phrases such as 'raising aspiration' and 'raising cultural capital' which implies a deficit in working-class people, I have framed the discussion in terms of 'desire'. I consider how my very early engagement with the cultural resources of my parents ignited in me a desire to connect with the world through the thinking, feeling and willing domains (Biesta, 2020). I finally reflect on some conclusions about the ways in which educators can think about their students' cultures.

How Is the Working Class Identified in Educational Discourses?

Bernstein's (1958, pp. 160–161) definition of class was that the middle classes were defined by educational achievement, employment in skilled or non-manual work and their attitude towards achieving long-term goals. He compared the individualism of the middle classes with the collectivism and communities of the working classes (Broadhead & Gregson, 2018). Reay (2002) argued that class always counts when people progress to higher education. She identified different working-class factions based on their attitudes to risk, challenge and fitting in to higher education. She pointed out that middle-class cohorts of students were often represented as fragmented whereas working classes were homogenised within policy and academic discourses. Within her work, Reay found working-class students, who chose the risk of higher education rather than striving to 'fit in', were atypical.

Wilson (2016) described 'working class' as a fluid grouping as members have very different experiences of poverty. Penney and Lovejoy (2017) argued for a distinct social group called the welfare-class within the working-class category, for those who are reliant on the welfare system. Penney and Lovejoy (2017) applied welfare-class to academics who, during their studies or precarious and part-time employment, are dependent on welfare support.

The current list of protected characteristics in the UK Equality Act (2010) does not include social class. However social class is still present in educational policies and debates, for example the concerns raised about the low participation of working-class boys in higher education (Baars, Mulcahy, & Bernardes, 2016). One way of understanding who the working classes are can be through a set of indicators that will not all apply in every case.

Baars et al. (2016) drew up a list of indicators based on the work of Goodman and Gregg (2010), Sharples, Slavin, Chambers, and Sharp (2011), Mongon and Chapman (2008), and Cassen and Kingdon (2007).

- Free school meal (FSM) eligibility
- Parental occupation
- Household income (either the lowest quintile or below 60% of the median)
- Parental uptake of state benefits
- Groups experiencing limited social mobility

Widening participation practitioners in higher education may also refer to other indicators, based on the need to report to organisations such as the Office for Students (OfS). These include Participation of Local Areas (POLAR) supplemented by Index of Multiple Deprivation (IMD). The POLAR approach allocates each ward into one of five ordinal quintiles based on the proportion of the resident population of young people who are eligible entering higher education at the age of 18 or 19. Quintile 1 would be an area of low participation and quintile 5 would be high. POLAR data are not synonymous with educational disadvantage or social class. It encapsulates information about the people living in a particular area and suggests the impact of underlying wider social factors operating in that area such as the quality of schooling, the labour market opportunities and young people's aspirations (Harrison & McCaig, 2015). IMD is a measure of relative levels of deprivation in neighbourhoods in England. The measure brings together 39 separate indicators across seven domains of deprivation including income, employment, health deprivation and disability, education and skills training, crime, barriers to housing and services and living environment (Noble et al. 2019).

These indicators and measures of socio-economic status focus on what the working classes do not have or do not do. It could be argued that they objectify the working-class subject and present a deficit model of working-class identity.

My Own Case

My early life as a child in the 1970s and 1980s is very pertinent to the topic of this chapter. I come from a small, provincial textile town in West Yorkshire. For the most part, my family and I lived in a three-bedroom council house. I did not realise at the time but it was actually a small space for two adults and three children.

Throughout my childhood we were relatively poor, although my parents made sure we had stability and the basic needs of life. My father worked as a gardener for the Salvation Army; his role like other agricultural workers was low paid. During the time when Margaret Thatcher was Prime Minister, he became unemployed along with my grandfather and my uncle. I remember being aware and worried about the scale of male unemployment and a fear of becoming part of what Penney and Lovejoy (2017) would call the welfare classes. There was little tradition of women working outside the family, but my mother broke the mould in the late-1980s, returning to education to train to be an administrator. Subsequently, she gained a job in the local health centre and became the bread winner of the family. I wonder how much my own interest in access and education and research was informed by my mother's brave decision to go back to learning.

During the 1970s and throughout my compulsory education, I was eligible for free school meals (FSMs) if I did not walk home for 'dinner'. This became a tremendous source of shame during my years at grammar school (I passed the 11 plus to everyone's surprise). My mother scrimped and saved so I could have a new uniform rather than second-hand, demonstrating the importance of working-class respectability (Skeggs, 1997). When I tried it on, it felt so stiff and strange but I was glad to have it. I remember two girls being mocked because their grammar school uniforms were pre-owned; it is surprising how children can pick up on these things.

Times were challenging during my secondary education. I was well aware I did not fit in with my middle-class peers and I did experience some bullying (from pupils and a member of the staff). However, most of the teaching I experienced in the grammar school was very good and inspiring. The deputy head mistress, Miss Hirst (a female academic), was a role model and she encouraged me to consider going to university or art school. I also respected my art teacher, Miss Taylor, who I felt I had an affinity with.

If today's measures associated with widening participation were applied to my case, it can be seen that I lived in an area of low participation, I received FSMs, my family had low socio-economic status and I would be the first in my family to go to university (Baars et al., 2016; Cassen and Kingdon (2007); Goodman & Gregg, 2010; Mongon & Chapman, 2008; Sharples et al., 2011). The realisation that the odds had been against me achieving in academia was and is very sobering. Yet I had a desire to be an artist from very early on in my childhood and later as a teenager to be an academic – I was adamant I would not be a mother and I would not be a secretary which my father hinted I should aspire to. The next sections investigate where this desire originated from by drawing on the work of Bourdieu (1973, 1986, 1990), Goldthorpe (2007), and Biesta (2017, 2020) and applying them to my own story.

Cultural Capital

One approach is to consider the working-class subject through the lens of Bourdieu's frameworks of habitus, depositions and cultural capital in order to understand why class is important in transitions to higher education (Reay, Crozier, & Clayton, 2010; Reay, Davis, David, & Ball, 2001). However, there are some criticisms of this concept and Goldthorpe's (2007) notion of cultural assets and resources could prove to be also relevant.

In the 1960s, researchers working within the sociology of education field began looking at educational attainment in relation to social class and ethnicity. Examples include Bernstein's (1961, 1965) work on the linguistic codes of children and Jackson and Marden's (1963) study of working-class children selected for the grammar school. Later, Bernstein (1975) demonstrated how visible (formal schooling) and invisible pedagogies (1960s' child-centred or progressive education) both advantaged middle-class children. Free secondary education had not raised attainment for all pupils. Therefore, culture and modes of socialisation as well as economic constraints were recognised as being important factors in educational inequalities. Researchers became interested in the cultural or subcultural influences on children's attainment. Within this context, the work of Pierre Bourdieu relating to cultural capital springs from these debates and continues to have a massive influence in how educational inequalities are understood. For example, in 2019, the United Kingdom's educational inspectorate, the Office for Standards in Education, Children's Services and Skills (Ofsted) created a new inspection framework that requires schools to develop their students' cultural capital (Nightingale, 2020).

Bourdieu and Passeron (1977, 1979) drew upon statistical data to demonstrate the extent of social inequalities in France. They conceived of cultural capital rather than cultural values or cultural resources (Goldthorpe, 2007). The notion of cultural capital appears to explain social class inequalities in educational attainment as well as being part of a wider theory of social reproduction.

Bourdieu (1986) recognised 'forms of capital' and their importance in social reproduction through processes that were advantageous to the dominant classes. In addition to economic capital there are other capitals such as cultural and social that operate together to create and sustain privilege.

Cultural capital is embodied in the individual through their dispositions and competencies that give them access to cultural capital in its objectified form of cultural artefacts. Furthermore, cultural capital is institutionalised in the criteria of cultural and academic evaluation, leading to the qualifications that provide opportunities for the holders. Culture of the dominant classes is recognised and legitimised by institutions.

In addition, social capital is the formal and informal networks of family, friends, colleagues and acquaintances that advantage members of that network.

The capitals are convertible and transmissible through families. Wealth, property and cultural objects can be bequeathed to offspring, preserving the privilege through generations. But families also pass on dispositions, knowledge and competencies to their members as well as facilitating social connections. Bourdieu (1973, 1986) argued that processes of socialisation made the transmission of cultural capital more secure and irreversible than the transmission of economic capital.

Bourdieu (1990) described 'habitus' as the system of socially constituted dispositions that the individual acquires in early life that determine their orientation to the world and their conduct in it. Transmission within the family and social context of cultural capital in its embodied manifestation is understood to be a major part of the habitus formation.

Habitus is formed by 'domestic' factors and developed further by the individual's experience of their class conditions. Bourdieu claimed that the habitus was resistant to other influences and so school and other educational institutions would have limited potential to change it. So, from Bourdieu's perspective, there is little scope for individuals to be re-socialised by the education system.

Bourdieu (1973) thought the content of culture was arbitrary and that there was no intrinsic superiority of what is taught in schools and colleges. What is taught and how it is taught are based on the interests of the dominant classes. What counts as cultural capital is what best reproduces the unequal distribution of social power and privilege over generations.

The degree of similarity between cultures or subcultures in which children are socialised and those that predominate in schools and colleges is seen to advantage some groups and disadvantage others. For the dominant classes, there is a degree of continuity between home and education through common modes of speech, style of social interaction and aesthetic orientation (Goldthorpe, 2007). Working-class children experience school as an alien (and in some cases hostile) environment where they feel out of place. Goldthorpe (2007) pointed out that Bourdieu's position assumed that working-class children, other than a few special cases, would fail to reach higher levels of the education system. Any working-class pupil or student who did succeed would be seen as the exception.

Bourdieu's theories around social reproduction and forms of capital appear to be a convincing explanation as to why inequalities resist change through educational interventions. However, there are some criticisms of this approach.

Goldthorpe (2007) points out that in practice some of Bourdieu's assertions about education can be challenged. For example, in the United Kingdom, the expansion of the secondary school system has made some impact on social mobility (Halsey, Heath, & Ridge, 1980); therefore, schools create cultural capital and do not simply reproduce it. Also, the idea that habitus is formed in the family and cannot be re-constituted in education is called into question. The notion that those working-class subjects who do succeed in school and beyond are unusual can also be challenged. The expansion of the tertiary educational sector infers that there has been some increase in working-class students entering higher education (Arum, Gamoran, & Shavit, 2007; Schofer & Meyer, 2005). There are still gaps and educational inequalities; however, the working classes and people from under-represented groups in higher education do take up opportunities and succeed. Working-class people who do well in education and later in academia should not be written off as insignificant or sporadic anomalies.

Goldthorpe (2007) argued that different class conditions do not give rise to such distinctive and steadfast forms of habitus as Bourdieu would suppose. Even the most disadvantaged classes with little access to 'high' culture and values that are favoured in education can still prevail. Some cultural resources do exist in families and schools can be agencies of re-socialisation that complement family influences in the creation and transmission of cultural capital (Halsey, Heath, & Ridge, 1980).

The criticisms that are sometimes aimed at Bernstein's structuralism (Broadhead & Gregson, 2018) can also apply to Bourdieu's general project of social reproduction. The theories can appear deterministic, ahistorical and static (Thompson, 1978). Processes of socialisation are described as if they endlessly reproduce the same power relations and any change is illusionary or unusual. This approach does not easily explain the transformation of systems nor does it explain the agency of pupils, families, students and educators.

O'Shea (2014) was also critical of the way the notion of cultural capital is applied to students from certain social groups, for example those students who are first in their families to go to university. By saying that these people 'lacked' the right kind of cultural capital was representing them as being in deficit, rather than the fault being with the educational systems they were entering. O'Shea favoured an approach developed from critical race theory by Yosso (2005) as a critique of Bourdieu's cultural capital. It was argued that although first-in-the-family students may not arrive in higher education with white, middle-class cultural capital of privileged students, they did come with other kinds of capitals (aspirational, navigational, social, linguistic, familial and resistant). This perspective suggests that although students maybe disadvantaged in education, they are not passive bodies and do call upon their own cultural resources to succeed although that success may be harder to obtain.

When considering Ofsted's recent focus on developing cultural capital, it is import to revisit Yosso's (2005) question, 'Whose culture has capital?' Will students from under-represented backgrounds be inculcated into the dominant culture to fit into educational systems, or will schools, colleges and universities adapt to value the cultures of those who they educate? (Nightingale, 2020). Goldthorpe (2007) suggests that thinking about the cultural assets and resources a working-class subject has may provide a more nuanced and less deterministic account of why some working-class subjects do succeed in education and in the arts.

Art as a Cultural Resource Rather Than Cultural Capital

Bourdieu perceives the canon of art as cultural capital embodied in cultural objects that are legitimised through institutions (including educational ones) that play a role in social reproduction of inequality. My own story is initiated by encounters with cultural objects collected by my parents and displayed in our home. When I reflect on my early years, I think it was the cultural resources in my parents' home that created my desire to be an artist that was not stymied by the lack of cultural capital associated with my particular habitus.

Biesta (2017) conceptualises art in a way that opens up possibilities for transformation, 'Rather than asking what it produces – ask what does it mean? Rather than asking what does it make – ask what does it make possible?' (p. 13). He goes on to claim that the arts allow people to express their own voices and identities. It enables people to find their own talents and create their own meanings. Biesta (2017) introduces an ethical dimension to his understanding of art, arguing that it needs to evoke the right voice, the right identity and the right creativity; otherwise there is a danger that the expression could be racist, bigoted, destructive and/or egocentric.

What is significant to Biesta (2017) is not necessarily the aesthetic experience of the art, but the existential quality of what or who is expressed. Art can suggest how people can exist well, individually and collectively, in the world and with the world. Art can potentially reveal what might be right and good in everyone's lives.

Importantly, for Biesta (2017) education and the arts empower people to be the subject of their own actions, intensions and responsibilities and not the object of what others would decide about their lives. This is a different understanding of art to Bourdieu's that it promotes the agency of people and encourages them to stand outside established social structures and think critically.

Desire is created through our connection with the world. Biesta (2015) argues that people need to understand that the planet cannot give them everything they want, therefore desire needs to be limited. People should be in the world but not be the centre of it, Biesta (2015) refers to this as a 'world-centred' approach.

Subjects need to exist in a 'grown-up' way by being in dialogue with the world materially and socially. Biesta (2017) writes that the subject is not who we are but how we are. What people do and what they refrain from doing. When people encounter the world in order to fulfil their desires, they will, most likely, encounter resistance. This causes three possible responses:

(1) Frustration makes people push harder. However, ambition and intensions are in danger of destroying what they encounter.
(2) Withdrawal – people could destroy their existence in the world.
(3) People can stay away from these two extremes. Stay in the middle ground and continue being in dialogue and existing with the world.

Thus, 'to be grown up we must accept a middle ground in coming to terms with desire' (Naughton & Cole, 2017, p. 4). This does not mean suppressing desires because they are the driving force of life, but making them become a force for living with the world in a grown-up way. People should not give up on their desires altogether but consider which aspects of desire are positive and which are destructive for the self, other living beings and the planet.

Art can be understood as an exploration of desires.

> Art makes our desires visible, gives them form, and by trying to come into dialogue with what or who offers resistance, we are at the very same time engaged with the desirability of our desires and in their rearrangement and transformation.
>
> (Biesta, 2017, p. 18)

Biesta (2020) argues that to exist is to connect with the world through different modalities. The senses such as vision, touch and sound reveal fundamentally different ways of being in dialogue with the world. Biesta (2020) draws upon the work of the Swiss pedagogue Johann Heinrich Pestalozzi (1746–1827) who proposed that the world is understood through the head, the hands and the heart that align to thinking, willing and feeling.

The world is the object of thinking; humans are always thinking about the world. However, they create an idea of the world rather than the world itself.

There is a discrepancy between the world and the ideas of the world. This can lead to frustration when resistance is encountered when humans try to impose their desires on the world.

However, Biesta (2020) argues that the work of the hands brings people closer to what is real; what is material, what is physical with its own integrity and pace. He goes on to say that,

> The domain of the hands is the domain of willing, of wanting something, of wanting to exist, in and with the world. To come into dialogue with the world is the question of the formation of the will – it is the question of adjustment, rearrangement and transformation of our will power so that it can help us come in dialogue with the world (p. 79).

Whereas thinking distances and willing connects, the domain of the heart, feeling, is about the care and love humans have for the world. It is the ways in which they are affected and touched by the world. Feeling draws us towards it.

Art comprises the work of the head, the work of the heart and the work of the hands and is important in relation to how people exist in the world.

Bourdieu's notion of cultural capital explains the classed dimensions of the arts. The art objects and practices that are celebrated (part of the western canon) are the ones that represent the interests, tastes and aesthetics of the dominant class. If working-class people are disadvantaged in education and their cultural objects are not recognised as having merit, how do working-class people engage with the arts?

Biesta (2017, 2021) has argued that the arts allow people to be in dialogue with the world through thought, feeling and willing and should be fundamental for all people, not just the privileged. One argument is that working-class people understand the world through their sensual experiences of their everyday lives (Unwin, 2009). The craft and artistry of vocational roles exist within workplaces where workers engage their heads, hands and hearts (for example hairdressers, cake-decorators, builders, engineers). Unwin (2009) describes her early life where she connected with the world through the 'aesthetics of everyday life' recognising the sensuality of working with food, fabrics, wood, bricks and concrete, 'Vocational education and valuing the artistry of skilled people was part, therefore, of my life in and outside the home, in my community, and even in the novels I read' (Unwin, 2009, p. 7). She continues to talk about her recognition that those skilful occupations associated with the working classes were defined in education and employment policy discourses as 'low' or unskilled. Educational systems and family expectations direct people into either studying the arts or studying vocational subjects dependent on their social class. Education does have an impact on habitus and desire as Goldthorpe (2007) suggests, but that impact could be to reinforce social class occupational norms as well as to challenge them. The case of artist/academic Professor Sheila Gaffney provides an example of someone who felt marginalised within 'high' art institutions, but was able to celebrate her class identity through her creative practice. She can be seen as one of Bourdieu's 'unusual' cases, coming from a working-class background and succeeding in her arts education and later in arts academia.

Gaffney (2017) writes about being an Irish, working-class, female sculptor. She explains the complexities of being subject to the class relations that are embodied in the cultural capital of the dominant classes whilst at the same time having the desire to create art herself:

> My own frame of respectability is the canon [works of art that are of indisputable quality] of British Sculpture. The saved scaffolds assemble and I hoard them to help me make strategy to intervene in territories, find form for expressing anger, assert my demand for recognition and the acceptance of a different voice within this canon.
>
> (Gaffney, 2017, para 20)

Gaffney expresses the contradictory position many working-class artist/ academics find themselves in. They recognise the artistic canon excludes them as its works are legitimised through institutions that support the interests of the dominant classes. Their work does not belong in the canon and yet at the same time some working-class artists yearn to be included – but on their own terms. Gaffney's sculptural practice responds to the resistance experienced when engaging with the world. Biesta (2017) described this encounter as leading to feelings of frustration. As Biesta (2017) noted, Gaffney has the option to withdraw from the art world, but instead she is motivated to push back and remain in dialogue with the canon. Through her will she demands her place as an artist, understanding that her inclusion will modify or even destroy the canon in its current form.

Furthermore, Gaffney is able to articulate how her classed sensibilities inform the making of her work. Her dispositions and cultural capital that are derived from her own habitus are embodied within her work.

> This self as subject is not some sort of uncontrollable oozing of expression through art materials. In my current works that I call *photoworks* [...] I employ my own strategy to ensure this does not occur, and begin making the sculpture using analytical drawing and measuring methods to interrogate a family photograph of myself as a child. The photograph provides me with a register of classed and gendered subjectivity, situation, place and an internalized knowledge, which I source as I use the data extracted from the image, to model in wax and distil the form of the child I remember being in that moment of time. This is how, bringing forward an analysis of my *self* within the sculpture, I use my own agency and lived experience alongside and within my material manipulations.
>
> (Gaffney, 2017, para 21)

Through her art practice, Gaffney is able to stand outside the institutions of academia and the art world to critically think about her marginalised position and internal knowledge about being a classed and gendered subject. However, the materiality and physicality of her practice as well as her sensibilities also spring from her classed and gendered subjectivity. Her sculpting wills the works and their meanings into being. Her will also confirms that Gaffney exists in the world. Gaffney also feels that her anger, desire and frustration draw her towards her practice and the wider art world. It is possible to see how cultural capital and habitus do reproduce social inequalities within the world; however, Biesta (2017, 2020) and Gaffney (2017) also demonstrate how the arts can give agency to working-class artists/academics. Where they find resistance to their desires to be artists they do not withdraw but remain in dialogue with the world through their creative practices.

My Encounter With Salisbury Cathedral

When I was four years old, about 50 years ago, there were two framed prints on the wall of my parents' 'front room' of works by John Constable (1776–1837), Salisbury Cathedral (1825) and Dedham Lock and Mill (1820). My mother later, when remembering them, confused the latter painting with *The Hay Wain* (1821). This was probably due to *The Hay Wain* being an iconic image of the idyllic English countryside (Pevsner, 1978). In addition to the Constables, there was also a print of a painting by Edwin Landseer (1803–1873) called *Suspense* (1834) depicting a dog waiting for its master and another print of *A Child's World* (commonly known as Bubbles) (1886) painting by Sir John Everett Millais (1829–1896). These images reflected the taste of an English lower working-class couple living in the late 1960s to the early 1970s. Interestingly my father (a manual and/or agricultural worker all his life) loved nature and did read the works of the Romantic poets such as George Gordon Byron (1788–1824). So even though my father left school well before he was 16 with no formal qualifications, he did have cultural assets (Goldthorpe, 2007).

When asking my mother (my father has since passed away) about how and why they chose these images on the wall, she told me,

> We collected coupons for them in the late 1960s– from buying tooth paste I think. When we had enough they sent them to us in the post. Then we got them framed. We both decided to do this because we liked them.

I have a vague recollection of the prints arriving and when my parents opened the package the prints were separated by tissue paper. Unfortunately, the pictures have long since been given to a charity shop so I am unable to find out anything more about the tooth paste company or the actual printers. Fig. 1 is a photograph from the family album, showing my mother holding my sister. A partial view of the Salisbury Cathedral print can be seen on the wall behind my mother's head.

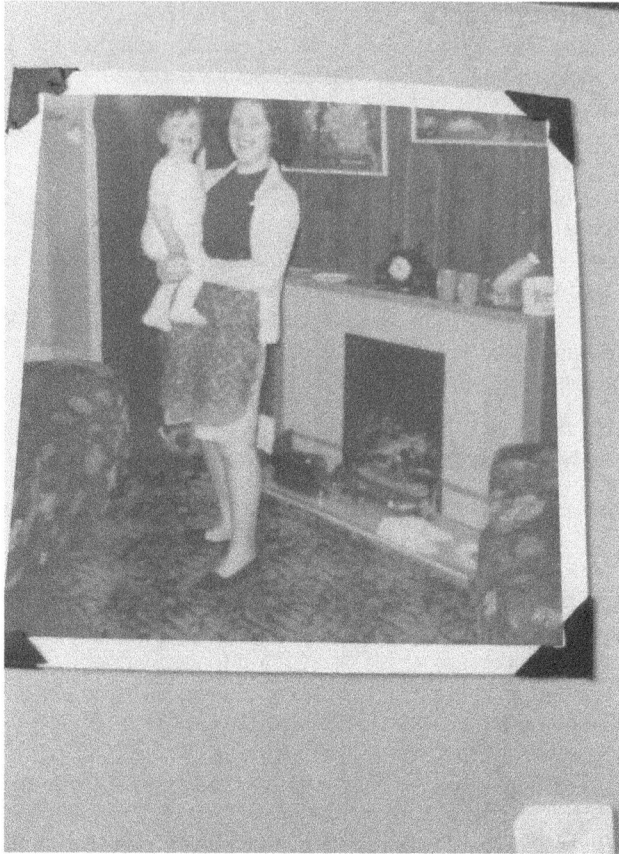

Fig. 1.   Photograph of Mother and Sister in the Front Room (1971).

We spent most time in the 'front room'. As a very young child, I would spend hours staring at these prints in awe. I have a very clear and powerful memory from when I was four, soaking up the details from Salisbury Cathedral with the intention of reproducing it at the 'play group' run in the neighbouring St. Andrew's Church (although my parents were not church goers). The architecture rendered with such detail, the trees that framed the spire, the clouds in the sky and the cows drinking from the small lake all fascinated me. There was a couple standing in the cathedral's grounds, a man was pointing something out to a woman in a bonnet and I used to wonder where they were going and what they were talking about. My father told me this was a painting (not a print) by Constable and he was an artist. Benjamin (2010) would argue that the uniqueness and authenticity of the art object in time and space is lost when it is reproduced. The fact that I was looking at a mechanical reproduction of the original painting was not relevant to me nor my father.

The idea that an artist was capable of re-creating the textures of bark and leaves on the trees, the reflections in the water and the intricate pale stone tracery was astounding to me. Barrell (1980, p. 22) writes of how Constable wanted the viewer to totally believe in his rendering of the Suffolk countryside, even though it was an idealisation. Constable met his aim for me as a four-year-old child viewer.

As we left the house that day to go to play group, I tried to keep Salisbury Cathedral in my memory, hoping that I too could reproduce it. I remember standing in front of the easel in the local church hall with the other kids running around and shouting while a helper tied an apron on me. The strange, sweet, smell of the coloured paint blocks was in my nostrils. The helper left me to my own devices. I was determined to paint like Constable. But unfortunately, I now remember the frustration and disappointment in my attempts in recreating the intricacies of the building that ended up as a chaotic grey splodge. Somehow the brush would not do as I wanted and my memory of the image was more elusive than I had anticipated. I wanted to try again but my allotted time at the easel was over and I had to move to the next activity. I believe this was the first significant incident that created my desire to be an artist even though there was no one in my family or in my local community who painted. Of course, there were many other critical incidents in my becoming an artist and later an academic. However, John Constable with help unknowingly from my parents was my first art teacher.

The power of Constable's image ignited in me a desire to create and to be an artist that stayed with me throughout my life. When I was a little older, maybe six or seven, my parents took me to visit my great aunt Sally, she asked me, 'What do you want to be when you grow up, a teacher?' I proudly replied, 'I want to be an artist'. I was very surprised to see the expression on her beaming face change to one of doubt and disapproval. I did not understand that response but it did not deter me from my goal. I wonder now if she did not think it would be a respectable occupation.

Much later I had more encounters with John Constable and Salisbury Cathedral. My art teacher, Miss Taylor, organised for her A-Level art group to go to Leeds Polytechnic to listen to a lecture on Constable. I also visited the Victoria and Albert Museum (V&A) on a school trip where I saw the original painting of Salisbury Cathedral. It was like seeing a familiar but much improved version of an old friend. I was struck by the larger size of the finished work and that it appeared to glow. The painted surface seemed so much richer and more tactile than the print version. The Constable's sketchbooks on show revealed more of his working processes and evidence that he was a successful professional painter.

Fig. 2 is of Christ Church, Staincliffe, an oil on paper that I painted from sketches I drew from the adjoining field in response to Miss Taylor's brief 'Fences and gateways'. It can be seen that I have borrowed some of the elements of Salisbury Cathedral; the architecture, the trees, a suggestion of cloud, the small figure in the mid-distance and a cat in the foreground instead of the cattle.

In the mid-1980s, when I was being interviewed with my portfolio for entry onto an arts degree, I became aware (perhaps too late) that not all forms of art

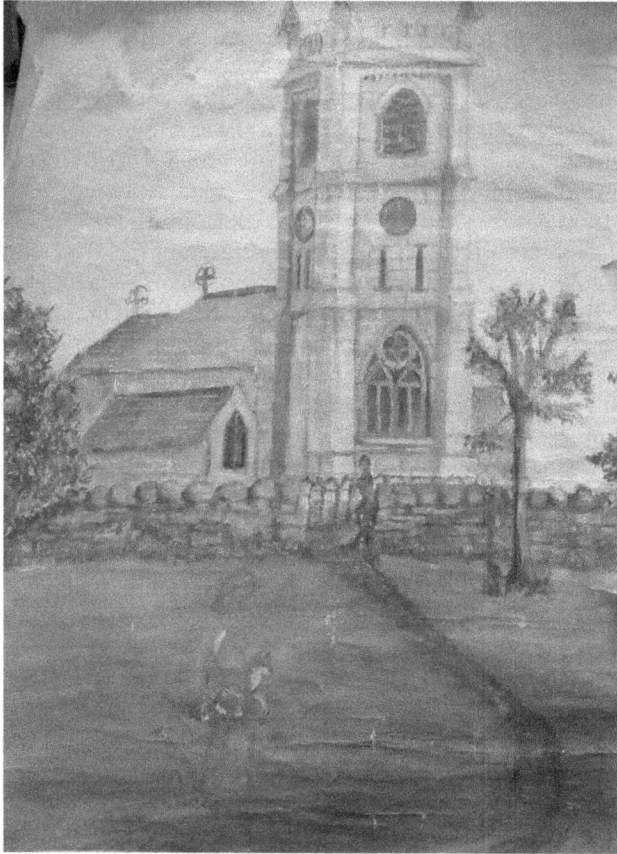

Fig. 2.   Painting of Christ Church Staincliffe by Samantha Broadhead
(1980).

were equally valued. John Constable maybe part of the canon of British art; however, his work was perceived as conservative, traditional and even 'chocolate box' by my interviewers (although I would challenge that now). The cultural objects that had currency in university art departments and art schools had their roots in Modernism. Salisbury Cathedral had become a beloved old relative who causes one embarrassment when introduced to new, sophisticated friends.

During my Pre-BA Foundation Course at Batley School of Art and my undergraduate degree in visual arts at Lancaster University, I did not reference Salisbury Cathedral. Instead, I became enamoured with the installations of Helen Chadwick (1953–1996) and Mary Kelly (1941) and the feminist writings of Rozsika Parker (1945–2010).

Who Was My Educator?

The images created by John Constable were seen as radical during the nineteenth century; his works were favoured by the French Impressionists (Crooker, 1965). Constable's paintings, large scale sketches and note books are housed in the V&A and other examples can be seen in many significant galleries. His work is part of the canon of English landscape painting along with that of Thomas Gainsborough (1727–1788) and J.M.W. Turner (1775–1851).

In the early 1970s, Constable's popularity and the subsequent printed reproduction of key paintings gave my family not only access to the images but also the means to embed them within the home (Benjamin, 2010). It must be remembered that we were not a wealthy family so for my parents to have these prints framed must indicate the extent to which they valued them.

My first encounter with Salisbury Cathedral was primarily visual and it allowed me, as Biesta (2017, 2020) describes, to be in dialogue with the world. I experienced the emotions of awe and then affection towards the image and connected it to my parent's knowledge. It was significant that my father told me that the print had been created by an artist. I thought about the image and had a desire to recreate it.

Of course, what we think about the world is not the world itself. So when I tried to paint Salisbury Cathedral, I experienced the frustration that Biesta (2017) noted we experience when we find resistance to our desires. Very early on I learned there is a discrepancy between the material world and the work of ideas. The connection I had with the brush, paint and paper on the easel led me to be in dialogue with the world in a very physical sense. Through my hands, I was trying to will something into being and I did not succeed. The frustration of not having the required skill could have led me to withdraw from art altogether, but instead it increased my ambition.

When thinking about the notion of cultural capital, it can be seen that my parents were not aware of contemporary art, or even the modern art from the early twentieth century. Their taste was not quite right for those in academia who legitimated cultural products and practices for the interests of the elites. But they did give me the cultural resources upon which I could build my own artistic journey. Gaffney (2017) talks about her 'scaffolds' that help her find expression and Salisbury Cathedral was, for me, a scaffold that led me to experience a sense of agency at four years old. This is why I recognise John Constable as my first art teacher.

As Biesta (2017) argues, it is not the actual painting that I tried to create that was important, but the role that action played in my becoming an artist; the significance is existential not aesthetic. There were other touchpoints in my relationship with Salisbury Cathedral throughout my childhood and teenage years that were facilitated by school through trips and lectures. The role my teacher, Miss Taylor, played was also significant as she encouraged me to paint and reinforced the knowledge I had started to discover for myself. I also recognise that neither my parents nor my school tried to dissuade me from being an artist. Miss Hirst and Miss Taylor actively encouraged me.

I have never considered myself nor my family as religious, so it is surprising to me that many references to churches appear in my story. The impact of institutions such as the Church of England, the family, the educational system and the art world have all had an influence on my becoming an artist/academic. But that influence is complex. They endorse the cultural capital of the dominant classes so that it has currency and exchange value. These institutions also regulate the normative behaviour of members from different social classes. But do they simply reproduce class power relations? It seems to me that they have at times enabled me to engage with learning and the arts, but at other times they have thwarted my progress.

My own case seems to illustrate Goldthorpe's (2007) argument that the model of cultural capital does not satisfactorily explain the successes of working-class people in arts education. My parents by exposing me to the work of John Constable gave me the cultural resources for becoming an artist/academic in spite of not having the economic, social and cultural capitals of the dominant classes.

The later realisation that John Constable was not considered a sophisticated source of inspiration evoked in me a different understanding of the art canon. It was not universal nor permanent but subject to changes in the tastes of the elites who managed it. Furthermore, the art canon was based on exclusion as practitioners from some social groups were not represented in it. My thoughts took a critical turn when, as an undergraduate, I became interested in feminist art theory and practice.

Some Conclusions

While reflecting on my own story, I wonder if Ofsted's focus on cultural capital needs to be carefully reconsidered. This is because it can assume a deficit in people who do not have the 'right kind' of cultural capital. It implies a notion that could undermine the work of educators, that working-class people and other under-represented groups are pre-destined not to succeed. A more innovative approach would be to look at the richness of the cultural assets and resources people do have. It is also easy to make assumptions about people's interests and desires based on their social background when their lives are much more complex and nuanced. Educators should get to know students as individuals so they can support their interests and aptitudes, some of which they may be surprised by.

Those young people from working-class backgrounds who have a desire to be creative should not be dissuaded from studying the arts. There are many possible careers in the cultural industries and what families need is good quality advice and guidance that is well informed about career trajectories in the arts.

My story also suggests that failure is not necessarily demotivating. In some cases, it can drive ambition. It is how 'failure' is managed by students, teachers and schools that is important. Resistance to one's desires is not really failure; it can promote critical thinking and lead to a more meaningful connection with the world.

References

Arum, R., Gamoran, A., & Shavit, Y. (2007). More inclusion than diversion: Expansion, differentiation, and market structure in higher education. In *Stratification in higher education—A comparative study* (pp. 1–35). Stanford, CA: Stanford University Press.

Baars, S., Mulcahy, E., & Bernardes, E. (2016). *The underrepresentation of white working class boys in higher education: The role of widening participation.* London: Kings College. Retrieved from https://www.cfey.org/wp-content/uploads/2016/07/The-underrepresentation-of-white-working-class-boys-in-higher-education-baars-et-al-2016.pdf. Accessed on November 23, 2021.

Barrell, J. (1980). *The dark side of the landscape: The rural poor in English painting, 1730–1840* (p. 22). Cambridge: Cambridge University Press.

Benjamin, W. (2010). The work of art in the age of its technological reproducibility [first version] (M. W. Jennings, Trans.). *Grey Room*, 39, 11–37. Retrieved from https://www.jstor.org/stable/pdf/27809424.pdf. Accessed on November 24, 2021.

Bernstein, B. (1958). Some sociological determinants of perception: an enquiry into sub-cultural differences. *The British Journal of Sociology*, 9(2), 159–174.

Bernstein, B. (1961). Social class and linguistic development: A theory of social learning. *Education, Economy and Society*, 288, 314.

Bernstein, B. (1965). A socio-linguistic approach to social learning. In J. Gould (Ed.), *Penguin survey of the social sciences* (pp. 144–168). Harmondsworth: Penguin.

Bernstein, B. (1975). Class and pedagogies: Visible and invisible. In A. Halsey, H. Lauder, P. Brown, & A. Stuart Wells (Eds.), *Education: Culture, economy, society* (pp. 59–79). Oxford: Oxford University Press.

Biesta, G. (2015). Wereld-gericht onderwijs: Vorming tot volwassenheid. *De Nieuwe Meso*, 2(3), 54–61.

Biesta, G. (2017). What if? Art education beyond expression and creativity. In C. Naughton, G. Biesta, & D. R. Cole (Eds.), *Art, artists and pedagogy: Philosophy and the arts in education* (pp. 11–20). Oxon: Routledge.

Biesta, G. (2020). *Letting art teach: Art education 'after' Joseph Beuys* (2nd ed.). Arnhem: The Netherlands.

Biesta, G. (2021). *World-centred education: A view for the present.* Oxon: Routledge.

Bourdieu, P. (1973). Cultural reproduction and social reproduction. In R. K. Brown (Ed.), *Knowledge, education and cultural change* (p. 178). London: Tavistock.

Bourdieu, P. (1986). The forms of capital. In I. Szeman & T. Kaposy (Eds.), *Cultural theory: An anthology* (pp. 81–93). Chichester: Wiley-Blackwell.

Bourdieu, P. (1990). *The logic of practice.* Stanford, CA: Stanford University Press.

Bourdieu, P., & Passeron, J.-C. (1977). *Reproduction in education, society and culture.* London: Sage.

Bourdieu, P., & Passeron, J.-C. (1979). *The inheritors: French students and their relation to culture.* Chicago, IL: Chicago University Press.

Broadhead, S., & Gregson, M. (2018). *Practical wisdom and democratic education: Phronesis, art and non-traditional students.* Cham: Springer.

Cassen, R., & Kingdon, G. (2007). *Tackling low educational achievement.* York: Joseph Rowntree Foundation.

Crooker, M. J. A. (1965). *The influence of French impressionism on Canadian painting (T)*. University of British Columbia. Retrieved from https://open.library.ubc.ca/collections/ubctheses/831/items/1.0104772. Accessed on November 23, 2021.

Equality Act. (2010). The Stationery Office Limited, London. Retrieved from https://www.legislation.gov.uk/ukpga/2010/15/introduction. Accessed on November 23, 2021.

Gaffney, S. (2017). The sickness of being disallowed: Premonition and insight in the "artist's sketchbook". *OAR: The Oxford Artistic and Practice Based Research Platform*. Retrieved from http://www.oarplatform.com/sickness-disallowed-premonition-insight-artists-sketchbook/

Goldthorpe, J. H. (2007). "Cultural capital": Some critical observations. *Sociologica, 1*(2), 1–22.

Goodman, A., & Gregg, P. (Eds.). (2010). *Poorer children's educational attainment: How important are attitudes and behaviour?* (pp. 76–92). York: Joseph Rowntree Foundation.

Halsey, A. H., Halsey, A. H., Albert Henry, H., Heath, A. F., & Ridge, J. M. (1980). *Origins and destinations: Family, class, and education in modern Britain*. Oxford: Clarendon Press.

Harrison, N., & McCaig, C. (2015). An ecological fallacy in higher education policy: The use, overuse and misuse of 'low participation neighbourhoods'. *Journal of Further and Higher Education, 39*(6), 793–817.

Jackson, B., & Marsden, D. (1963). *Education and the working class*. London: Routledge.

Mongon, D., & Chapman, C. (2008). *Successful leadership for promoting the achievement of white working class pupils*. University of Manchester/NUT and NCSL.

Naughton, C., & Cole, D. R. (2017). Philosophy and pedagogy in arts education. In C. Naughton, G. Biesta, & D. R. Cole (Eds.), *Art, artists and pedagogy: Philosophy and the arts in education* (pp. 1–10). Oxon: Routledge.

Nightingale, P. (2020). 'As if by osmosis': How Ofsted's new deficit model emerged, fully formed, as cultural capital. *Power and Education, 12*(3), 232–245.

Noble, S., McLennan, D., Noble, M., Plunkett, E., Gutacker, N., Silk, M., & Wright, G. (2019). Ministry of housing, communities and local government. In *The English indices of deprivation*. Retrieved from English Indices of Deprivation 2019: research report (publishing.service.gov.uk). Accessed on July 01, 2022.

O'Shea, S. (2014). Transitions and turning points: Exploring how first-in-family female students story their transition to university and student identity formation. *International Journal of Qualitative Studies in Education, 27*(2), 135–158.

Penney, E., & Lovejoy, L. (2017). Navigating academia in the 'welfare-class'. *Journal of Working-Class Studies, 2*(2), 54–65.

Pevsner, N. (1978). *The Englishness of English art*. Harmondsworth: Penguin Books.

Reay, D. (2002). Class, authenticity and the transition to higher education for mature students. *The Sociological Review, 50*(3), 398–418. doi:10.1111/1467-954X.00389

Reay, D., Crozier, G., & Clayton, J. (2010). 'Fitting in' or 'standing out': Working-class students in UK higher education. *British Educational Research Journal, 36*(1), 107–124.

Reay, D., Davis, J., David, M., & Ball, S. (2001). Choices of degree or degrees of choice? Class, 'race' and the higher education choice process. *Sociology, 35*(4), 855–874.

Schofer, E., & Meyer, J. W. (2005). The worldwide expansion of higher education in the twentieth century. *American Sociological Review, 70*(6), 898–920.

Sharples, J., Slavin, R., Chambers, B., & Sharp, C. (2011). *Effective classroom strategies for closing the gap in educational achievement for children and young people living in poverty, including white working-class boys.* London: C4EO.

Skeggs, B. (1997). *Formations of class and gender: Becoming respectable.* London: Sage.

Thompson, E. (1978). *Poverty of theory.* New York, NY: Monthly Review Press.

Unwin, L. (2009). *Sensuality, sustainability and social justice: Vocational education in changing times.* London: Institute of Education; University of London.

Yosso, T. J. (2005). Whose culture has capital? A critical race theory discussion of community cultural wealth. *Race, Ethnicity and Education, 8*(1), 69–91.

Wilson, N. (2016). *Home in british working-class fiction.* Oxon: Routledge.

Chapter 11

Class Is a Verb: Lived Encounters of a Minority Ethnic Academic Who Self-Identifies With Aspects of Working-Class Cultures in the United Kingdom

Stephen Wong

Abstract

This chapter makes the assertion that social class is a verb, which is to say, an individual's class identifications are not fixed and ascribed at birth but must be understood as something that is practised and lived. In an era in which hyper mobility is the norm among a growing segment of the global population, social class identifications are increasingly fluid, context-dependent and could only be understood in relation to 'other' social class categories. By taking a discourse analytic approach to closely look at the episodes of my interactions with a range of interlocutors in my biographical trajectory across multiple contexts, this chapter provides accounts of the complexities of my class identifications as an academic in the UK higher education (HE) sector. Following Marxist scholarship in general, this linguistic autoethnography shows how class is not depicted as an attribute of people that is stationary in contemporary stratified societies. It argues that class must be understood as a social relation, as evolving in the social interactions with human subjects and the cumulative relationships that people engaged with, all arising out of the economic order in societies. Second, the interactional episodes highlighted in this chapter also shows how social class is interconnected with other identity inscriptions, such as gender, ethnicity, race and nationality. As such, this chapter shows how the nature of social class identifications in contemporary times are impacted by an individual's alignments with a range of social categories.

The Lives of Working Class Academics, 155–171
Copyright © 2023 Stephen Wong
Published under exclusive licence by Emerald Publishing Limited
doi:10.1108/978-1-80117-057-420221011

Keywords: Class cultures; identities; institutional habitus; social interactions; linguistic autoethnography; discourse analysis

The utterance 'I'm a working-class Chinese man from a small seaside town in Malaysia' is my habitual response to questions about my identity as a foreign national who occupy positions as an academic in higher education (HE) institutions in London. This chapter offers the reader some examples and discourse analyses of the contexts in which I deploy the utterance. To understand the problem of class identifications, the speech events in this chapter show why it is crucial to critically analyse human subjects' experiences of self-identifications of class, ethnic and national categories during their encounters with the 'others' in their biographical trajectories. In contemporary times, hyper mobility is the norm among a growing segment of the global population, and this has impacted on traditional understandings (e.g. the notion of one country, one homogenous group of people who share one language and one culture) of identity categories. Due in part to the effects of globalisation and post–Cold War movement of people, contact between languages and cultures has intensified. As a result, the certainty with regard to questions like 'Who is the other?' and 'Who am I?' are increasingly difficult to answer. What I'm trying to articulate here is that the diversification of diversity is commonplace, leading the anthropologist Steven Vertovec to coin the term 'superdiversity'. Superdiversity is a term which signifies relatively recent dimensions of social, cultural and linguistic diversity evolving from post–Cold War migratory and mobility patterns (Vertovec, 2007). In this context, the notion of social class, ethnic and national identifications is multi-faceted and is indexicalised by class ascriptions specific to place. As I have also shown elsewhere (Wong, 2018), a putatively homogenous group of people align and disalign with a range of ethnic, linguistic, religious and cultural identities as a resultant effect of the itineraries travelled in their biographical trajectories. Taking the notion of superdiversity and my own personal biographical trajectory as the starting point, I provide a critical reflection of the ways in which the intersection of my place of origin, ethnic background and travel itineraries contours my fluctuating self-identifications and ascribed social class categorisations as an ethnic minority academic in the United Kingdom. In the following passages, I will also show how personal lived experiences are permeated with political/cultural norms and expectations, and that an in-depth self-reflection is crucial to firstly, identify and secondly, to question the intersections between the self and social life. My self-reflections in this chapter reveal my experiences of 'figuring out what to do, how to live, and the meaning of [my] struggles' (Bochner & Ellis, 2006, p. 111). In a sense, this chapter also demonstrates *why* the notion of social classes isn't only a matter of history, a relationship with tradition, a discourse of one's roots and routes travelled but that it emerges from practices. In other words, instead of a reductive understanding in which social class as something that is fixed and ascribed at birth, I demonstrate how the interplay of my habitus and ownership of different forms of capital (Bourdieu, 1984) shapes my fluctuating self- and ascribed identifications with different aspects of social class categorisations. In this chapter, the ways in which I identify with social classes (especially working class) during my social interactions show how the notion of class is often vague and emergent. In this sense, class identities are never stationary but should be understood as something that is processual, reproductive and dynamic, inevitably situational but always relational. As Skeggs points out, working-class people are conscious of how they are perceived and assessed by 'middle-class institutions and authority' and, 'are fully aware of how cultural distinction and classification work in the interests of the powerful – legitimating inequalities so that privilege cannot be contested' (Skeggs, 2012, p. 283). For me, lived class culture is prosaic and is embodied by *how* the possession of one's available forms of capital indexicalise their social class categorisations.

At this juncture, it might be useful to, firstly, interrogate the definition of social class in advance of a critical analyses of my lived class experiences. The encyclopaedia Britannica defines social class as '...a group of people within a society who possess the same socioeconomic status... the concept of class as a collection of individuals sharing similar economic circumstances has been widely used in [Government] censuses and in studies of social mobility' (Encyclopaedia Britannica, 2019). In this definition, class is understood as the amount of material or economic assets that are in possession by individuals. Individuals who own similar amounts of capitals are then categorised into particular social classes. While this definition is used in government censuses, it is simplistic, deterministic and isn't nuanced enough to capture the complexity of social class identifications. For a more sophisticated understanding of class, I would have to rely on general Marxist scholarship. However, as noted by Gray and Block (2014), while Karl Marx's ruminations often inform conversations about class, he did not offer a concise definition of class. To get a better grip on the intricacies of class, scholars aligned with the Marxist school of thought, for example, Vladimir Lenin who in his reworking of Marxism to Russian everyday life in the early twentieth century offered a clearer definition:

> Classes are large groups of people which differ from each other by the place they occupy in a historically determined system of social production, by their relation (in most cases fixed and formulated in law) to the means of production, by their role in the social organization of labour and, consequently, by the dimensions and method of acquiring the share of social wealth of which they dispose. Classes are groups of people one of which can appropriate the labour of another owing to the different places they occupy in a definitive system of social economy.
>
> (Lenin, 1947/1919, p. 492)

What is salient in the above definition, and in Marxist scholarship generally, is the fact that social class is not depicted as a characteristic redolent of certain groupings of people nor as a stationary position in stratified societies, but instead, as a relational notion that emerge in the social spheres in which individuals rub along with others and the cumulative relations that people build on, which emerges out of the economic order in societies.

Like Marx, Max Weber meditated about economic orders in industrialised societies and the ways in which class and class position are relational. That said, Weber's thinking about the meaning of economic order diverged from Marx's articulations. In Marx's view, economic order was articulated in terms of the connections between capital and labour, and to him, this connection led to the abuse of labour by those possessing capital. Weber, however, saw the economic order as a market. In this market, stratification and inequality emerge resulting from the barter of resources by people with inequitable access to and ownership of these resources. As such, in Weber's perspective, '[c]lass situation' and 'class' refer only to the same (or similar) interests which an individual shares with others', takes into account 'the various controls over consumer goods, means of production, assets, resources and skills which constitute a particular class situation' (Weber, 1968, p. 302). In this light, Weber's thinking about class did not only focus on production but also includes economic exchange arising after production, for example, consumption.

In thinking about how the notion of social class had manifested in affluent Western societies, Pierre Bourdieu's importantly notes how:

> .... class or class fraction is defined not only by its position in the relations of production, as identified through indices such as occupation, income, or even educational level, but also by a certain sex-ratio, a certain distribution in geographical space (which is never socially neutral) and by a whole set of subsidiary characteristics which may function, in the form of tacit requirements, as real principles of selection or exclusion without ever being formally stated (this is the case with ethnic origin and sex). A number of official criteria: for example, the requiring of a given diploma can be a way of demanding a particular social origin.
>
> (Bourdieu, 1984, p. 102)

What Bourdieu articulates is the fact that there are capitals beyond economic capital. Importantly, Bourdieu (1984) proposed that cultural capital, which he views as the ownership of recognised knowledge, could be creatively exchanged or used to create other capital categories such as 'educational capital', 'linguistic capital', 'artistic capital' and so on. Conversely, Bourdieu shows how social capital, viewed as the deployment of cultural (and economic) capital, is utilised in the form of power derived from certain social relations which enables some individuals to achieve success in their life trajectories. In Bourdieu's (1984, p. 114) view, these capitals are measurable and should be realised 'as the set of actually useable resources and powers' that individuals in possession of these capitals could draw upon. Crucially, one could see how these capitals or resources are inequitably distributed across individuals who take part in practices across a variety of fields. These are domains of social practices that are shaped by certain perspectives and patterns of consumption, for instance, type and level of education, preference for opera or hip hop, football or rugby. In this light, class is depicted as a social relation which emerges in the everyday practices of individuals. These routine, everyday practices, then become embodied in the human subject to form a class *habitus*. It is also important to note that the set of internalised dispositions is not in a state of stasis but instead, it constantly evolves as a result of partaking in situated social practices that are contoured by institutions and global economic forces.

Finally, I also want to bring the reader's attention to the sociolinguist David Block's (2012a, 2012b, 2013) very useful list of key dimensions associated with class as an identity inscription which I will draw upon in the analysis of my narratives and encounters in which class plays a part.

In Table 1, Block (2012b) persuasively shows how markers or dimensions of class as he calls them, delineate an individual's social class categorisation. Instead of preformed categories that focus on economic circumstances, Block includes a range of dimensions that one must account for in any analysis of class. Informed by preceding definitions and thinking about social classes, the following passages offer evidence to support my overarching argument about class is a verb. Next, I offer a short discussion about the salience and nature of autoethnographies, followed by a narrative of my roots, routes taken and some examples of interactions in which I self-identified, was ascribed and denied entry into certain social class categories and experiences of being mis-read by my interlocutors.

Table 1. Key Dimensions of Class (Block, 2012b, p. 194).

Dimension	Gloss
Property	This refers to one's material possessions, such as land, housing, electronic goods, clothing, books, art etc.
Wealth	This refers to disposable income/money and patrimony (e.g. what owned property is worth in financial terms).
Occupation	This refers to the kind of work done across a range of job types, such as blue-collar manual labour vs. white-collar knowledge-based labour, or service sector jobs vs. manual jobs etc.
Place of residence	This can refer either to the type of neighbourhood one lives in (is it identified as poor, working class, middle class, an area in the process of gentrification, or upper class?) or the type of dwelling (individual house, flat, caravan etc.).
Education	This refers to the level of schooling attained and the acquired cultural capital one has at any point in time. There is close link here to Bourdieu's notion of cultural capital.
Social networking	This refers to the often unspoken reality whereby middle-class people tend to socialise with middle-class

Table 1. *(Continued)*

Dimension	Gloss
	people, working-class people with working-class people and so on. There is a close link here to Bourdieu's notion of social capital.
Consumption patterns	This might refer to behaviour patterns like buying food at a supermarket that positions itself as 'cost-cutting' vs. buying food at one that sells 'healthy', organic and expensive products. Or it might refer to buying particular goods (e.g. food, clothing, gadgets) in terms of type and brand.
Symbolic behaviour	This includes how one moves one's body, the clothes one wear, the way one speaks, how one eats, the kinds of pastimes one engages in etc.
Spatial relations	This refers to living conditions such as physical mobility (does the person frequently travel abroad?) or the spatial conditions in which one lives (size of bedroom, size of dwelling, proximity to other people during a range of day-to-day activities).

The Question of Autoethnography as a Scientific Method of Analysis

First, a preamble about the salience and nature of autoethnographies. The value of autoethnographies has gained some traction in the past few of decades and the eminent anthropologist James Clifford (1997) wrote in *Routes: Travel and Translation in the Late Twentieth Century*:

> A certain degree of autobiography is now widely accepted as relevant to self-critical projects of cultural analysis… Writing an ethnography of one's subjective space as a kind of complex community, a site of shifting locations, could be defended as a valid contribution to anthropological work (p. 88).

Following Clifford's proposition, I will be 'self-critical' of the vignettes and lived experiences of subjective spaces and shifting locations that I share with the reader. The kind of deep, self-reflective analysis would be categorised as autoethnography (Ellis & Bochner, 2000). In this vein, autoethnographies are very much individualised, divulging texts in which researchers share 'their own lived experiences, relating the personal to the cultural' (Richardson, 2000, p. 931). Further, according to Ellis and Bochner (2000, p. 739):

> ... auto-ethnographers gaze, first through an ethnographic wide-angle lens, focusing outward on social and cultural aspects of the personal experience; then they look inward, exposing a vulnerable self that is moved by and may move through, refract and resist cultural interpretations.

Informed by the critical elements of autoethnography, the subsequent sub-sections offer accounts of my narratives of roots and routes travelled as I encounter, refract and resist the discourses of class, ethnicity and cultural interpretations.

The Discourse of Roots

To kick off this section, I offer a narrative of why I don't 'feel' middle class even though I am currently employed as an academic in the United Kingdom. I attained my PhD in the field of language, discourse and communication from a Russell Group institution when I was in my late 40s. Soon after, I managed to occupy the paradigmatically bourgeoisie positions as senior lecturer of Education Studies at a post-1992 institution and as lecturer of Applied Linguistics at a Russell Group university. By securing this occupation, I felt that all my hard graft regarding my education has paid off and the fruit of my labour is the prestigious career of an academic I sought after. At this juncture, the reader might challenge my disalignment with certain aspects of the middle classes. While I'm paid a middle-class salary to perform middle-class things, I don't fully think of myself as a middle-class person. Although I possess a slice of social capital due to my membership of a network of colleagues who confidently 'feel' middle-class, I simply do not think of myself as an entirely middle-class person because I do not consume 'high culture' such as the opera and classical music and I do not know how to make distinctions between art produced in the renaissance vs neo-classicism periods. I do not practice the symbolic behaviour that is closely con-nected with dimensions of the middle classes. I was educated in a state school in a postcolonial context, and importantly, I do not speak with an English public-school accent. I listen to jazz and hip hop, I read beat poetry and so on. My educational background and tastes in music and literature are crucial points to stress because as I've alluded in the above, class isn't only an objective entity but instead, is constituted by a question of identifications, practices, perceptions and feelings as Bourdieu argues, '[t]aste classifies, and it classifies the classifier' (Bourdieu, 1984, p. 6). That said, I'll be deluding myself if I claim to be an uncomplicated card-carrying member of the working classes, even if I'm tempted to do so at times, if only to enjoy the reactions that it can trigger among my mostly middle-class colleagues. Beverly Skeggs lacerating remark, 'Who would want to be seen as working-class? (Perhaps only academics are left)' (Skeggs, 1997, p. 95) warns against pretensions of being the underprivileged. There is also the warning by Bestwick (2020) about granting free access to people to self-identify as working class:

...risks collapsing vastly different economic and cultural experiences into a homogenous melting pot of 'working-class' narratives, where already privileged voices are privileged again, producing further barriers to access for the less privileged among the extended community of working-class people.

(Bestwick, 2020, p. 266)

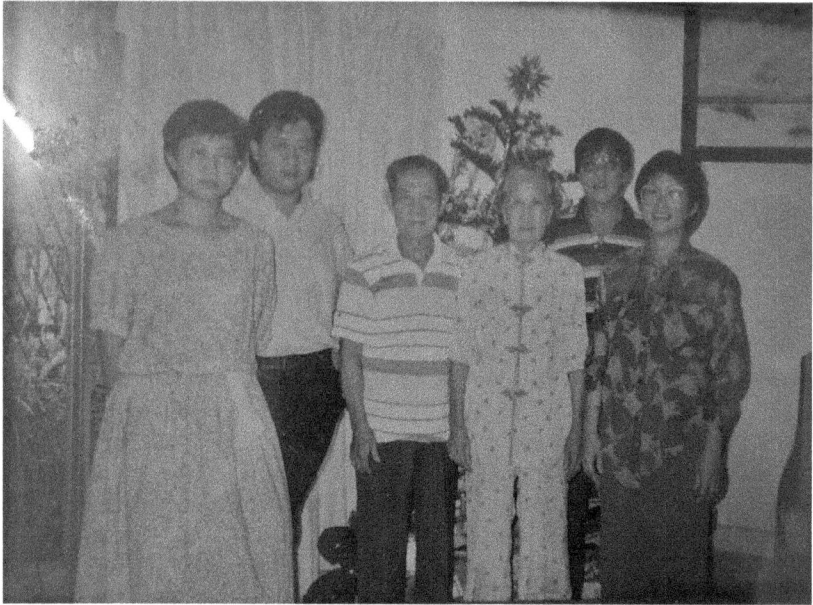

Christmas in 1985 – The Author With His Sister, Grandparents, Father and Mother in Malaysia

However, to disregard a person's self-identification also risks ignoring important aspects of working-class disadvantage, for example, the 'affective' or feeling that might resonate among individuals despite the affordances of upward class mobility (Skeggs, 2012). As such, this chapter shows why I do not feel a strong sense of belonging in the British middle classes despite my access to a variety of capitals that Bourdieu points out as markers of class.

Let me start by offering the reader a narrative of my roots as a way to explain why I don't feel middle class in the British context. I grew up in Malaysia as a third generation Malaysian of Chinese heritage, where I lived for about 25 years of my life. In the Malaysian context, my upbringing isn't redolent of the working classes as I was brought up in a relatively privileged home environment in a small town on the east coast of Malaysia. The privileges that my sister and I enjoyed are the result of the hard graft by my grandparents' and parents' generations. My paternal and maternal grandparents migrated to Malaysia during the 1930s to escape the communist revolution in China. As first-generation immigrants from the Guangdong province in China, my grandparents worked hard to make ends meet during the British colonial rule and then during the Japanese occupation of Malaysia during the Second World War. My memories of my paternal grandmother are filled with images of her chain-smoking Benson and Hedges cigarettes and drinking copious amounts of strong black coffee while she reminisced about her life as a child of a rich landowner in China before the Communists seized her father's assets. As a child, she lived a privileged life; she attended private schools and smoked opium in her early teens – with the approval of her parents as it was a typical cultural practice among the elite in her community. At the advent of the communist revolution, a matchmaker approached her father and promised to marry her off to a rich merchant in Malaysia. Hoping for a better future for her daughter, my great grandfather bought into the matchmaker's offer and agreed to send my grandmother to Malaysia. However, when she arrived in Malaysia with gold bars and necklaces hidden in her orifices and sewn in her clothes, she discovered that my grandfather wasn't a rich merchant but instead, worked as a porter in a soy sauce factory. With expectations of a life of luxury dashed, she worked as a labourer in a rice farm for six cents a day. She also recalled harrowing tales about how she had to hide my aunts from being sexually assaulted by Japanese soldiers during their occupation of Malaysia during Second World War. Now, as can be seen from the narrative, the first instance of downward class mobility resulting from her travel itinerary was experienced by my grandmother; she has been downgraded from being a member of the bourgeoisie in southern China to a day labourer in a rice farm in Malaysia. The social and cultural capital she enjoyed such as smoking opium and attending private schooling that indexicalise her as a member of the elite in China have lost its currency at the point of her arrival.

My father was a second generation Malaysian Chinese, and as the eldest son of a family of eight children, he was not able to complete his primary education in the 1950s because he had to work since he was 10 years old to help feed his siblings. Apart from flipping through the pages of newspapers, I've never seen him read a book. Initially, he worked as a shopkeeper's assistant and then as a car salesman. My father's siblings were also firmly entrenched in working-class professions, one of them was a construction worker, salesman, housecleaner, seamstress and one of my aunts worked as a clerk in an office. My father worked hard; he was a frugal and enterprising person who saved up enough money to become a moderately successful businessman who part owned a lucrative paint distributorship business and an upscale Chinese restaurant. My mother is an intelligent person who achieved excellent results in her O levels examinations and was offered a place in a Malaysian university but because she fell in love with my father who proposed marriage, she decided to train as a secondary schoolteacher instead. After graduating, she taught English at a state school until retirement. While my parents' occupations would be classified as middle-class professions, they demonstrated working-class ethics of being frugal and that the only way to achieve success is to work hard. These ethics were instilled in my sister and me from an early age. Crucially, my mother also transmitted the importance of educational and linguistic capital to us by ensuring that we acquired English and encouraging us to become voracious readers from an early age. On most weekends, my mother took us to the local library to borrow and read books by Enid Blyton and classic children literature such as *The Wizard of Oz* and *The Chronicles of Narnia*. While my father might not possess educational and linguistic capitals, he took us to upscale restaurants for Sunday dinners, which is an uncommon experience among my peers at the state school I attended. As such, the consumption patterns which we experienced would firmly entrench us as members of the middle classes in the Malaysian context. We also enjoyed annual holidays in Singapore during the 1970s in which we stayed in nice hotels and shopped at glitzy malls. These lived experiences relate to spatial, wealth, property and social dimensions of a particular class as pointed out by Block (2012b). Further, my mother's encouragement for us to read, be proficient in English and the provision of material resources by my father would firmly entrench my practices and identity as a member of the middle classes in the Malaysian context. In a sense, my habitus is constituted by social and cultural capital that has a strong emphasis on the importance of education, the consumption of English literature and the belief that hard work always pays off. As the above suggests, my lifestyle and material affordances provided by my family cements me as belonging to the middle classes in Malaysia, and in this context, I *feel* middle class in relation to many of my peers in school. Having given the reader a sketch of my roots, I now turn to how my self-identification with class shifts during my encounters and lived culture resulting from my engagement in a range of social spheres in the itineraries of my biographical trajectory.

The Significance of Routes in the Formation of Classed Self-Identifications

After I completed my GCSE 'O' levels, I obtained a scholarship to study Economics at a Midwestern university in America. It was here that I realised that the economic, social and cultural capital that indexicalise me as a middle-class person in Malaysia had lost its value. Let me expand on what I mean here. While I consider myself to be a proficient speaker of English, my Malaysian or 'non-native' English accent does not have the same currency or prestige in America, specifically in Kansas. My Malaysian accent gives the impression that I speak 'bad' English. Further, the auditory and visual markers of difference from the mostly white American students created the assumption that I'm not proficient in English and probably, by extension, lack intelligence. Oftentimes, my American classmates spoke unnaturally slow to me, perhaps they assumed that by doing so, I would understand the message that they were trying to convey. It was also here that I realised that the economic and cultural capital that I possess does not equate with dimensions of middle class that were valued by the students at the university. Here, middle-class students typically belong to the social network of fraternity or sorority organisations, dimensions of property and wealth are marked by the ownership of nice cars and the dimension of spatial relations are the practice of holidays in which the students ski at Colorado or to visit Daytona during spring break holidays. These dimensions of class were not available to me, I had to work hard as a chef for the campus cafeteria and during the summers, I worked in a floppy disk factory in Cape Cod, Massachusetts to earn money for my living expenses. My inability to enter the social realms of fraternity organisations and lack of economic capital to indulge in practices of middle-class American students prevents me from self-identifying as a middle-class student in this context.

Upon the completion of my undergraduate studies, I worked as a stockbroker for a major investment company in Wall Street, New York, for about 5 years. My relative success in securing employment with an influential global firm allowed my partial access into the network and social realms of some of the richest people in America. What I meant by 'partial' is also due to the fact that I did not attend an Ivy League institution in which most of the members of my social network graduated from. Added to this marker of difference is my ethnicity and nationality, because most of the people in my network are white Americans who have lived cultures that are different from mine. To give an example of what I meant by partial access, while I habitually partook in the ritual of after-work dinner and drinks with my colleagues, I was never invited to weekends at their holiday homes at the Hamptons – an area which privileged Americans own their holiday homes. The firm did not select me to provide service to the wealthiest clients of the firm. As such, social categories such as class must also be understood in relation to ethnicity and race. While I performed as well as, if not better than, some of my colleagues, preferential treatment was reserved for the white and privileged colleagues who obtained degrees from Ivy League institutions. In this light, while I possess the symbolic markers of middle-class America such as my occupation, income and self-presentation as regards to body language, clothing and living in an upmarket location, the effects of my race, schooling and upbringing has affected my membership into certain middle-class social spheres. In this light, membership into the elite middle classes in America is impacted by national and ethnic categorisations that create social inequity.

To continue the narrative of my route, the next destination on my itinerary was my return to Malaysia. In the early 1990s, my father was going through a series of health issues and following the advice of my mother, I returned home. In Malaysia, I had to help wind down my father's businesses before he passed away. After a period of mourning, I secured a position as a stockbroker on the Kuala Lumpur Stock Exchange. Here, I mostly continued where I left off in New York as the nature of the occupation is somewhat similar but in a different context. In Kuala Lumpur, I felt more middle class than in America while I definitely do not belong to the aristocratic classes, my status as someone with a US university degree together with experience in working at Wall Street was very well-received by my well-heeled managers, colleagues and clients. Some of my clients were CEOs of multinational corporations and government ministers. I entertained these high-flyers at fine restaurants as I was given an enormous expense account to use up every month. Further, in the Malaysian context, the consumption of high culture was not a significant marker of the privileged classes as the possession of economic capital trumps cultural capital in the assessment of social class cate-gorisations. During this time, I certainly enjoyed the trappings of wealth, I was able to buy a large house in a desirable location, I drove an expensive car and I received preferential treatment at most upscale restaurants – all key dimensions of middle-class practices in Malaysia. However, the terror attack in New York on 11 September 2001 triggered a global stock market crash which had a severe impact on my personal finances. Almost overnight, I lost all the material wealth that I accumulated because I had to sell my house, my flashy car and most of my assets to pay off the debts to the stock brokerage firm that was incurred by myself and my clients. The event had a severe impact on my life and made me reflect upon my career as a stockbroker and to think about the things that matter to me as a human subject.

After I came to terms with my financial losses, I decided that the world of high finance was not the route for me to take. Not knowing what to do, I decided to visit a female friend who was settled in London as a practising chartered accountant. After spending some time with her in the city, we fell in love, and I decided to settle down here. As I have decided not to return to the corporate world, I had to contemplate the next move in my career. The question of 'what to do?' took a while to answer because while I have a university degree, it was narrowly focused on economics and finance. Initially, I thought about opening a Chinese takeaway outlet because I had received many compliments about my cooking skills, but after researching the nature of the business and the start-up costs in London, I decided not to risk the remaining economic capital that I possess. While reading the Metro newspaper for job vacancies one day, I saw an advertisement for a Certificate in English Language Teaching to Adults (CELTA) course in a North London college. As I considered myself to be a proficient speaker of English, I thought this accreditation might provide an avenue for me to be gainfully employed as an English teacher in London. I enrolled in the full-time one-month course at the college, and it was probably one of the most difficult educational experiences I had encountered because I had never been taught or learned about teaching skills before. At the college, I noticed the apprehensive looks that the instructors and fellow classmates gave me, probably as a resultant effect of the combination of my ethnicity and accent that marks me as a non-native English speaker. In this social sphere, I was positioned as an outsider, and I also noticed that the instructors and my classmates initially spoke in a simplified English register with me during our conversations. I had to demonstrate that I possess the required linguistic capital to gain access or to be considered as a member of this community of practice. Due to all my perseverance and hard work, I managed to achieve a merit result at the conclusion of the course. Feeling proud of my achievement, I began to apply for jobs that are advertised by colleges that offer English as a second language (ESOL) courses in London. I probably applied for more than 50 positions in various colleges and was offered two interviews in which I was unsuccessful. One of the interviewers told me that the applicant they chose was more qualified than me. Feeling distraught, I saw an advertisement for a Master of Arts in English Language Teaching qualification at a post-1992 institution in East London. Thinking that this might be the route for me to take to teach in the ESOL sector, I made an appointment with the pro-gramme leader to discuss aspects of the postgraduate degree. During our con-versation, he asked me about my interest in the programme and I relayed what transpired during my job interview. He smiled and said my lack of success was probably because I'm not a native English speaker. His words made me realise that while I have the required qualifications, my accent and ethnic background negatively impacted my success with my job search. However, he strongly encouraged me to enrol in the programme because he believed that I would gain from the experience and be more equipped to secure gainful employment as an ESOL teacher. Over the period of my studies, he became my mentor and friend. He had immense belief in my modest academic skills and frequently encouraged me to continue to enrol in a PhD degree before I had even completed the MA degree. By taking his advice to read a range of journal articles and books during the MA programme, I became fascinated with key topics within the fields of sociolinguistics, cultural studies and sociology. The important insights emerging from the intersection of the fields compelled me to make the decision to apply for a candidacy of PhD. That was an exciting period, as my successful application to be supervised by one of the most highly regarded international scholars in the field of interactional sociolinguistics at a Russell Group institution in London brought me great joy. After years of hard graft, I passed the viva examination with glowing comments by the examiners. With this qualification added to my cultural capital, I managed to secure a fractional fixed-term lectureship at a world-leading

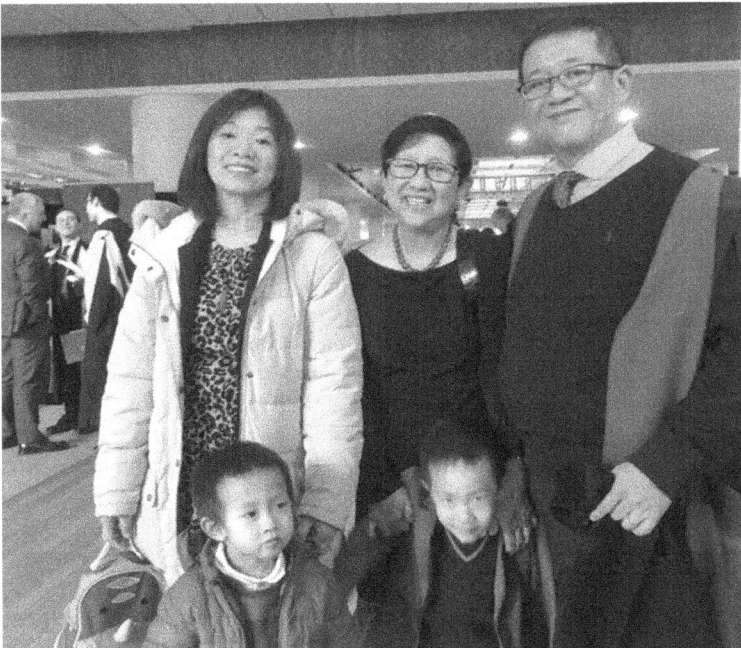

The Author With His Mother, Partner and Sons During His PhD Graduation Ceremony in 2017

institution for education. It was certainly a momentous achievement for me, and the joy was shared with my partner and family. However, while the PhD gave me status and cultural capital, for some inexplicable reason, I still do not feel like I belong to the middle classes in the British context. The following vignettes might persuade the reader to share my sentiments in this regard.

At the conclusion of the British Association of Applied Linguistics (BAAL) conference at the institution I work, a group of academics from our department and acclaimed scholars from other Russell Group and Ivy League institutions from America gathered for a ritual drinking session. After we had consumed more than a case of some lovely Pinot Noir, the voices and laughter were amplified, no doubt fuelled by the alcohol in empty stomachs. A colleague who was recently promoted to a tenure-tracked professorship mentioned how he and his partner will have to pack their suitcases late into the night to make the morning flight to Martha's Vineyard in Cape Cod, America. In a semi-drunken stupor, I expressed to him that I've visited the place during my undergraduate studies in the late 1980s. 'Aha! did you stay at "The Lodge"?' he asked. The Lodge is an upmarket, exclusive holiday let that is highly sought after by the rich and famous and is owned by the Kennedy family. I replied, 'No, I worked there as a waiter during my summer holidays to save money for my tuition fees. I'm just a working-class Chinese boy from a small seaside town in Malaysia'. Upon hearing my response, he turned red in the face, struggled to continue the conversation, and mumbled something about the pristine beaches before shifting the topic to work-related matters. Here, my interlocutor – who attended public schools and graduated from Oxbridge – assumed that I share similar quantities of economic, social and cultural capital with him. While we might be insiders in a particular academic social sphere, my lived experiences as a person with working-class ethics from Malaysia and as a student who had to work hard to save money in America positions me as an outsider in this context due to my lack of economic capital to enjoy a holiday at Martha's Vineyard. The encounter above is an illustrative example of the effect of economic capital in creating class distinctions. While we share somewhat similar amounts of social capitals, we were differentiated by our ownership of dissimilar amounts of economic capital. Having deliberated upon the importance of the possession of economic capital as a marker of class, the following vignette shows how my linguistic capital was impacted by my ethnicity and place of origin.

At a colleague's book launch at the above institution, the usual preamble about potential impact of the publication ended, and staff members and guests proceeded to enjoy a selection of fine finger foods and wines. During this event, I took the opportunity to congratulate the author, an eminent scholar in the field of bilingualism and education. She possesses a gravitas of the obligatory four-star research publications and multiple single- and joint-authored books. Well known for her cutting remarks and for making her PhD supervisees cry outside her office, she asked, 'How long have you been in the UK, Steve?' At that moment, I have been in the country for about 12 years and that was my response. 'Oh, you speak so well, how did you manage to learn the language so quickly?' When I told her that my mother was an English teacher in Malaysia and that I've spoken the language since birth, she looked surprised and said, 'Oh, yes, no wonder you speak so well'. She then proceeded to thank me for sharing some of my research data for her publication. In this instance, it was surprising to say the least when a professor of bilingualism studies made a particular assumption of my linguistic capital because of my ethnicity. In this way, her evaluation of my cultural capital with regard to linguistic registers was impacted by my ethnic background and place of origin. Further, the phrase 'you speak so well' connotes the idea that my visible markers of ethnic difference would somehow affect my oracy. The preceding encounters are examples of why I don't 'feel' middle class in the academy, I don't possess similar amounts of property, symbolic behaviour and spatial relations dimensions (Block, 2012b) that many of my colleagues own. Having shown the reader how I was mis-read in particular ways within my social network, the following shows how I was prevented from claiming a working-class identity during encounters with my colleagues.

During my induction into the Russell Group institution, I was provided with a professional mentor who offered invaluable advice about the internal departmental practices of marking, teaching and MA dissertation supervision. She is a person of modest background from the Midlands and was the first person in her family to enter HE. She achieved remarkably well and occupies a position as Professor in the field of languages in education. During one of our many interactions, she asked about my educational experiences in Malaysia. I shared my experiences of attending state schools in Malaysia and how I had to work hard during my university days in America. At a point in this conversation, I tried to explain my humble origins by uttering 'I'm just a working-class Chinese boy from a small seaside town in Malaysia' but with her eyes narrowed, she replied, 'There are many things I could say about you, Steve, but working-class isn't one of them'. I wanted to defend my statement, but her facial expression spoke volumes. In this final vignette, I will share with the reader a recent conversation with my current line manager. He was the programme leader and academic mentor at the post-1992 institution where I gained my MA degree. This speech event relates to this very chapter. During a staff appraisal for me, he said that my performance over the year under review had exceeded the goals that were set for me but remarked about my lack of publications. This is very important aspect of my occupation and is essential if I wanted to apply for a promotion within the department. I acknowledged his observation and responded by saying that I was in the process of writing a chapter for a book about the lived experiences of working-class academics in the UK HE sector. His response was immediate, 'Good God, Steve, why are you contributing to this book?'. I responded with my typical utterance about being a working-class Chinese person from Malaysia, but he said, 'One wouldn't think that you're a working-class person, Steve'. In the vignettes earlier, both my professional mentor and line manager evaluated me as a person who belong to the middle classes. Perhaps due to my possession of varying amounts of social and cultural capitals, my attempts at self-identifying with aspects of the working classes were denied by members of my social network. Class dimensions as outlined by Block (2012b) such as occupation, education, social networking, symbolic behaviour and spatial relations position me in particular categories during evaluations by my interlocutors. As such, class identities are fluid, it's not simply a free market in which one could choose to identify oneself but, rather, is contingent on class evaluations by the *other*.

To conclude this chapter, I maintain my overarching argument that class is a verb and that class identifications shift according to the context and social sphere one engages in. As I have shown in the preceding, the notion of class is mostly elusive, always relational, and evolving. In my itineraries of mobility, my accumulated forms of capital at times mark me as a working-class person and, at other destinations, firmly entrench myself as a member of the middle classes. While I still do not feel entirely comfortable enough to claim a middle-class identity due to my patterns of consumption and area of residence in London, I have also shown how my social and cultural capitals bar me from claiming a working-class identity even though I 'feel' and am guided by aspects of working-class sensibilities such as being frugal and my belief that the key to success is to work hard. In super-diversity, class, ethnic, national and linguistic identities have become even more complex and as I have clearly shown earlier, self-identifications are processual, dependent on one's roots and are the resultant effects of interactions in a range of social spheres that individuals have experienced in their biographical trajectories.

References

Beswick, K. (2020). Feeling working class: Affective class identification and its implications for overcoming inequality. *Studies in Theatre and Performance*, *40*(3), 265–274.

Block, D. (2012a). Economising globalisation and identity in applied linguistics in neoliberal times. In D. Block, J. Gray, & M. Holborow (Eds.), *Neoliberalism and applied linguistics* (pp. 56–85). London: Routledge.

Block, D. (2012b). Class and SLA: Making connections. *Language Teaching Research*, *16*(2), 188–205.

Block, D. (2013). *Class in applied linguistics*. London: Routledge.

Bochner, A., & Ellis, C. (2006). Communication as autoethnography. In G. J. Shepherd, J. St. John, & T. Striphas (Eds.), *Communication as....: Perspectives on theory* (pp. 110–122). Thousand Oaks, CA: Sage Publications, Inc.

Bourdieu, P. (1984). *Distinction*. London: Routledge.

Britannica, T. Editors of Encyclopaedia. (2019, September 20). Social class. Encyclopedia Britannica. https://www.britannica.com/topic/social-class. Accessed on April 3, 2022.

Clifford, J. (1997). *Routes: Travel and translation in the late twentieth century*. Cambridge, MA: Harvard University Press.

Ellis, C., & Bochner, A. P. (2000). Autoethnography, personal narrative, reflexivity. In N. Denzin & Y. S. Lincoln (Eds.), *Handbook of qualitative research* (2nd ed., pp. 733–768). Thousand Oaks, CA: Sage.

Gray, J., & Block, D. (2014). All middle class now? Evolving representations of the working class in the neoliberal era–the case of ELT textbooks. In N. Harwood (Ed.), *English language teaching textbooks: Content, consumption, production*. Basingstoke: Palgrave Macmillan.

Lenin, V. I. (1947/1919). A Great beginning. In *The essentials of Lenin in two volumes* (p. xxx). London: Lawrence and Wishart. Retrieved from http://www.marxists.org/archive/lenin/works/1919/jun/19.htm. Accessed on October 2, 2012.

Richardson, L. (2000). Writing: A method of inquiry. In N. Denzin & Y. Lincoln (Eds.), *Handbook of qualitative research* (2nd ed.). Thousand Oaks, CA: Sage.

Skeggs, B. (1997). *Formations of class and gender: Becoming respectable.* London: Sage.

Skeggs, B. (2012). Feeling class: Affect and culture in the making of class relations. In *The Wiley-Blackwell companion to sociology* (pp. 269–286). New York, NY: John Wiley & Sons.

Vertovec, S. (2007). Super-diversity and its implications. *Ethnic and Racial Studies, 30*(6), 1024–1054.

Weber, M. (1924/1968]). *Economy and society (Vols. 1 and 2).* Berkeley, CA: University of California Press.

Wong, S. (2018). *South London Somali ethnicities in superdiversity.* PhD thesis, King's College London, British Library ETHOS. Retrieved from https://ethos.bl.uk/OrderDetails.do?uin=uk.bl.ethos.778177

Chapter 12

Reading the Posh Newspapers

Teresa Crew

Abstract

In this chapter, I use an autoethnographic approach to explore my everyday experiences as a senior lecturer at a UK-based university. My academic trajectory covers over 20 years when I, a working-class person with no qualifications, entered university. I outline my journey from student to academic. My day-to-day experiences of being a working-class academic (WCA) have been generally positive, but I've still encountered micro-aggressions, and feelings of isolation. This chapter also illuminates the cultural wealth that I bring to academia by virtue of my working-class heritage before ending with some points for reflection.

Keywords: Working-class academic; classism; autoethnography; capital; 'fitting-in'; cultural wealth

Introduction

Academia is one of the few places in which I have experienced a curious combination of being a minority and subjected to heightened visibility (i.e. hyper-visibility). Statistical data partly explains this: only 14% of academics in the United Kingdom identify as being working-class academics (WCA) (Friedman & Laurison, 2019). There is a continual loss of working-class talent as institutional, financial and cultural barriers sift out disadvantaged cohorts from academia at every opportunity. Research, like the classic study by Ryan and Sackrey (1984), tells us that the academy is not a welcoming environment to WCA. Classed microaggressions, from students and colleagues, are typical for WCA (Haney, 2015; Sykes, 2021; Warnock, 2016). Warnock (2016) found that WCA experience a dual sense of alienation where they do not 'fit' in with their colleagues, and at the same time struggle to maintain close relationships with their working-class friends and family (p. 28). As such, Dews and Law (1995) note that there is a sense of being 'neither here nor there', so much so that 'the working-class academic

The Lives of Working Class Academics, 173–185
Copyright © 2023 Teresa Crew
Published under exclusive licence by Emerald Publishing Limited
doi:10.1108/978-1-80117-057-420221012

never fully moves in' (p. 130). The contemporary literature highlights further difficulties, such as impostor syndrome (Breeze, 2019; Gravois, 2007; Long, Jenkins, & Bracken, 2000), academic precarity (Courtois and O'Keefe, 2015; Michell et al., 2015) and the influence of the type of institution on one's experience (Binns, 2019).

Even though the literature mainly focuses on examples of where WCA are judged harshly for their working-class traits and values, research does point to what WCA bring to academia. For instance, Walkerdine (2021) argues that WCA offer 'both an understanding of othering and discrimination', something I have found WCA bring to their teaching (Crew, 2020, 2021). While WCA experienced isolation and at times have felt inauthentic within their academic community, Pifer, Riffe, Hartz, & Ibarra (2022) noted that in some cases this led to a stronger identification with their families. Research by Lee (2017) refers to the potential for WCA to mentor students, to be academic role models and also to contribute to a diverse campus environment. My own research identified the various forms of capital and funds of knowledge that working-class cohorts offer the academy. In this chapter I adopt an autoethnographic approach, whereby my own lived experience, derived from my working-class heritage becomes the topic of investigation.

Autoethnography as a Research Method

Heider (1975) first used 'auto-ethnography' to describe the practice of people in Indonesia giving an account of their own culture. Autoethnographies 'are highly personalized accounts that draw upon the experience of the author/researcher for the purposes of extending sociological understanding' (Sparkes, 2000, p. 21). According to Adams, Holman Jones, and Ellis (2015), autoethnography is a qualitative research method that: (1) offers a deep and careful self-reflection on the intersections between the personal and the political; (2) shows 'people…and the meaning of their struggles'; (3) balances intellect, emotion and creativity; and (4) strives for social justice (p. 2). In short, autoethnography is an observational, participatory and reflexive method that places the self within a social context (Campbell, 2016). Using personal narratives in academic scholarship can be seen as self-indulgent and egotistical due to their focus on the self (Coffey, 1999). Stahlke Wall (2016), a reviewer of autoethnographic manuscripts, provides a fairer critique, stating that this method provides the value of lived experience while maintaining scholarly rigour. This chapter covers a period of almost 20 years, covering my journey into and through HE ('getting in' and 'getting on') as both a student and graduate, before focusing on my (ongoing) experiences as an academic. I focus on three main areas:

- Can an academic be working class?
- The difficulties I have experienced as a working-class academic
- The benefits I bring to the academy as a working-class academic

'Getting in' and 'Getting on'

I was born in 1972 to working-class parents from large cities (Liverpool and Nottingham). For most of my childhood I lived in Runcorn, Cheshire, on a social housing estate. My class biography is mixed in so much that it includes periods of long-term unemployment and a reliance on welfare benefits, often called the 'underclass' (a term I detest as it divides people into the deserving and underserving poor). Alongside this, I have elements of the aspirational working class as my maternal grandparents rented a corner shop and some of my uncles were able to go to university. My biography also includes examples of traditional working-class occupations as my dad and some of my uncles worked 'down the mines' in Nottingham, as well as in various low-skilled employment in various factories, hotels and shops. My mum stayed at home with my brother and I when we were young, but in my teens she began to work as a contract interviewer for various organisations. As a sign of things to come, my mum would often complain about the researchers she worked for and would always tell me 'you could do this job, you could explain things much easier than these researchers'. I was good at school, a B student most of the time, an A student every so often, but there was no active planning to go to university like there is in many middle-class families. I was rebellious at school so I eventually left school with no qualifications. I went on to do various manual roles such as waitressing and working as a chambermaid, but I was always a critical thinker who read voraciously. I became a mum at 21 and 23, which was wonderful. I loved my time with my daughters, but wanted to make sure they saw education in a positive light. Inspired by films such as *Educating Rita* and *Working Girl*, I grew more interested in going to university. I didn't have a particular career in mind – that wasn't for 'people like me' – I just wanted to be able to read the 'posh' newspapers. But I kept putting it off as I had no one who I could speak to about what university was like, and I wasn't sure how I would fit it in around my daughters' school. I remember mentioning my plans about university to someone I worked with, she laughed her head off, and then she announced to rest of the waitresses in the café where I worked that I thought I was better than everyone else. That embarrassed me so much that I didn't mention it for another few years and university remained a pipe dream. But when I turned 30, a desire for my children to have better choices than I had started to dominate my thoughts, and so I decided to give university a try.

As I was in receipt of welfare benefits, I was eligible for financial support to study with the Open University (OU). The flexibility of the course meant I could fit it around my daughters' school. I loved the OU but wanted the typical university experience, so a few days before university started in 2003, I joined Bangor University to do an undergraduate degree in Criminology. There is a huge sense of anxiety and unease inherent in the working-class experience of university (Ryan and Sackrey, 1984), so for the first 18 months I felt sick, constantly on edge, thinking I'd be asked to leave as I was unsuitable. There was a lot I didn't know, but I had what Yosso (2005) terms as 'aspirational capital'. This form of capital refers to the ability to maintain hopes and dreams even in the face of real or perceived difficulties. While financial, social and academic barriers hindered each phase of my academic journey, I was driven by a determination that nothing was going to stop me from gaining a first-class honours degree. I was fortunate enough to get a scholarship to do my master's. My scholarship was vital as I could not have otherwise afforded to have paid for postgraduate study. It's important that when people tell their story, they also mention their economic or social capital, or even if they had pieces of luck. If I had not been awarded the scholarship, I doubt very much I would be here now writing this chapter because I did not have the finances to pay for a master's, but if I did I would have felt selfish spending more money on myself when I had a young family.

Beyond Graduation

Financial barriers meant I needed to work full time alongside my master's. I was fortunate enough to gain graduate-level employment as a researcher, a housing officer and a communications officer, to name but a few positions for my local council and charities. I now know that I was, again very fortunate, to have found graduate employment as the impact of class disadvantage does not begin or end with an undergraduate degree as graduates from disadvantaged socioeconomic groups are generally more likely to be unemployed and less likely to be in graduate employment (See Boliver, 2011, 2013; The Sutton Trust, 2011). I graduated into the 2008 recession, which meant that the local graduate labour market consisted of short-term, temporary research and project manager posts, advertised by employment agencies. This was a stressful period, exacerbated by my need to earn money and my epilepsy. While I was never unemployed, my 'working-classness' felt even more emphasised as there were clear social divisions between myself and the people I worked with. My colleagues were all similar, 'people with privilege, who grew up in big houses, who went to restaurants and on holidays abroad' (O'Neil, 2020). They all seemed metaphorically large due to their advantages, while I felt small and insignificant. My postgraduate education meant I was often given higher level tasks than my pay grade, but this was for the benefit of the children of my middle-class employers. For instance, one employer asked me to help her son to write reports 'just like you do'. I inadvertently ended up training him to take over my role.

The many material points of difference between my colleagues and I stood out. I lived (and still do) in rented accommodation on a working-class housing estate and had (and still do) friends from there. People in management positions would give me well-meaning advice to 'work on my presentation' i.e. middle class speak that suggested I should sound more like them so I could 'fit' the graduate role better. While I didn't feel intellectually inferior to my colleagues, I felt hyper-visible due to my support for working-class people. For instance, I would get increasingly angry when many of my colleagues would discuss 'clients' or 'service users' (whichever term was in vogue at the time) as these people in need would be discussed in disparaging ways. I had so many uncomfortable discussions with colleagues, for example, reminding them that 'people on benefits' were not scroungers or lazy or stupid. A conversation about the parliamentary expenses scandal in 2009 was particularly telling. I was working in local government at the time, and I expressed my utter disgust about how easy it had been for MPs to misuse the expenses regime for personal gain. I was aghast with my colleagues' views as they appeared more comfortable with an MP claiming expenses for their gardening or for a house they did not live in, than there being a rise in the level of benefits or an increase in the hourly wage. It's worthwhile noting that this time in my career served me well for when I started working as a lecturer as I was adept at conducting research. So, while many academic peers have had a seemingly advantaged, classic linear trajectory, from undergraduate to postgraduate study, to a lecturer or researcher position, this can mean they have little experience outside of academia. My trajectory, in comparison, was fraught with difficulty, but my experiences of working in local councils and charities make me a much more experienced academic, and enable me to give students very practical career guidance.

The following sections now focus on my experience – which is ongoing – as an academic.

What do You Mean by a 'Working-Class' Academic?

I've been asked the above question countless times. Wakeling (2010) provides a solid critique of whether academics can be working class, stating that one could not compare academia to other 'solidly' working-class occupations such as a cleaner or supermarket checkout assistant' (p. 38). I see the value in this commentary as my partner works as an NHS cleaner, so there is an obvious salary differential between us, and he does not have the same level of autonomy that I do in my workplace. The COVID-19 pandemic highlighted a further advantage, that people in professional occupations like mine have the ability to work from home. While the pandemic was initially seen as 'the great equaliser', my partner was an essential worker, so he has 'served on the frontline', leaving him exposed more significantly to the risk of infection. There also is an obvious level of prestige I have as an academic, yet it's been a source of amusement to both of us that societal gender biases have meant he has often been mistaken as being the recipient of the 'Dr' title that I hold.

Economic advantages do not mean that I leave the landscape of my class background behind, as a working-class identity is distinct from socioeconomic status, whereby credentials such as connections and culture are just as important as any financial assets. I have built small networks in academia, but my social capital lacks the 'wealth' of those from privileged backgrounds. Although my social contacts do include lecturers and researchers, my main networks comprise of care workers, couriers and people working in customer service – all of whom, sadly, may not have the knowledge to help me to gain research funding or a promotion. My cultural capital is varied. I consume highbrow cultural items such as academic books and works of art (objective cultural capital) and also possess elite educational qualifications ('institutionalised' cultural capital), but my 'embodied' cultural capital always 'displays' my class background. While I can 'decode' the cultural capital of the dominant culture by using the 'right' language and mannerisms, my natural speech and behaviour is informal, and I tend to revert to that when I am relaxed, or when I am nervous. This gives me an ease with students as I am professional, but I cut out the bullshit. My preference to watch a play than visit a pub may be used as an example of my store of cultural capital, but I have consumed highbrow art and books from a child. When people ask me about being a WCA, I remind people that I can 'consume' sophisticated culture, and still be working class, ideas to the contrary just perpetuate well-worn stereotypes of working-class people. Furthermore, my class trajectory meant I entered university as an undergraduate student in 2003 aged 31 and then became an academic 10 years later.[1] So for the vast majority of my life I have been employed in working-class occupations, such as waitress, chamber maid, sales assistant, with working-class people. Admittedly I have financial advantages, but I'll always be playing cultural catch up to my middle-class colleagues. Thus, I define a WCA as someone perceives their 'background/upbringing to be working-class and continues to identify in this way' (Crew, 2020, p. 7).

The Difficulties of Being a Working-Class Academic

My experience within my institution has been overwhelmingly positive, but from the very start I've been aware of my class difference. I was originally offered a 'fees only' scholarship after completing my master's degree, to go on to do my PhD. This was a fantastic offer as the funding body, which provided the scholarship, only fund an average of 500 PhDs per year. Yet as this award did not include a monthly stipend, I had no choice but to turn it down. This was an upsetting period in my life as I remember thinking that even when working-class people have the educational ability, external forces will often disadvantage you. I thought I'd not get this chance again but luckily, the next year, after working with my supervisors to fine tune my application, I was awarded a fully funded PhD scholarship. While this is a very prestigious award, the basic UK Research Council stipend equates to earning less than the minimum wage (Cornell, 2006). So again, financial issues impacted on my PhD journey, and I needed to work full time alongside my PhD – something that my supervisor gently reminded me was actually against the rules of my scholarship. The problem was that I could not have financially afforded to have completed my PhD without further financial support. But working full time alongside my PhD and still finishing within three-and-a-half years exacerbated my epilepsy and has led to other long-term health issues. My experience is typical as academics in a study by Gill and Donaghue (2016) reported 'chronic stress, anxiety, exhaustion, insomnia and spiralling rates of physical and mental illness' (p. 91), while a survey by Gorczynski, Hill, and Rathod (2017) found that 43% of academic staff exhibited symptoms of at least a mild mental disorder. Respondents in my own study referred to a variety of physical problems such as headaches, weight gain/loss, digestive issues, as well as constant aches and pains (Crew, 2020, p. 59), all issues I have experienced in this strange environment.

Ingram and Abrahams's (2015) typology is very useful in understanding how people experience new and secondary social fields. It is a useful device to unpick my habitus as each 'type' has been a suitable descriptor at various times throughout my academic career. For instance, if I consider my taste in books, food and where I shop, I often hide this part of me by not talking about it with people who share my working-class heritage. Hiding these indicators of my diversity would be seen as an abandoned habitus. As one's habitus adapts to new social fields (Bourdieu, 1990, p. 57), when I teach, I'm confident, I feel at ease, so if a member of my family was listening I would more than likely 'sound like me'. While the two fields of home and work are opposing, they are integrated, otherwise known as a reconciled habitus (Ingram & Abrahams, 2015, p. 148). On the other hand, when I present to colleagues, I have a resurgence of imposter syndrome and I worry about my legitimacy. I have described myself as a patchwork quilt, with each 'square' representing the old and the new 'me'. While past and present embrace me, I can be awkward in each setting. It's painful feeling 'different' in each field. I should admire what I've achieved but instead I fixate on 'dropped stitches'. While the structuring forces of each field are incorporated, the habitus cannot be reconciled, otherwise known as a destabilised habitus (Ingram & Abrahams, 2015, p. 148).

When I'm with people I don't know from my community, I can feel myself sounding stiff and I struggle to breathe correctly. I swear more than is needed. Yet, I feel so distant from academia. I see words and no action, precarious employment as the norm, diversity that is a tick-box exercise, poor mental health, bullying and abuse. When I reflect on my life now, I can see how much I've moved away from good friends since I went to university. I miss them, I just want to be home, and after all, I only ever wanted to be able to read the posh newspapers. My habitus is divided from this new field (re-confirmed habitus) (Ingram & Abrahams, 2015). But then just as I feel like I'm not suited to academia, I'm at an open day and I see someone I vaguely know, and I can tell she is nervous. She spots me and says she wants to do a degree, and that she's glad I'm here as she didn't realise people like us went to university. Then I know I am in the right place. I realise I have two 'versions' of me, an adaption to both fields, what Abrahams and Ingram (2013) terms a 'chameleon habitus'.

Accentism is cited as an example of how academia is not an especially welcoming environment for working-class scholars. Edwards (2019) interviewed 20 academics from Russell Group institutions and found accentism was rife as every respondent had negative experiences. Respondents in my own study reported being stigmatised for their 'Northern' or 'Welsh' accents (Crew, 2020, p. 71). While I have not heard comments about my accent, I've been excluded from opportunities when others from traditional academic backgrounds, who sat in my company, have been invited. The latter serves to remind me of the nepotism in academia, to the point where the same academic editors in journals and on research committees, cite their friends publications and ignore new publications (unless of course it is written by their friends). While I have a thick skin, microaggressions like this serve as a reminder of my second-class status in academia.

The most common issue I have faced in academia is microaggressions, defined as 'everyday verbal, non-verbal and environmental slights, snubs or insults, whether intentional or unintentional, which communicate hostile, derogatory or negative messages to target persons based solely upon their marginalised group membership' (Sue, 2010). I do have a number of examples of incidents that mainly seem to occur at conferences. Thankfully as I was a mature student, and now academic, I've been able to manage these negative incidents, but I am not immune to the impact of such behaviour. One example is when I was subjected to 'hyper-attention' at a conference. My presentation appeared to be received well within the room, but outside, when I am trying to leave for my train, I am relentlessly interrogated by two academics who correct me on my terminology and ask if I had heard about the work of Pierre Bourdieu (even though he is a renowned sociologist, and his work was in my presentation). The questioning is incessant, scornful and feels bullying. There are people around, but no one thinks to help me. I leave to get a taxi and frantically write a message explaining myself, wanting to let them know I'm not stupid, and I do know about the work of Pierre Bourdieu. I hear myself meekly apologising for having given the wrong impression. I sit on the train feeling stupid, overwhelmed and angry. But then thankfully, I stop myself and read an extract of an article that always reminds me of what I am facing in academia as a working-class academic:

> It's hard work defending ourselves and protecting our profiles against those who judge us, look down on us, sneer and laugh at us. They laugh when we get it wrong, when we try to be like them – when we don't know about wine, geography or politics. They deride us when we wear big gold earrings, speak loudly, laugh loudly, or swear; our honesty is misrepresented as stupidity, they shout over us, they silence us, and they use big words to intimidate us. They wait for us to say the 'wrong thing', to make a mistake, to get confused, to feel scared; they shout at us 'you are stupid', 'you are aggressive', 'you should be locked up', 'you should be sacked'.
>
> (McKenzie, 2015, para 5)

While Lisa's article is an upsetting read as it reminds me of the times when thoughtless academics have embarrassed me, knowing there was someone like Lisa was the perfect antidote for me on that long journey home. As Lisa said:

> Who would be a working-class woman? To be honest, only a working-class woman. We are the only ones who have the balls for it.
>
> (McKenzie, 2015, para 4)

She's right, I've got balls. I've got the balls to be kind to other academics, to be collegiate, to not want to shame or embarrass them!

The Benefits that the Working-Class Academic
Offer to the Academy

Discussions of my outsider identity should be offset by an acknowledgement that my working-classness is an attractive status that offers the academy something that is not like the norm. In Crew (2020) I highlighted that the WCA respondents had various funds of knowledge that made them sources of support to their students and an embodiment of what was possible. Interview data also identified a 'working-class academic pedagogy', a teaching approach with social justice at its heart, it engaged with students from a strength's perspective, embraced shared experiences and encouraged students to be co-creators of knowledge (p. 133). They also displayed various examples of the type of community wealth described by Yosso (2005). The task of reflecting upon and articulating my own assets has been the most difficult aspect of this autoethnography. I recently listened to part of an interview that I did, as it was included in a colleague's presentation. I sat there cringing throughout as I heard my voice and I sounded 'full of myself'. This feeling would typically be ascribed to imposter syndrome. Yet while the literature on this subject is interesting, especially the work of Addison, Breeze and Taylor (2022), I feel my embarrassment is mainly due to feelings of difference i.e. 'I don't sound like other academics' and my experiences of classism. However, as research on WCA continually positions us as 'less than' in comparison to elite or middle-class academics, examples of working-class forms of capital, adds much needed texture to this field.

Reflexive methods like autoethnography can be used to demonstrate the multiplicity of an identity. One asset I have is familial capital which is a further resource that I have drawn upon in HE. This form of capital refers to my extended familial and community networks and can manifest as caring and nurturing. Research by Shapiro (2018) on youths with a refugee background found several of her participants described how their family members instilled a sense of community responsibility. I have this same ideal with regards to the working-class people I encounter in HE, that desire to do community service by supporting them through academia. I tell students that I am the first in my family to go to university and that I am a WCA so that they know they are not alone. I'm also upfront about the positives and negatives of my university and graduate experience. This form of capital serves me well with students as memories of these difficulties and of important milestones have never left me so I *think* I know what to say to students when they go through tough times. I don't mind letting them know about jobs I've not gotten, or funding bids that have failed. I'm always up for a coffee and am sympathetic to the difficulties they may have, but I also know when to give some tough love.

My linguistic capital is demonstrated in the way in which I communicate with my students. My students have often commented on how 'normal' I sound, and not like a traditional lecturer due to the way in which I explain lecture or seminar material in an accessible manner. Part of my pedagogy utilises a Freirean approach as I avoid asking students to just memorise and repeat my ideas without understanding the meaning behind them (1970, p. 71). This approach has been demonstrated most recently in a module I have written, which encourages students to develop an awareness of how social divisions permeate the social order both publicly and privately which at times leads to differentiation, exclusion and disadvantage. One of the assignments I have set is to ask students to combine academic literature with an autoethnography about the social divisions they have needed to overcome/are still overcoming. I hope this reflexiveness will help them not just understand about their own inequalities, but their advantages and where others have disadvantages.

As universities have a history, and in many ways still do, of being unsupportive and hostile to people from disadvantaged backgrounds, I've used my navigational capital to manoeuvre through these classist institutions. In Manzo et al. (2018), the health care workers indicated that they felt they had a sense of responsibility to take action to address the disparities in their community. I understand this because, at heart, I am an academic who feels guilty that I have 'made it'. As such I feel I have a responsibility to support students, especially those who are the first in their family to get to university. My navigational capital has included practical methods such as embedding employability and study skills in my teaching, offering internship opportunities and bringing in speakers who are 'visible' example of class and other differences. I've also encouraged my students' academic success by writing many letters of recommendation. The latter is typical academic housekeeping, but the desire behind this example of navigational capital is to help other working-class people into professional jobs.

Resistance is key to my research and teaching as I challenge the ways that various 'groups' such as Roma, Gypsy Travellers, the long-term unemployed and, of course, how the 'working class' are portrayed. I've used this form of capital to challenge the typical administration roles that are carried out according to one's gender. Having undertaken senior pastoral care roles in the school, I'm conscious that this is a form of academic housekeeping that is not carried out equally, often being the preserve of female academics. I raised this with colleagues in executive meetings and discussed it with students in my gender module. While I have not resolved the propensity for students to consider women as their first port of call, the school management has been active in ensuring there is a more even division of labour in these academic roles. O'Shea (2016) discussed resistance capital as countering the constraints around 'what is possible' (p. 72). This echoes my own resistance capital, as for me university has enabled me to resist the deeply entrenched, societal roles that are typically expected of working-class women, for instance, pursuing a profession as opposed to focusing solely on caring responsibilities. Moving forward I hope my daughters and my working-class students too can resist the expectations placed upon them due to their class heritage.

Final Thoughts

Using an autoethnographic approach, I have offered an account of the personal and professional experiences of a working-class academic at a UK higher education institution (HEI). This chapter serves as a reminder that recognising class inequalities is vital. It allows us to consider ways to be inclusive and encourages action. It is hoped that this personal account of how it feels to encounter microaggressions encourages reflection i.e. if you have observed microaggressions, what form of supportive action could you have taken? The positive experiences I have had far outweigh the negative ones, but when I have been on the receiving end of a microaggression, I could have done with a friendly face. This chapter has also drawn upon the work of Yosso (2005) and the themes within my own research to reflect the assets that I, as a working-class academic, bring to academia. We have long heard about the deficits of working-class people, so a more balanced portrayal is long overdue. I end with some points for reflection:

- How do you support disadvantaged groups in HE?
- Have you observed microaggressions against others? If so, what is your reaction?
- What is your cultural wealth?

Note

1. Chapter 2 of my book goes into more depth, describing the four main features that define people as being a working-class academic: working-class family background, uneven access to capital, a lack of a safety net to 'manage' academic precarity and a disrupted habitus (Crew, 2020, p. 32).

References

Abrahams, J., & Ingram, N. (2013). The chameleon habitus: Exploring local students' negotiations of multiple fields. *Sociological Research Online*, *18*(4), 21. Retrieved from http://www.socresonline.org.uk/18/4/21.html

Adams, T. E., Holman Jones, S., & Ellis, C. (2015). *Autoethnography*. Oxford: Oxford University Press.

Addison, M., Breeze, M., & Taylor, Y. (Eds.), (2022). *The palgrave handbook of imposter syndrome in higher education*. London: Palgrave.

Binns, C. (2019). *Experiences of academics from a working-class heritage: Ghosts of childhood habitus*. Cambridge: Cambridge Scholars Publishing.

Boliver, V. (2011). Expansion, differentiation, and the persistence of social class inequalities in British higher education. *Higher Education*, *61*(3), 229–242.

Boliver, V. (2013). How fair is access to more prestigious UK universities? *British Journal of Sociology*, *64*(2), 344–364.

Bourdieu, P. (1990). *The logic of practice*. Cambridge: Polity Press.

Breeze, M. (2019, March 11). Imposter syndrome as a public feeling. *The Sociological Review*. Retrieved from https://www.thesociologicalreview.com/imposter-syndrome-as-a-public-feeling. Accessed on November 19, 2021.

Campbell, E. (2016). Exploring autoethnography as a method and methodology in legal education research. *Asian Journal of Legal Education*, *3*(1), 95–105.

Coffey, A. (1999). *The ethnographic self*. London: Sage.

Cornell, B. (2006). *PhD life: The UK student experience*. Higher Education Policy Institute. Retrieved from https://www.hepi.ac.uk/wp-content/uploads/2020/06/PhD-Life_The-UK-Student-Experience_HEPI-Report-131.pdf

Courtois, A., & O'Keefe, T. (2015). Precarity in the ivory cage: Neoliberalism and casualisation of work in the Irish higher education sector. *Journal for Critical Education Policy Studies, 13*(1), 43–66.

Crew, T. (2020). *Higher education and working-class academics. Precarity and diversity in academia.* London: Palgrave Macmillan.

Crew, T. (2021). Navigating academia as a working class academic. *Journal of Working Class Studies, 6*(2), 50–64.

Dews, B., & Law, L. (1995). *This fine place so far from home: Voices of academics from the working class.* Philadelphia, PA: Temple University Press.

Edwards, K. (2019, June 10). Gerraway with accentism – I'm proud to speak yorkshire. *The Guardian.*

Freire, P. (1970/2000). *Pedagogy of the oppressed* (30th anniversary ed.). New York, NY: Bloomsbury.

Friedman, S., & Laurison, D. (2019). *The class ceiling: Why it pays to be privileged.* Bristol: Policy Press.

Gill, R., & Donaghue, N. (2016). Resilience, apps and reluctant individualism: Technologies of self in the neoliberal academy. *Women's Studies International Forum, 54*, 91–99.

Gorczynski, P., Hill, D., & Rathod, S. (2017). Examining the construct validity of the transtheoretical model to structure workplace physical activity interventions to improve mental health in academic staff. *Emergency Medical Services Community Medical Journal, 1*(1), 2.

Gravois, J. (2007, November). You're not fooling anyone. *The Chronicle of Higher Education, 54*(11), A1.

Haney, T. (2015). Factory to faculty: Socioeconomic difference and the educational experiences of university professors. *Canadian Review of Sociology = Revue canadienne de sociologie, 52 2*, 160–186.

Heider, K. G. (1975). What do people do? Dani auto-ethnography. *Journal of Anthropological Research, 31*(1), 3–17.

Higher Education Funding Council for England (HEFCE). (2015). Differences in employment outcomes: equality and diversity characteristics. Bristol: HEFCE.

Ingram, N., & Abrahams, J. (2015). Stepping outside of oneself: How a cleft- habitus can lead to greater reflexivity through occupying "the third space". In J. Thatcher, N. Ingram, C. Burke, & J. Abrahams (Eds.), *Bourdieu – The next generation: The development of Bourdieu's intellectual heritage in contemporary UK sociology.* Oxon: Routledge.

Lee, E. (2017). "Where people like me don't belong": Faculty members from low-socioeconomic-status backgrounds. *Sociology of Education, 90*(3), 197–212.

Long, M., Jenkins, G., & Bracken, S. (2000). Imposters in the sacred grove: Working class women in the academe. *Qualitative Report, 5*(3), 1–15.

Manzo, R. D., Rangel, M. I., Flores, Y. G., & de la Torre, A. (2018). A community cultural wealth model to train promotoras as data collectors. *Health Promotion Practice, 19*, 341–348.

McKenzie, L. (2015, October 5). Who would be a working-class woman in academia? *Higher Education* Retrieved from https://www.timeshighereducation.com/lisa-mckenzie-who-would-be-working-class-woman-academia

Michell, D., Wilson, J. Z., & Archer, V. (Eds.), (2015). *Bread and roses: Voices of Australian academics from the working class.* Rotterdam: Sense Publishers.

O'Neil, D. (2020). On being a working class academic. *Working Class Academics.* Retrieved from https://workingclass-academics.co.uk/on-being-a-working-class-academic-by-deirdre-oneill/

O'Shea, S. (2016). Avoiding the manufacture of 'sameness': First-in-family students, cultural capital and the higher education environment. *Higher Education, 72,* 59–78.

Pifer, M., Riffe, K., Hartz, J., & Ibarra, M. (2022). Paradise, nearly forty years later: The liminal experiences of working-class academics. *Innovative Higher Education.*

Ryan, J., & Sackrey, C. (1984). *'Strangers in paradise': Academics from the working class.* Boston, MA: South End Press.

Shapiro, S. (2018). Familial capital, narratives of agency, and the college transition process for refugee-background youth. *Equity & Excellence in Education, 51*(3–4), 332–346.

Sparkes, A. (2000). Autoethnography and narratives of self: Reflections on criteria in action. *Sociology of Sport Journal, 17,* 21–43.

Stahlke Wall, S. (2016). Toward a moderate autoethnography. *International Journal of Qualitative Methods, 15.* doi:10.1177/1609406916674966

Sue, D. (2010). *Microaggressions in everyday life: Race, gender, and sexual orientation.* Hoboken, NJ: Wiley.

Sykes, B. (2021). Academic turning points: How microaggressions and macro-aggressions inhibit diversity and inclusion in the academy. *Race and Justice, 11*(3), 288–300.

The Sutton Trust. (2011). *Degrees of success: University chances by individual school.* London: Sutton Trust.

Wakeling, P. (2010). Is there such thing as a working-class academic? In Y. Taylor (Ed.), *Classed intersections: Spaces, selves, knowledges.* Farham: Ashgate.

Walkerdine, V. (2021). What's class got to do with it? *Discourse: Studies in the Cultural Politics of Education, 42*(1), 60–74.

Warnock, D. (2016). Paradise lost? Patterns and precarity in working-class Academic narratives. *Journal of Working-Class Studies, 1*(1), 28–44.

Yosso, T. (2005). Whose culture has capital? A critical race theory discussion of community cultural wealth. *Race, Ethnicity and Education, 8,* 69–91.

Chapter 13

Thames Estuary Academic

Jo Finch

Abstract

In this chapter, I reflect on the impact my Estuary English accent has had on me, both personally and professionally as a former social worker, now social work academic, and the impact it appears to have on others. From parental chastisement for dropping my 'T's, attributions of being 'Cockney' and 'Essex', with associated assumptions made about my educational background, class and indeed my very moral character. My accent appears at times, to disrupt some peoples' presuppositions – about who or what I am. I discuss some of the linguistic features of my accent and some 'critical accent incidents'. I reflect on the challenges of managing academia as someone with an accent that I argue, is underpinned by gendered and classist assumptions. I argue why a critical focus on accentism remains important, generally and within social work education. The chapter utilises theory from a wide range of disciplines, including cultural theory, linguistics, education studies and autoethnography.

Keywords: Estuary English; accent; class; gender; assumptions; cockney; essex; vajazzle

Introduction

In this chapter, I reflect on the impact my accent has had on me, both personally and professionally as a former social worker, now social work academic, and the impact it appears to have on others. From parental chastisement for dropping my 'T's, attributions of being 'Cockney' and 'Essex', with associated assumptions made about my educational background, class and indeed my very moral character.[1] My accent appears, at times, to disrupt some peoples' presuppositions – about who or what I am. Indeed, I wondered if I was approached to contribute to this book because of assumptions made about my class because of my accent. My accent may suggest, therefore, that I am from a working-class background, although as I go on to discuss, my class identity is complicated.

The Lives of Working Class Academics, 187–202
Copyright © 2023 Jo Finch
Published under exclusive licence by Emerald Publishing Limited
doi:10.1108/978-1-80117-057-420221013

In this chapter I discuss some of the linguistic features of my accent and some 'critical accent incidents' as I have termed them. I reflect on the challenges of managing academia as someone with an accent that, as I go on to argue, is underpinned by gendered and classist assumptions. In writing this chapter, I have stepped outside my usual social work academic comfort zone and traversed across disciplinary boundaries in a very unorganised manner, dipping inexpertly into biography, autoethnography, linguistics, education studies, sociology, political geography and cultural studies to name but a few. I cannot therefore claim expertise in all of these disciplines. This chapter, therefore, is somewhat a sur-reptitious journey of discovery – I did not know where this chapter was heading.

It is also important to acknowledge at the outset however, while I have experienced accent prejudice, as a white person, I continue to retain a level of privilege and power, not afforded to many global majority people; so whilst this chapter is intended as a reflective account about my experiences as a perceived working-class lecturer, it is in no way comparable to the endemic racism global majority people are subjected to everyday. I have, nonetheless, found ideas such as internalised oppression helpful in understanding my own experiences. I begin with a brief rationale as to why an exploration of accent and accent prejudice remains important.

Who Cares and So What?

Given how many regional accents there are in the United Kingdom, the decline of Received Pronunciation (How the British Monarchy speaks) and the numerous accents we now hear on television alongside accents from the United Kingdom's long and rich history of immigration, does accent matter? As the chapter dis-cusses, my accent, Estuary English, has been argued by some as evidence of traditional class divides becoming lessened, and a more democratic form of speech emerging. I would argue however that the research evidence is clear that ones's accent can have a material impact on how one is perceived and as such judgements will be made. Lippi-Green (2012) writing in an American context, argues that accent discrimination serves to perpetuate existing structural inequalities and power relations. Some interesting studies have focused on accent and employability. For example an American study found that while ethnicity was not a factor in rating employability, a 'heavy' accent was (Carlson & McHenry, 2006). Research by Dixon, Mahoney, and Cocks (2002) found that having a Birmingham accent, known as a Brummie accent, would indicate guilt of a crime. The same study also demonstrated the impact of race and accent, with the strongest judgement of guilt being given to a Black man with a Brummie accent suspected of a blue-collar crime. An American study, by Cantone, Mar-tinez, Willis-Esqueda, and Miller (2019), found that jurors were more likely to give a guilty verdict when judging Mexican American and Black American defendants, compared to white defendants, particularly so when the defendants had a strong and stereotypical accent. Derwing and Munro (2009) argue that people with non-native accents are often discriminated against and subject to harassment. Accent clearly then is important to focus on, not least as a social work academic focusing on issues of social injustice.

In terms of higher education and accent, an article in *The Guardian* newspaper in 2020, reported that students from working-class backgrounds attending universities in England, particular Russell Group Universities, were suffering from classism, with their backgrounds criticised, their accents mocked and derided, and in some cases their intellectual ability questioned (The Guardian, 2020). One student interviewed in the article said:

> Since moving down south a month ago, I can think of at least 10 occasions when my accent, being a relatively strong one from Birmingham, has been brought up and mocked in conversation. Most notably, my peers in politics modules specifically have said they'd never have guessed I'd want to take a subject like politics, and that I should speak more eloquently if I want to be taken seriously.
>
> The Guardian Newspaper, 24/01/22

Accent therefore, is important to consider in the context of oppression and discrimination, as well as identity in all its forms. I now move on to discuss my experiences of speaking with a distinct accent.

School

I was aware from a young age that accent, and how one spoke, could be weaponised, used to categorise people, exclude people and something I needed to worry about. I grew up in Crawley, West Sussex, which is located in the South of England. Crawley is a New Town, built in the late 1950s.[2] Often, people from London moved to the town, with the lure of housing and plenty of jobs. My parents were originally from Kent however, and often appeared concerned about my developing 'Crawley' accent. I often recall being told, 'don't drop your Ts' and 'speak properly'. I recognised that in this particular accent system, consonants would often be missing from the beginning of words, so happy would be 'appy', Ts would disappear from the middle of words, so butter, was Bu-err and 'th' was often pronounced as an 'F', so 'I think so' would be 'I fink so'. I described the Crawley accent at that time, as a watered down version of cockney – a traditional accent coming from a particular part of East London. I therefore developed some of these 'watered down cockney features', which I latterly found out was called Estuary English. My accent however was certainly not as strong or pronounced as some of my school peers and I was often called posh. I did after all pronounce 'Th' as 'th' and would not drop consonants from the start of words although as my parents commented, I would 'drop my Ts'.

In terms of class, this was not something I would understand personally (and very painfully) until I went to university as an undergraduate. In a new town like Crawley, with significant amounts of council housing (social housing), and with lots of jobs due to its proximity to Gatwick airport, class divisions were very subtle – all secondary schools in the town were comprehensive schools. While my parents owned their own home, unlike the majority of my secondary school friends who lived in council houses bigger than my own, any divisions about housing type disappeared very rapidly when former Conservative Prime Minister (1979–1990), Margaret Thatcher, enacted her policy, 'The Right to Buy Scheme', which enabled council house tenants to buy their house at a significant discount.

Thames Estuary English

I therefore speak with an accent that others have labelled, and which I have now embraced, Thames Estuary English, which, as the literature reveals, remains a somewhat contested and debated term, but continues to be a topic of linguistic academic study, both nationally and internationally. The term 'Estuary English' was first used by Rosewarne (1994), where an attempt was made to define this accent and the distinct linguistic features were identified. Rosewarne's definition remains very broad indeed, perhaps unhelpfully so, but is as follows:

> Estuary English is a variety of modified regional speech. It is a mixture of non-regional and local south-eastern pronunciation and intonation. If one imagines a continuum with Received Pronunciation and London speech at either end, EE speakers are to be found grouped in the middle ground.
>
> (Rosewarne, 1994, p. 3)

The estuary reference refers to the River Thames which flows into London and then into the English Channel, with Kent on one side of the river and Essex on the other. Coggle, writing in 1993, argued that Estuary English served as a useful bridge, which allowed traditional class distinctions to be lessened, for example, those with upper class accents could adopt some or all of Estuary English features, what he termed moving down market, while those with traditional cockney accents could move up market by discarding some aspects of Cockney and adopt linguistic features more associated with received pronunciation. He also argued that Estuary English was replacing much of the regional variations in the home countries, i.e. Hampshire, Essex and Kent. Coggle (1993) claimed further that Estuary English may have some street credibility because it was 'urban' rather than rural. Nonetheless negative, and essentially classist, attitudes towards estuary English were highlighted in his book and included delightful comments such as:

> The sad thing is that suburban speak is so anaemic in comparison with the glorious pungency of what went before (1992, p. 88).

> The sounds of English get even more depressing....It [Estuary English] is London of course, but debased London: Slack-jawed, somnambulant London, not the sharp, vivacious chatter of real Cockney.
>
> (Coggle, 1993)

I feel that adapting a South London accent involves mumbling and using the wrong words, and eventually it limits the ability to express oneself (1992, p. 91).

Coggle's book is a celebration of Estuary English however and includes a quiz to test how Estuary English one really is. I scored 43 which according to Coggle reveals 'I almost certainly qualify as a user of Estuary English' (1992, p. 13). Coggle remains hopeful that despite ongoing prejudice about the accent, its rapid geographical and social spread would mean that the accent would become a 'common ground for the coming together of British society' (1992, p. 87). My experiences might suggest otherwise as I go on to discuss.

Davies (2016) in an article on jokes defines Estuary English as a 'variety of lower class South-Eastern English that sounds as if it has Cockney ancestry' (2016, p. 260). Indeed academics have explored the linguistic features of this accent (for example, Hickey, 2007; Rosewarne, 1994;), researched the differences between Estuary English and cockney (for example, Wells, 1994), debated whether it is an accent or dialect (for example, Maidment, 1994; Wells, 1997) and explored regional variations in Estuary English (see, for example, Przedlacka, 2001).

As someone who does not have any familiarity with the academic discipline of English language and linguistics, this has been challenging journey, not least trying to find a way of describing a glottal stop, a distinct feature of Estuary English, and a feature of my everyday speech. While I can demonstrate a glottal stop in action however, I certainly cannot write about it in a technical way, but at best, in my own words, it is not fully pronouncing the consonant at the end of certain words, so for 'cat' – the T at the end of cat is only half formed. Estuary English is therefore an accent and a way of speaking, using syntax that would be considered non-standard English and as such grammatically incorrect. So, in Estuary English syntax, I know nuffink (nothing) about linguistics! So the parental reminder to speak properly as a child, concerned the accent, using correct grammatical form and avoiding using colloquialism – 'have not', instead of 'aint'. For example 'I do not have any money' instead of, 'I aint got no money'. As I go on to discuss later however, I have learnt to 'code switch' depending on the environment I find myself in.

Returning back to Estuary English, as a perceived 'lower-class accent' it has consistently received negative media and public attention as highlighted by Coggle in 1992. Indeed, during the early stages of the writing of this chapter, Lord Digby, a former UK government minister, posted a number of negative Twitter comments about a female TV sports presenter and former footballer, Alex Scott's accent, during her commentary of the Olympics. He specifically noted disapproval at 'dropping her Gs' at the end of words, i.e. 'swimmin', 'fencin', 'rowin' which in his view, spoiled her commentary (Anderson, 2021). I noted the furious debate that subsequently ensued on Twitter, with many posts of support, but also many who criticised her accent. In the tweet exchanges the issue of class also arose with Lord Digby @Digbylj tweeting:

> Alex Scott, please don't play the working class card...Not sounding a g at the end of a word is wrong: period. It's not a question of class, its not a question of accent, it's a question of elocution. Don't let it spoil your otherwise excellent performance.

Likewise, Stacey Dooley, a UK TV presenter, has long been criticised for her accent, and as reported in a tabloid newspaper (Fleet, 2020), Dooley commented that she 'is really not arsed' what people think of her accent, after an online Twitter follower suggested she needed to have elocution lessons.[3] In another newspaper Dooley described the 'obsession' with her accent, which she found 'fucking boring' (Barr, 2019). She has also been accused of being a 'mockney', i.e. putting on a cockney accent, as she is from Luton, and exaggerating the features of her accent over time.

Stacey Solomon, who originally appeared on *The X-Factor*, a very popular singing competition show, coming third in 2009, similarly discussed in a newspaper, peoples' preconceptions about her because of her Estuary accent. Such preconceptions focused on her apparent stupidity and lack of education. For me however, there is a striking gendered aspect to speaking with such an accent. Indeed, Jamie Oliver, a TV chef originally from Essex, and Damon Albarn, a musician, while both being accused of being 'mockneys' (Crystall, date unknown) have certainly not experienced the same level of criticism and derision, nor assumptions made about their intelligence, taste and moral character. Indeed, there is a tradition of 'Essex girl' jokes, which portray young Essex women with strong Estuary English accents, as uneducated, working class, lacking taste (dyed blonde hair and white stiletto shoes) fake and being sexually promiscuous (Carter, 2019). Skeggs (2004) has commented, for example, that the Essex girl has become the 'condensed signifier of the epitome of the white working class woman in the UK' (2004, p. 112). Indeed, an augmented reality TV programme, called *The Only Way Is Essex*, known affectionately as TOWIE, has further cemented the Essex girl stereotypes to some degree, i.e. blond (or dyed blonde hair), heavily made up, fake (as in having had plastic surgery, botox etc.), wearing expensive designer clothes, and are in and out of difficult relationships (Nunn & Biressi, 2013). On the other hand, some of the colloquialisms used by the actors in the programme have now become common parlance in the UK context, for example 'well jell', 'reem' and 'vajazzle'.[4-6]

University

I studied for a degree in Politics, in what is now termed an 'old university' in the North East of England. My Estuary English accent was a clear marker that I had attended a state school. At this university, there were not many of us from state schools, with the majority of state-educated students formerly attending grammar schools, and even less from comprehensive schools. Those of us with 'state school accents' from across the country, nonetheless found each other, and we rallied against the 'majority others' who were pejoratively termed the 'agrics', 'sloanes' and the 'ra-raas'. We criticised the volume of their speech, their posh drawl, their confidence and we were shocked at the rugby team's antics.

Class differences had never before identified themselves so starkly to me, and I realised I had a complete lack of cultural and social capital as a first generation higher education learner from a comprehensive school in Crawley. If only I had known about Bourdieu's work at that time, I could have located my confusing experiences in something tangible, rather than fumbling around, feeling terribly homesick for three long years, and either being accused of being one of those rich 'southerners' or else a cockney. I was neither of course, but the journey from being one of the posher ones at school (but not the poshest) to a cockney and 'state educated' in this new institution was tough. I recall being accused of 'fiddling the finance forms' so I could get a full grant – this from someone with a strong Northern working-class identity, who did not receive a grant because her parents were both senior teachers. Some other students would ask me 'what school had I attended', assuming if I was at university I must have attended a well-known Public (private) School. I used to respond to such questions by saying 'its unlikely you would have heard of the name of my Comprehensive School!' My university tutor told me, 'people like me', i.e. from comprehensive schools, had been given much lower A level grade offers as a way to increase participation. I wondered if I should have felt grateful?

When I first arrived at the university accommodation, there was a conversation about what series of BMW cars their dads preferred! They asked me – I responded, that I did not have a dad (at that point he was no longer in my life) but that my Step-Dad drove a Nissan Micra! I therefore felt confused about class, identity, accent and why I was subject to such diverse perceptions about who I was. I lost my voice, confidence and felt othered. I did not know the rules of academic engagement, how to reference or what to do in a lecture or seminar. I lost confidence to talk in seminars and doubted my intellectual ability to be in that institution. I noticed behaviours that were alien to me, i.e. the rugby team antics, I knew that if my male friends at home engaged in such behaviours, i.e. vandalising the coach on the way back from a rugby match, then rather than it all being 'jolly good japes', they would have been arrested for criminal damage. I discovered new foods, mangetout was a vegetable I had never seen previously!

I remember writing a letter to my former sociology A level teacher in my first year, telling him about my confusing and alienating experiences. I was angry with my school that they had not sufficiently prepared me for this environment – why had they supported me going to such a university when I probably would have felt more comfortable in the Polytechnic. He wrote back and said parents had paid a lot of money for their children to be at university, so it was inevitable there would be a lot of privately educated students from privileged backgrounds there! At school I had felt cared for, liked, nurtured and was pushed academically and intellectually. I had imagined university would be like my school but in fact, it felt like an educational conveyor belt – it felt transactional and distant – not least when sitting in large lecture halls, thinking 'what the fuck am I doing here?' My eyes were therefore forced wide open to confront very directly issues of class, privilege and discrimination – it was a good education, albeit an extremely painful and lonely lesson – but one that has informed my pedagogical practices today. I would never want any student in a classroom where I am teaching (note not lecturing) to feel the way I did.

Accent, Social Hierarchy and Education

Ascherson (1994) in a rather controversial newspaper article, argued that:

> ...for at least a century, accent in England has been two things: a vertical indicator about geographical origins, and a horizontal caste-mark separating 'top people' from the rest.

Accents can also be liked or not liked, for example the media often reports surveys, albeit it not academically robust, of what is Britain's favourite accent and conversely what is the least favourite accent. A poll reported in 2022, for example, cited a Birmingham accent as Britain's least favourite and an Irish accent as the most favourite – interesting as Ireland, of course, is not in the United Kingdom. The poll found that Scouse (Liverpool), Mancunian (Manchester), Cockney (London) and Glaswegian accents ranked low on the list, while received pro- nunciation, Welsh, Yorkshire, West Country and Geordie (Newcastle) were placed highly on the list (McCallig, 2022). More robust academic studies have been undertaking research into accent preferences and one in particular noted gender differences (see, for example, Coupland & Bishop, 2007), with women being more likely to value stronger accents than men.

Honey (1989) argues that there are three factors that have helped accents gain their position in the social hierarchy. The first factor is the 'strength' of the accent, for example an accent deemed to be moderate rather than strong. The second factor concerns how educated the accent portrays its speaker to be, and the third factor concerns geography, i.e. is the accent rural or urban? What Honey does not consider is the intersectionality of class, gender and race. As noted previously in this chapter, a woman with an Estuary English accent appears to be more critiqued than men with such accents. Indeed, David Beckham, a famous and very rich, now ex-footballer married to one of the Spice Girls, Victoria, has not been derided because of his Estuary English accent.

It is interesting however to follow up on Honey's (1989) notion of accent being a signifier of education, possibly because of the connotation of being working class and having poor educational outcomes. As the *The Guardian* article dis- cussed earlier revealed, accent was related to perceptions of intelligence as one student commented:

> You'll never get anywhere talking like that, it makes you sound stupid. 'You need to try and flatten your Yorkshire accent'. That was a member of staff in my third year of university. I tried to not to cry, and sort of managed, crumbling completely when I left the room. What could I say to that? They must be right. They knew what they were talking about.

The danger is, of course, that such elitist attitude and perceptions about accent will follow people into the workplace and into other aspects of their lives.

Being a Social Worker

I qualified as a social worker and then worked in a number of London Boroughs. I do not recall there being negative experiences or reactions to the way I spoke. Perhaps having a distinct accent helped me form relationships with the diverse families I worked with. Maybe some of them saw me as 'one of them' and maybe others would always see a social worker as other, to be feared and loathed. My relatively young age was more of a problem I felt than accent, in creating rapport with families where I was clearly much younger than the parents. Given the diversity of accents in the teams I worked with and the people I engaged with – accent did not preoccupy me, rather the social injustices the families I worked with faced on a daily basis. The inner London borough I worked in as a newly qualified social worker had significant disparities between its rich and poor residents. I noticed how middle-class parents operated (some would bring their lawyers along to social work meetings) and were treated very differently. I remember all too starkly a middle-class parent, who refused to let me enter her house, although she let the child protection police in, and I was left sitting on the doorstep. It was clear her daughter was suffering neglect and some degree of emotional abuse, yet this deemed to be an 'eccentric' Mother and we subsequently received supportive letters from 'important' people about the family and the investigation was closed. This was class privilege in operation, and I began to critically question whether social work was actually helping families, and by helping, I mean empowering them to change their lives meaningfully, or else was the profession merely tinkering around the edges, our job being to mitigate the worst effects of capitalism. In other words, were we nothing more than agents of the state, essentially policing working class and/or global majority people and their families? The care versus control issue has of course been a debate ever since the very inception of the profession (Finch & Parker, 2020) but the notion of a social worker as a sinister, surveilling and controlling state actor remains. Certainly it is something that with my cowriter David McKendrick, we have subsequently written about using the example of the policy called PREVENT, a strategy to identify and protect people at risk from being drawn into extremism and terrorism.

The research in social work is clear that the profession is far from what its values purport, some key examples include, an over-representation of black and dual heritage children in the care system (Bywaters, Kwhali, Brady, Sparks, & Bos, 2017), with associated poor outcomes in later life, an over-representation of Black men being detained under the Mental Health Act and over-medicated (Keating, 2007), and a lack of diversity in the profession itself, which despite being a majority female profession, is mostly led by white men (Turner, 2017).

There is also a similar demographic amongst social work professors with a disproportionate number of white men.

From Social Worker to Lecturer

My journey from front-line practitioner to social work lecturer in a college of Further and Higher Education was rather serendipitous. I had previously moved from South London to the London Borough of Barking and Dagenham, an outer London Borough situated to the North East of Central London. I was pregnant, had bought a property with my partner and did not intend to return to my social work post in South London. The shock of being a new Mother prompted me to begin working as a freelance off-site practice educator for the college.[7] I then eventually applied for a Lecturing post at the college, where I taught social work to undergraduate students for eight years. The Further Education culture permeated the Higher Education provision in a positive way, so lengthy lecturer exposition was frowned upon and there was a focus on learning objectives, assessing learning as one went along, and the importance of writing good learning outcomes. I learnt my craft of 'teaching' while utilising my former social work group work skills. The college was diverse in its student body as well as its educational provision. Staff were diverse in some respects, and one heard Estuary English, Cockney and Essex accents, although global majority colleagues were few and far between.

Going Back to University

Given such negative experiences as an undergraduate I found myself returning nonetheless to university to undertake a variety of courses, not least I trained as a social worker at the London School of Economics. I felt much more comfortable in this environment as I had more cultural capital and my fellow students, in social work and on other programmes, were from diverse backgrounds, so there was diversity in accent. Class differences, while present, were no longer so stark and as social work students, there was some sense of shared values, namely an understanding of structural disadvantage and which groups were likely to be subject to discrimination.

However, this comfortableness I experienced at a London university (and indeed two others I attended) whilst initially training, then working as a social worker in London disappeared when I attended a university in the South of England to undertake a part-time doctorate in social work. I was confronted with the limits of my knowledge of grammar, the anxiety of having to unlearn and no longer being able to 'wing it' as I had done in previous studies. One distinct accent incidence stood out however when a fellow student in a class I was undertaking a group work task with, thought it ok to mock my accent by doing a grotesque EastEnders impression of me and making reference to it.[8] I said, 'That is not how I speak, I do not have a cockney accent'. He continued again with his impression of my accent, and I told him I did not feel comfortable with him doing impressions of me. The lecturer intervened at this point and made some bland comment about the student's own accent – he was French. I made sure to avoid this student again although I chastised myself for not being more assertive about how he had made me feel.

Inherent in this exchange was, of course, classism on his part; he often chose not to socialise with the student group and when I had asked about it, he commented that our values were very different. He was also a member of staff, and involved in this exchange, was clearly his need to feel superior to me, a woman who was much younger than him, indeed I was the youngest in my cohort. I also was aware that he failed a PhD previously and so this was perhaps his 'second chance'. The classist nature of the interaction however hurt and upset me, and perhaps unconsciously reawakened my Mother's chastisement of my accent 'slips', dropping my Ts, using glottal stops. It also reawakened a comment my dad had made one day when teachers mentioned the possibility of going to university, that I would not get into university because of the way I spoke.

Nonetheless I enjoyed my doctorate immensely, not least because for me, it was respite from the demands of a 2 year old child and I felt I was reawakening my brain, and I enjoyed having a private space in my brain to think about my study.

Being a Social Work Academic

After 8 years of working at the college, and just as I submitted my Doctorate in Social Work Thesis, I moved to a post-92 university. I cannot recall when I felt I then moved from Social Work Lecturer to social work academic and indeed, I still balk at the term 'academic'. My first attempt to get an article published was extremely painful and I was not sure I would make it as an academic. I did not understand the journal format, what was required or how I would even have the writing skills to manage such an arduous task. Luckily, with some good reviewers, support from my former doctoral supervisor and encouragement from my mentor, it finally was published.

Being an 'academic' is very exposing however and in my early days as a lecturer I was surprised at the emotional impact teaching had on me, not least being subject to students' transferences and projections. There is something about writing for publication which makes one feel even more exposed, alongside the pressure to publish. This chapter, for example, while conforming to some features of academic writing, is autoethnographic in nature and reveals personal stories about me. I was worried I would come across as too 'moany', or 'poor me, people have been nasty because of my accent' but my accent is part of my identity, I cannot be something else, nor do I chose to lose my accent.

It is clear that academics from all disciplines have to manage the demands of academic speak, in terms of writing for publication, lecturing and other knowledge exchange activities while engaging in our everyday languages and cultural practices. Practices such as 'language' or code 'switching' are perhaps common practices in academia anyway, depending on disciplines and in everyday parlance I certainly do not speak like I write. I knew this anyway, but it was brought home during the height of the COVID pandemic, when my younger son overheard my lecture online. He said he did not recognise my voice, that it 'didn't sound like my mum'. Instead, he said I sounded like Teresa May, a former UK Conservative Prime Minister! I sound nothing like her of course, but what he meant was that I sounded 'posher', used academic conventions in my speech patterns and had a more authoritative tone.

Nonetheless ensuring my teaching practices, and to some extent my writing practise, are accessible is something very important to me, not least because being a social work academic has additional challenges. There is a conflict between social work values, i.e. being accessible, good communication skills, engaging and developing relationships with people from a wide variety of backgrounds, actively promoting social justice and challenging discrimination and oppression, with the traditional values of Higher Education, namely cultures and practices based on white middle-class male sensibilities. At a recent doctoral conference I attended at the University of East London, for example, despite the diversity of students and presenters in terms of protected characteristics, there was still a reliance on dead white middle-class male theorists, i.e. Bourdieu and Foucault to name but a few. Likewise social work, despite its rhetoric, still utilises theory and research from mostly white, male middle-class academics, although the focus on decolonising the curriculum will hopefully begin to change the current status quo.

As a social work academic, working in post-92 universities, formerly in East London and now at Suffolk University, with students from a huge variety of backgrounds, my accent has not been an issue. However, I worked in a connected institution in another part of London where I taught a Master's dissertation module. I was greeted with 'how does it feel to work here when you come from East London'? I was immediately perturbed by this comment. I noticed the 'coming from East London'. Was working in East London meant I came from East London? Was an assumption being made about my accent and therefore my origins? Was there a mixing up of place of work with where I lived or had grown up? More concerningly did this comment imply I was supposed to feel grateful that I had been 'allowed' to teach in what this person clearly considered a more prestigious institution? I replied, 'You are lucky to have me'.

I experienced further comments from this person, he appeared surprised when I got good module feedback; he made assumptions I had not taught in a higher education institution before (I had taught 8 years elsewhere before coming to East London) and when a group of colleagues went out for dinner, there were comments made about my food and drink choice (pizza and beer). I did an exaggerated Estuary English accent in response, 'I ate wine, tastes likes piss innit', I noticed him wince in disgust and mimic 'innit'... Here was someone teaching social work students that clearly had not reflected on class and associated accents.

I wonder whether I have restricted myself to working in post-92 universities as my one attempt to apply for a job in an old university was not positive; I did not get the job after all, but I had not been sure whether to apply, would I fit in for example, and be subjective to accentism? What would the students think of me? Would I have to work harder to have any credibility? Would they think I was stupid? Similarly in having worked in one institution discussed earlier, albeit not in a permanent capacity, I felt like an outsider by virtue of accent, dress style and my social work identity which meant I was focused much more on external worlds than internal worlds, which in my job I had felt as a luxury – the people I worked with needed the basics of shelter, food and income after all.

Internalised Oppression?

I am now reflecting on the extent to which I may have internalised classism and accentsism, alongside parental memories that my accent was not quite good enough and that 'I would never get into university'. In fact, I have studied at six higher education institutions. In writing this chapter, have I perhaps focused on the negative experiences of accent rather than the majority of the times that my accent has not preoccupied me, or indeed preoccupied other people? Internalised oppression therefore was a theory initially proposed by Fanon (1965) and taken up later by many others. This is a process whereby one takes on, or accepts unconsciously the devaluation or inferiorisation of one's self and group. My own distaste at times towards Stacey Dooley's accent is precisely an example of this, that I have internalised my own accent oppression.

Class Identity

So, who am I? This chapter has somewhat skirted around the issue of how I perceive my own class identity. I feel somewhere between working class and middle class, straddled between these two identities but it's a continually shifting line that is often relational and situational. My current occupation clearly defines me as middle class, I receive sick pay and a pension, I own my own house. My children are middle class, although my partner, a senior NHS manager, has a working-class identity. I certainly describe myself as coming from an 'ordinary' background with limited money, but we certainly were not poor. I largely grew up in a single-parent household and wrote about this experience in a short blog for a social work project (Finch, 2016), where I traced the origins of becoming a social worker and the development of my political ideology, an awareness of global social injustice and my early feminist leanings. I started the main body of the chapter with a subheading entitled, 'Who Cares and So What?' Does it matter if I self-define as working class or not? Does it matter if other people make assumptions about my class identity? The answer to both these questions is, I do not really know.

Celebrating Accents, Diversity and Switching It Up

I would like to end this chapter on a positive, celebratory but equally cautionary note – the caution being that I need to actively reflect on my own class prejudices or distaste towards particular accents. I have to admit to having inwardly 'winced' at Stacey Dooley's accent, and so as a social work academic, I should challenge accentism, and call out its associated classism and gendered undertones, both upwards and downwards. I recognise my own inverted class snobbery and my behaviour at my undergraduate university to mock and despise the 'ra-rass' and the 'Sloane rangers' was of course unacceptable. I recognise I need to do more in terms of teaching social work students about all aspects of class and to reflect on accents, as one possible identifier of class, and what they might mean for us individually in terms of identity as well as how society discriminates against certain accents and classes of people.

I recognise my ability to code-switch, i.e. the ability to turn on or turn off my Estuary English depending on what the situation requires. Truth be told, I sometimes turn it on full blast, to deliberately provoke people. Living in London however is a constant reminder of the many thousands of accents (and languages) that exist; so rather than be part of the problem by internalising my own experiences of accentism, I chose instead to embrace my Estuary English, to accept my accent will change depending on the situation at hand, and to celebrate my glottal stopping!

Notes

1. Essex is a large county that borders North and East London.
2. New Towns in the United Kingdom developed in the post-war era under the powers of the New Towns Act (1946) and the first wave were intended to relocate populations in poor, bombed-out areas and to address housing shortage issues. Crawley is located 28 miles away from London, and so many of its original inhabitants came from London.
3. Can't be arsed means I cannot be bothered or care.
4. Very jealous.
5. Brilliant, cool, good or fashionable.
6. A beauty treatment in which a woman's vaginal pubic hair is adorned with crystals, glitter or other decoration.
7. An off-site practice educator is someone who goes into a variety of social work agencies and assesses social work students in these settings.
8. *EastEnders* is a long running TV soap opera on BBC1. The *EastEnders* refers to people who live in a part of East London.

References

Andersson, J. (2021, July 31). BBC presenter Alex Scott challenges lord who says her accent 'spoils' coverage: 'I'm working class and proud'. *The Independent*. Retrieved from https://inews.co.uk/sport/olympics/bbc-presenter-alex-scott-olympics-lord-digby-jones-accent-working-class-proud-1129788. Accessed on April 1, 2022.
Ascherson, N. (1994, July 8). Britain's crumbling ruling class is losing the accent of authority. *Independent Sunday*. Retrieved from https://www.phon.ucl.ac.uk/home/estuary/ascherson.htm. Accessed on April 1, 2022.

Barr. (2019, July). Retrieved from https://www.independent.co.uk/life-style/stacey-dooley-accent-strictly-come-dancing-glow-up-cosmopolitan-interview-a8854231. htmlTheIdpendenceonUSnday,*th July

Bywaters, P., Kwhali, J., Brady, J., Sparks, T., & Bos, E. (2017). Out of sight, out of mind: Ethnic inequalities in child protection and out-of-home care intervention rates. *British Journal of Social Work, 47*(7), 1884–1902.

Cantone, J. A., Martinez, L. N., Willis-Esqueda, C., & Miller, T. (2019). Sounding guilty: How accent bias affects juror judgments of culpability. *Journal of Ethnicity in Criminal Justice, 17*(3), 228–253. doi:10.1080/15377938.2019.1623963

Carlson, H. K., & McHenry, M. A. (2006). Effect of accent and dialect on employability. *Journal of Counselling Employment, 43*, 70–83.

Carter, A. (2019). 'Essex girls' in the comedy club: Stand-up, ridicule and 'value struggles'. *European Journal of Cultural Studies, 22*(5–6), 763–780.

Coggle, P. (1993). *Do you speak estuary? The new standard English – How to spot it and speak it.* London: Bloomsbury.

Coupland, N., & Bishop, H. (2007). Ideologised values for British accents[1]. *Journal of SocioLinguistics, 11*, 74–93. doi:10.1111/j.1467-9841.2007.00311.x

Davies, C. (2016). How jokes change and may be changed: Simplifying, transforming and revealing. *Tertium Linguistic Journal, 1*(1&2), 253–265.

Derwing, T. M., & Munro, M. J. (2009). Putting accent in its place: Rethinking obstacles to communication. *Language Teaching, 42*(4), 476–490.

Dixon, J. A., Mahoney, B., & Cocks, R. (2002). Accents of guilt?: Effects of regional accent, race, and crime type on attributions of guilt. *Journal of Language and Social Psychology, 21*(2), 162–168. doi:10.1177/02627X02021002004

Fanon, F. (1965). *The wretched of the earth.* New York, NY: Grove Weidenfield.

Finch, J. (2016). "Yellow star" in social work in 40 objects. Retrieved from https://socialworkin40objects.com/2016/07/11/yellow-star/. Accessed on April 20, 2022.

Finch, J., & Parker, J. (2020). The history and context of contemporary social work (including global social work). In J. Parker (Ed.), *Introducing social work.* London: Learning Matters, Sage.

Fleet, H. (2020). The express newspaper Stacey Dooley hits back at fan for criticising her 'awful' accent: 'I'm not really ar**ed'. Retrieved from https://www.express.co.uk/celebrity-news/1314440/Stacey-Dooley-twitter-accent-elocution-fan-bbc-documentary-strictly-come-dancing-latest. Accessed on April 20, 2022.

Hickey, R. (2007). Dartspeak and Estuary English advanced metropolitan speech in Ireland and England. In U. Smit, S. Dollinger, J. Hüttner, U. Lutzky, & G. Kaltenböck (Eds.), *Tracing English through time: Explorations in language variation.* Vienna: Braumüller,.

Honey, J. (1989). *Does accent matter?: The Pygmalion factor.* London: Faber and Faber.

Keating, F. (2007). African and Caribbean men and mental health, a race equality foundation briefing paper. Retrieved from https://raceequalityfoundation.org.uk/wp-content/uploads/2018/03/health-brief5.pdf. Accessed on May 3, 2022.

Lippi-Green, R. (2012). *English with an accent: Language, ideology, and discrimination in the United States* (2nd ed.). London: Routledge.

Maidment, J. A. (1994). Estuary English: Hybrid or hype? Paper presented at the 4th New Zealand conference on language & society, Christchurch, New Zealand, August 1994. Lincoln University. Retrieved from https://www.phon.ucl.ac.uk/home/estuary/maidment.pdf. Accessed on April 2, 2022.

McCallig, E. (2022). YouGov ranked the best and worst accents in the British Isles and it's sparked a row. *Indy500.com*. Retrieved from https://www.indy100.com/viral/yougov-accents-british-isles-sparked-debate-b1988176. Accessed April 1, 2022.

Nunn, H., & Biressi, A. (2013). Class, gender and the DocuSoap: The only way is Essex. In C. Carter, L. Steiner, & L. McLaughlin (Eds.), *The Routledge companion to media and gender*. London: Routledge.

Przedlacka, J. (2001). Estuary English and RP: Some recent findings. *Studia Anglica Posnaniensia, 36*, 35–50. Retrieved from http://www.phon.ox.ac.uk/files/people/przedlacka/sap36_jp.pdf. Accessed on April 1, 2022.

Rosewarne, D. (1994). Estuary English: The New R.P. *English Today, 37*, 3–7.

Skeggs, B. (2004). *Class, self, culture*. London: Routledge.

The Guardian Newspaper. (2020, October 24). UK's top universities urged to act on classism and accent prejudice. Retrieved from https://www.theguardian.com/education/2020/oct/24/uk-top-universities-urged-act-classism-accent-prejudice. Accessed on May 3, 2022.

Turner, A. (2017, October 23). Social work leaders' lack of diversity out of step with workforce. *Community Care*. Retrieved from https://www.communitycare.co.uk/2017/10/23/social-work-leaders-lack-diversity-step-workforce/. Accessed on May 2, 2022.

Wells, J. (1994). Transcribing estuary English: A discussion document. *Speech Hearing and Language: UCL Work in Progress, 8*, 259–267. Retrieved from http://citeseerx.ist.psu.edu/viewdoc/download?doi=10.1.1.62.7465&rep=rep1&type=pdf Accessed on April 1, 2022.

Wells, J. (1997). What is Estuary English? Retrieved from https://www.phon.ucl.ac.uk/home/estuary/estuary.pdf. Accessed on May 1, 2022.

Chapter 14

Concluding Chapter: Tackling 'the Taboo': The Personal Is Political (and It's Scholarly Too)

Michael Pierse

Having been privileged to have read all of the other contributions to this book, and having been buoyed, enthused, moved, energised and educated by the richness of the insights they articulate, I write the following as a concluding chapter. The purpose of this chapter is to draw together observations and themes across the volume, asking what they suggest in terms of potential future research *and action* within the academy. In the autoethnographic spirit of the rest of the book, I do so by way of a detour into my own journey into academia and some observations on the affective and intellectual trajectories of working-class students who are often failed, but also in many cases liberated and conscientised, by higher education (HE).

My principal area of research is representations of the working class in Irish literature, but I'm also interested more broadly in cultural production, in things like film, TV, festivals and popular culture; where do our notions about class come from and what kinds of ideas, stereotypes, ideologies and distinctions do we associate with class? Cultural representation can define people, enable them, or, as is often the case, limit their horizons. As someone who grew up in inner-city Dublin, the strong sense of disadvantage in my community began to be theorised more fully for me once I got to university and began to read working-class literature. That set me on a path to the research and teaching I do at university level today and like many of the academics in this volume, I thus have the blessing of something of a vocation: a job – and research path – that allows me to write and teach about deeply personal and emphatically communal concerns – about my class, its history, its representation and the role of systems, institutions and ideologies in shaping its experiences. Autoethnographic analysis of such journeys into the academy – in which the personal and political shape the scholarly and pedagogical – would seem, logically, apt, yet as so many of the contributors here have also suggested it can also feel either too intense or too self-indulgent. All the more reason that the present volume is fascinating. In exploring how

The Lives of Working Class Academics, 203–217

Copyright © 2023 Michael Pierse

Published under exclusive licence by Emerald Publishing Limited

doi:10.1108/978-1-80117-057-420221014

working-class academics are made – and how they generate so much hope (or as Crew terms it, in this volume, 'aspirational capital') as to excel in their disciplines – we get glimpses of how education can facilitate marginalised people in gaining a profound understanding of themselves and their society, leading them to roles in which they can in turn facilitate others in transformational activism. As Paulo Freire argued, 'it is necessary that the weakness of the powerless is transformed into a force capable of announcing justice. For this to happen, a total denouncement of fatalism is necessary. We are transformative beings and not beings for accommodation' (2021/1997, p. 6). These explorations also teach, however, about how that success can come following often difficult and painful experiences of exclusionary practices in educational settings. As Freire also observes,

> There is no such thing as a *neutral* educational process. Education either functions as an instrument that is used to facilitate the integration of the younger generation into the logic of the present system and bring about conformity to it, *or* it becomes 'the practice of freedom,' the means by which men and women deal critically and creatively with reality and discover how to participate in the transformation of their world.
>
> (2005/1968, p. 34)

In the writing of working-class lives, schools and universities are so often the sites of contradictory impulses. For example, in one of her most evocative poems, Paula Meehan captures powerfully the paradox of how education can both wound and motivate. She writes, in *The Exact Moment I Became a Poet* (2000, p. 24) of how her journey into her lifelong calling began in 1963, when a teacher in her inner-city Dublin school

> rapping the duster on the easel's peg
> half obscured by a cloud of chalk
>
> said *Attend to your books, girls,*
> *or mark my words, you'll end up*
> *in the sewing factory.*

For Meehan, that members of her own and her friends' families worked in this factory was less the cause of her ensuing anger – and hazy bewilderment, in that 'cloud of chalk' – than the way in which the teacher's admonition was phrased,

> that those words 'end up' robbed
> the labour of its dignity.

The alienation of the factory floor and that of the classroom are suddenly crystallised – as if in an Althusserian formula – as one and the same, in a brutalising system:

But: I *saw* them: mothers, aunts and neighbours
trussed like chickens
on a conveyor belt,

getting sewn up the way my granny
sewed the sage and onion stuffing in the birds.

Words could pluck you,
leave you naked,
your lovely shiny feathers all gone.

As we've seen from the present volume, such experiences of being shamed, undermined and alienated – 'sewn up', 'plucked' and 'trussed' – in an educational setting can produce lifelong aversions to the education system, yet paradoxically, as in Meehan's sense of this 'exact moment' as the source of her budding craft, they can also generate defiant determination and pride. And after all, as Meehan concedes, if only partially sardonically, 'the teacher was right/and no one knows it like I do myself'. Like the student educators who 'reported that they had little personal experience of disadvantage [which they felt to be ...] *alien, unfamiliar*, and *uncomfortable*' in White's research (Chapter 5) for this volume, Meehan's teacher may simply not have understood or possessed 'the language to talk about class'. Meehan did indeed attend to her books, ascending to the lofty position of Ireland Professor of Poetry five decades later, in 2013. Yet her poem also reminds us of the dignity of the so summarily discarded (by the teacher, and by extension by history, by society) women who came before her and the humiliations of an education system in which their labour was mechanically 'plucked' of its dignity. Meehan reminds us of how it feels to be categorised because of where or what you come from, those searing, emotive lines speaking to those who've known that sudden feeling of being excluded by a callous or careless comment that hurt. For her teacher, however, what she said about getting an education and not ending up in monotonous, low-paid work probably just seemed like solid, sensible advice. From her perspective, it might even have seemed like feminism: an attempt to rescue working-class girls from alienating factory labour. But the hurt caused also conveys the extent to which educators, even with good intentions, can be oblivious to exclusionary practices; ideologies that hurt and alienate can seem 'normal'. As Pierre Bourdieu once put it,

> The educational system helps to provide the dominant class with what Max Weber terms 'the theoricy of its own privilege' [...] through the practical justification of the established order which it achieves by using the overt connection between qualifications and jobs as a smokescreen for the connection – which it *records surreptitiously*, under cover of formal equality – between the qualifications people obtain and the cultural capital they have inherited – in other words, through the legitimacy it confers on the transmission of this form of heritage. The most successful

ideological effects are those which have no need of words, and ask no more than complicitous silence.

(1977, p. 188)

As the Irish sociologist of education Kathleen Lynch has recently observed, 'things that matter most are often the things we speak about least. They are the taboo subjects, kept hidden, and if spoken of are discussed in euphemisms or metaphors that hide the full truth. Social class is one such subject in Ireland' (2020). Common assumptions around class can seem so obvious, so commonsense that we spontaneously accept them, or they're spoken about in ways that hide their real, lived reality, but Bourdieu and Lynch, like Meehan, invite us to delve deeper, to ask if 'common sense' might not be so sensible after all.

In this context, educational approaches can, as also enlarged upon by the foregoing contributors, assume the common sense of a deficit model of working-class life and the logical corollary that the classroom ought to be corrective. In these situations, class itself is everywhere implicitly present but rarely explicitly discussed. Baker et al. point to the importance of educating and talking about class, and being self-aware in how we speak about class, in ways that clearly weren't part of Meehan's experience. As they write:

> Another silence that is typical of many educational settings is their failure to advert to the reality of social class. In cultural terms, schools are fundamentally middle-class institutions [...]. Their organizational procedures and mores assume a lifestyle and set of resources that middle and upper class households are most likely to possess. Parents and children who are outside this frame are variously defined by middle class teachers as culturally deficient or deviant [...]. Students are expected to have class-specific skills that the schools themselves do not teach [...]. The failure of schools to acknowledge the cultural dissonance that exists between their mores and practices and those of students from diverse class (and ethnic and racial) backgrounds exacerbates their educational failure and their sense of alienation from the education process itself [...]. The deeply classed culture of schools, and in particular of universities, is exacerbated by a lack of systematic education about social class.
>
> (2009, p. 144)

It is not simply, then, that educational settings often reproduce class shame and classist stereotypes in everything from casual remarks to institutional practices, but that the lack of a 'systemic education about social class' facilitates the ignorance in which such remarks and practices can pass as *unremarkable*, or even as the 'common sense' that produces that chalky cloud of confusion and shame for many working-class students. As Barker et al. argue, 'the failure to name social class inequalities has several indirect effects on the process and procedures of schooling. It leaves the attitudes of students and teachers in relation to class inequality untouched' (2009, p. 156). By writing about our experiences of class in educational settings, we bear testimony to the dangers of this systemic avoidance.

Awkward Voices and 'Intense Silence'

bell hooks broached this important issue in relation to her own experience of attending elite institutions in a US context, arguing that 'nowhere is there a more intense silence about the reality of class differences than in educational settings' (2003, p. 142). Those who break that silence by pointing to the obvious class inequalities in academic settings often appear as (and are treated as) awkward voices, as Crew discussed in this volume, and even when opportunities arise within institutions to discuss classism in education, those on the receiving end of class inequality can feel reticent about disclosing their relevant experiences, such is the impact of the habitual lack of discourse about class. As Sanders and Mahalingam note,

> This lack of discourse—manifested as taboos restricting discussions of money or economic status—prevents economically advantaged individuals from critically reflecting on their privileges, rendering those privileges invisible, and further renders economically disadvantaged individuals mute and unable to discuss their lived experiences.
>
> (2012, p. 112)

A number of years back, I was invited by the organisers of a topical seminar series to give a talk at my *alma mater*, Trinity College Dublin (TCD), on the subject of 'Social Class in Dublin: The Final Taboo'. The title was theirs, not mine, but it resonated with my experience as a former TCD student who had grown up in a different world precisely 17 minutes' walk away from this elite HE institution. As an undergraduate, I had made that walk daily from my home in Seville Place, in north inner-city Dublin, one of the most economically deprived areas in Ireland and an area synonymous with drug addiction and crime. On the programme for the event, a statement from the organisers read: 'There is a representative gap between the city in which Trinity resides, not least in terms of language, race and class, and the images and narratives of that city put forth in the broader culture.' For me, this was unequivocally true, not least of the university itself, though the opportunities opened up by that university would also set me on a path through academia, in which my positionality, socially, became part of my professionalisation: I later embarked on a PhD there about Irish working-class writing, which has subsequently sent me into an academic career. What I studied at university, and the kindness and encouragement of academics at TCD, played a significant role in broadening my range of opportunities, for all that I also keenly felt the fish-out-of-water imposterism that working-class students and academics (and many of the contributors to the current volume) have so often experienced and continue to experience in such hallowed institutions.

Coming back to TCD to talk about class dredged up a range of emotions and memories, and I asked organisers if I could speak to these – as both a scholar and on a more personal level – which they agreed was fine, but just as some of the scholars in this volume admit to uncertainty when asked to discuss the personal in the context of the professional, I hesitated. An obvious, difficult memory of exclusion emerged as I considered how I could approach that 'Final Taboo' of the event's title, but would it seem bizarre or unseemly, self-indulgent or unprofessional, to discuss my own emotional and intellectual journey through the academy in relation to the broader experiences of class in Irish HE? Was it proper to speak as both a professional concerned with representation and class and as an individual who had endured its 'hidden injuries'? (Sennett & Cobb, 1972) As Fourie concedes, citing Winkler, 'it is challenging for autoethnographers to take a deep look at their personal life and experiences but still stay focussed on culture – to decide if they are self-indulged narcissists or if they rather are self-reflexive, vulnerable scholars. To the latter I can add: who wish to make a difference?' (2021, p. 11) Academics who chart their personal journeys no doubt often repeatedly second-guess themselves in this way, partially the result of that silencing of class-related issues in educational settings described earlier. However, as the present volume illustrates, such combinations of scholarly rigour and personal, critical, reflexive introspection yield powerful lessons, and can prove cathartic for both those who recount those experiences and those who read them.

Coming to Trinity from a background of unemployment and poverty in inner-city Dublin, I had very mixed experiences within the institution, in terms of how class for me was *felt*, in relational and personal terms, keeping in mind E. P. Thompson's important qualification about class being a 'relationship, not a thing' (1980, p. 10). What Thompson meant of course is that class is about more than graphs illustrating divisions of wealth, nor can we properly conceive of it as something static, or essentialised; class is all about relationships – to wealth, to each other, to historic forces and also to representation. These relationships are far more than mere designators of social positioning; they are sometimes the origins of deeply personal traumas and life-defining wounds that go far beyond the economic per se. It is salutary to return to the words of Sennett and Cobb of five decades ago:

> Class society takes away from all the people within it the feeling of secure dignity in the eyes of others and of themselves. It does so in two ways: first, by the images it projects of why people belong to high or low classes – class presented as the ultimate outcome of personal ability; second, by the definition the society makes of the actions to be taken by people of any class to validate their dignity – legitimizations of self which do not, cannot work and so reinforce the original anxiety.
>
> (1972, p. 170)

More recently, scholars such as Diane Reay have shown how much all of this is experienced psychosocially – how much we internalise feelings of worthlessness and shame, even if, on an intellectual level, we may notionally reject them. Reay wrote, in one study of young British girls in educational contexts, that by the age of 10 they 'inhabit a psychic economy of class defined by fear, anxiety and unease where failure looms large [...] a place where they are seen and see themselves as literally "nothing"' (2005, p. 917). Many working-class people endure the scars of feeling – of being made to feel – this way. This is partly why an awareness of class can be so important in challenging class shame. As Skeggs and Loveday observed just a decade ago, in the responses of British working-class people to their demonisation in popular media,

> The people that populate this paper all had access to the language of class, even after thirty years of attempts to rhetorically eradicate the concept in Britain. The concept of class enabled them to understand the structural conditions by which they are positioned, and made it possible to deflect interpretations of structural injustice as their own responsibility and faulty psychology.
>
> (2012, p. 487)

I can still recall having this dual pull in my teenage years – in my emotional responses to my impoverished circumstances – between the 'fear, anxiety and unease where failure looms large' and the growing 'understanding of structural conditions' that helped me resist class shame. Educational attainment is another potential route out of that shame. As someone growing up in poverty, the son of parents who had experienced long-term unemployment, in a house with, for most of my youth (into the 1990s), an outdoor toilet and no washing facilities better than a tin bath that we shoved under the kitchen table, getting into TCD seemed like getting the keys to a world where I could be 'something'. Indeed, getting into TCD filled me with an unrealistic and naive sense of having already 'made it'. But I also carried with me those 'hidden injuries of class', with still-fresh memories of being followed around shops by security guards because of how I looked (tracksuited, short-cropped hair), of not feeling able to invite schoolmates to my house because of the embarrassing state of it, of constantly worrying about status symbols like clothes that we couldn't afford. I'd already fretted about being 'found out', long before I entered academia and discovered (without knowing the word for it) those feelings of imposterism common to those working-class academic 'amphibians' (Tokarczyk, 2014, p. 5) who move between worlds. Both of my parents had left education early and without qualifications. My father had become a carpenter after he emigrated to London in the 1960s, where he first worked as a general labourer on building sites, but as our sole earner he was often unemployed for long periods in the Dublin of the 1980s – a grim economic climate. We had no significant knowledge or experience of what a university was, and nobody I knew well was educated beyond second level. But education, for me, was vitally important in improving my material circumstances and my conscientisation. I started in TCD three years after Irish Labour Education Minister Niamh Breathnach announced the abolition of third-level fees. At the time,

Breathnach had said that 'abolishing fees will have a tremendous psychological impact' (O'Brien, 2008). For me it no doubt did. I had confidently told my guidance counsellor at school that I wanted to study at TCD, an aspiration that was met by a disbelieving (and in retrospect cruel) laugh; she had advised me to seek the extra points being offered by another university, for denizens of 'deprived areas'. I can still remember the juvenile satisfaction that my 18-year-old self took in telling her I'd made it to TCD. The university proudly advertised itself as an elite institution; one brochure blurb message from its Provost reminded prospective entrants of how its giant institution's small doors symbolised its (vaunted) exclusivity and the opportunities that lay in store for all who entered.

But other barriers, not all of them as visible or remediable as fees, remained once a working-class student entered through that narrow portal. One particular incident that drove this point home to me was the one I spoke of at the 'Final Taboo' event – an incident that had happened almost two decades earlier, in the early 2000s, and maybe 100 yards from where I was speaking at that event. As an undergraduate, I had arranged one day to meet a close friend – we'll call him Jimmy – who came from an inner-city flat complex, for lunch at TCD. Jimmy was an exceptionally bright young man who had long left school and worked various routine jobs, including as a courier, and like I had, part-time at that juncture, as a 'gotchie': a night security guard on building sites and office blocks. Like me, he was a left-wing political activist, and we shared a lot in common in our politics and upbringing. We arranged to meet at the 'Campanile' – an iconic bell tower in Trinity's front square, and I was standing at that building when I received a text from Jimmy to say that he'd been expelled from the university grounds, which I at first thought was a joke, typical of him. When I rang him, however, Jimmy sounded uncharacteristically upset. He said he had been ejected from the campus for no reason; he would never set foot in the place again. I suspect he couldn't bring himself to meet me elsewhere as he was by then too angry, or maybe, too shaken and ashamed. I was incensed and immediately made my way to the Head Porter's office. There, the official in charge of security explained that Jimmy was acting suspiciously. 'How?' I enquired. He'd been seen 'with a bag, loitering' in the square, was the reply. I asked the man to leave his office at the Front Arch – which to his credit, he did – and when we were outside I pointed to a range of people standing idly at buildings in TCD's Parliament Square, with bags on their backs. 'Are *they* suspicious?' I said. He nodded, conceding the point. The Head Porter was a decent man and brought me back into his office to elaborate that the staff who had evicted my friend were new and had made a mistake. 'I know why they threw him out', I told him. 'He looks like someone from the inner city. He looks working class.' A working-class Dubliner himself, he admitted that this seemed to be correct. There were a lot of bicycle thefts around TCD at that time and it was undoubtedly the case that Jimmy, with his haircut, his choice of clothing, and all those embodied things that came with his habitus (a certain bearing, look, and 'dead-wide' way of observing his surroundings), was deemed suspicious. His experience that day was another of those alienating and categorising events that the less well-off often encounter in educational settings; he had felt that confused anger of the 'cloud of chalk' in Meehan's poem. When I had started at TCD, I always wore clothes and no doubt a bearing that distinguished me as different and other, but as time went on, my ability to successfully code switch improved. I'd take my glasses off and walk in a certain way in my own neighbourhood, then drop the macho front and embrace another form of anxiety and pretence as I entered those narrow gates. But Jimmy was Jimmy: he didn't present differently on either side of the magic door.

Some years later and amazingly – considering his own lack of formal educational achievement to that point – Jimmy nonetheless ended up a student on a widening participation scheme in University College Dublin (UCD). I was delighted. He had a very difficult upbringing, with alcoholism and heroin addiction having destroyed lives in his family, as in many others in inner-city Dublin at that time. But Jimmy had firmly eschewed the addiction trap, was resolutely, fanatically anti-drugs – even to the point, as a mere teenager, of being well known in the late 1990s anti-drugs movement in Dublin. He had a great deal of unresolved anger issues about the deprivation of his childhood and the marginalisation of his community, but he was fiercely intelligent and someone who might, given the opportunity, buck the trend. Unceremoniously shunted out the door of one university, he was now commencing studies at another.

Chiming with some of the research presented in this book, however, other barriers to participation remained – barriers that belied UCD's notional commitments to 'access'. As Shukie observes in Chapter 9 of this book, 'the ironic recognition is that education, that route of transformation, becomes also the site of the greatest exposure and judgement'. Working-class students coming to university from outside formal educational structures can feel especially exposed and judged as they navigate the transition to HE. As recent research by Scanlon et al. has shown, university students from non-traditional backgrounds in Ireland can find their initial excitement at taking their first steps in HE can be overshadowed by fears of failure and not fitting in.

> Students described a mix of emotions in relation to their transition to HE, including a sense of euphoria at having 'made it' to university and the excitement of being on campus during the first few days of term. However, like Risquez, Moore, and Morley (2007–2008), we found that this 'honeymoon phase' was often overshadowed by feelings of insecurity (e.g. about academic mediocrity or failure) and disorientation in their new surroundings. [...] Anxiety about the social dimension of university life was a dominant theme in students' accounts of the period leading up to enrolment and their early weeks at university. Most of the young people in our study did not know anyone at university when they first started and were worried about the prospect of having to develop new friendships in unfamiliar surroundings.
>
> (2020, pp. 756–757)

The same study recommends 'that, for first-generation students, generic support programmes (e.g. peer mentors, orientation, study skills, etc.) need to be supplemented by more targeted supports' (p. 762). In Jimmy's case, there were, to my knowledge, no such targeted supports, and UCD became a profoundly alienating experience. I can recall him deciding, with little elaboration, that university was not for him. As Burnell Reilly writes in her chapter for the present volume, including 'learners from under-represented groups is a major step towards social inclusion', but 'if this new type of learner does not feel comfortable or included, or does not have any history in that arena then the effects will be felt'. Jimmy dropped out of UCD in his first year there, finding the course – and what was expected of academic essays and thinking – too challenging, the environment too alienating; he experienced a strong field-habitus clash (see Burnell Reilly and Akbar in this volume). And as Akbar notes, such drop outs of students can go 'unnoticed'. After his decision to leave university, Jimmy spiralled downward into addiction. He died two years later, in his sleep, in his early 20s. He had contracted pneumonia but had taken so much cocaine and heroin that he didn't even know he was unwell. The priest at Jimmy's funeral recalled that the last time he'd seen him, Jimmy was sitting on the steps of his flat complex reading the *Collected Works* of V. I. Lenin.

The Importance of Class in Class

My own trajectory as a researcher and academic who works on the representation of working-class life began inside classrooms, with helpful teachers and educators, both in my secondary school and at TCD. Universities in Ireland have, since the 1990s, embarked on various access initiatives which have proved successful in providing space for many other working-class students to excel. The Trinity Access Programme, for instance, set up in 1997, has had significant successes in retaining and preparing 'non-traditional' students for the rigours of university degrees (Keane, 2013). As Lynch discusses, class itself isn't discussed much in Irish formal education, but my own experience of discussing class *in* class was profoundly enabling. It was in TCD that I first encountered the concept of 'working-class writing', in Dr Aileen Douglas's module on 'British Working-Class Fiction'. This course was inspirational for me, in both my capacity to understand and analyse the dynamics of representation and class, and in my later career trajectory. Reading writers like Robert Tressell, George Gissing, Nell Dunn, Alan Sillitoe, Pat Barker and Irvine Welsh for the first time, I discovered a rich vein of brilliant portrayals of working-class experience that resonated in various ways with my own life. Part of our feeling at home in the university is the extent to which the institution acknowledges, takes action on – and produces research and teaching on – diverse issues that resonate with students' lives. In a 2017 comparative study of the experiences of working-class English and Irish university students, Fergal Finnegan and Barbara Merrill found that a high proportion of their Irish working-class respondents experienced 'a feeling of dislocation, or at least a sense of social distance, from the dominant culture in [the] universities' they attended, one describing the academy as 'a foreign country' (p. 318). In elite institutions, working-class students were particularly alienated: 'in some cases interviewees discussed going through the difficult and painstaking process of cultural adaptation' and, as Finnegan and Merill conclude, 'These accounts of fitting or not fitting in at university were often discussed as something which was *felt as embodied and as deeply emotional* by the students' (Ibid.; emphasis mine). My own experience was that one way the university allowed me to feel at home was by including the working class in the curriculum. As Sue Clegg observes, 'while theories that elaborate on the alternative sources of capital are important, therefore, they require greater elaboration in terms of how these capitals are mobilised in ways that enable students' epistemic access to the curriculum and not just the ability to resist the symbolic violence of the hidden curriculum' (2011, pp. 96–97). Rethinking the relevance of curricula to working-class students' lives – along with the targeted interventions recommended by Scanlon et al. above – can play a significant part in improving the university experience for the working class.

Seeking the Margins

bell hooks (1989) urges us to 'choose' the 'radical openness' (p. 22) of the margins. Those 'on the edge' develop 'a particular way of seeing reality', she argues – a 'sense of [society's] wholeness', which yields 'an oppositional world view—a mode of seeing unknown to most of our oppressors' (p. 20). By way of this sense of alterity and its implicitly dialectical, 'whole' worldview, the margins can para-doxically become enriching, 'much more than a site of deprivation. In fact [...] just the opposite: that is also the site of radical possibility, a space of resistance' (1990). One must *choose* the margins, even as that may seem an improbable, or even presumptuous, endeavour for those who move into foreign territories like academia:

> I located my answer concretely in the realm of oppositional political struggle. Such diverse pleasures can be experienced, enjoyed even, because one transgresses, moves 'out of one's place.' For many of us, that movement requires pushing against oppressive boundaries set by race, sex and class domination. [...] Moving, we confront the realities of choice and location.
>
> (p. 15)

The challenges and opportunities of these realities of choice and location recur throughout this book and proffer a range of insights into the present state and future possibilities for universities – and for academics from working-class backgrounds – to transform pedagogies, curricula, entrance mechanisms and people. How we 'position' ourselves is key.

As Shukie writes in Chapter 9, autoethnography problematises the normative position of the objective, dispassionate academic – is 'immediately challenging [to] the objectivity of a distanced neutrality preferred by much academic process'. But it is all the more challenging for the working-class person turned academic, following 'a lifetime of "chip on your shoulder" reproaches that silence any reflections of what has shaped me'. In her Preface, Burnell Reilly reminds us that autoethnographic methods provide not only the tools for gleaning powerful lessons from personal experiences but also a protective shield against accusations that the narrator of these experiences is either unreflexive or self-indulgent. It is also entirely logical that we should devote time to reflecting on the relationship between our life experiences and academic preoccupations, as good practice in scholarly rigour *and* a potential source of valuable information about how the academy can leave current and future students from excluded groups well placed to do likewise. Rowell and Walters' chapter (Chapter 4) is particularly illuminating in this regard: their 'experimental autoethnographic' approach, generating conversations between two early-career academics through artefacts and recollections, brilliantly teases out memories, conversations and contradictions that might otherwise have been lost – a wonderful model of sharing, probing, disclosure and discovery. Working-class academics sharing experiences in this way can evidently be personally cathartic and richly revealing, and Rowell and Walters suggest one way in which this book might encourage similarly rewarding interchanges into the future.

Moreover, this book reminds us of how damaging the exclusion of class is in diversity measures at HE. In Chapter 6, Akbar uses the analogy of a 'Rubik's Cube of Identity' to explore how intersections of classist and racist discourses operate to alienate and exclude – leading to 'an increased level of cognitive dissonance while trying to develop a more cohesive and personal identity'. Burnell Reilly's discussion of accentism, microaggressions, symbolic violence and code-switching illustrates the everyday discomforts experienced by fish-out-of-water students and academics (Chapter 8) – the kinds of discomforts that don't seem to feature much in university equality and 'allyship' training – which suggests that HE could do a lot more in this regard. Wong's experience (Chapter 11) of being repeatedly misidentified in class terms again exemplifies how poor the academy is in addressing these matters systematically. Wilson's recollection (Chapter 7) of her experiences of accentism in the lecture theatre are a reminder also of the dangers of HE managements' obsession with metrics, whereby students can impact career progression through evaluations of aspects of a lecturer's/tutor's delivery, including accent and communication, which undoubtedly provide opportunities for veiled forms of sexism and racism (Austin, 2021), and classism. As Wilson illustrates, it is also incumbent on universities to ensure that *students* are not disadvantaged by such prejudices (conscious or unconscious) among staff, especially given how difficult it is to identify and complain about 'covert racism' and 'microaggressions' that are 'very hard to evidence'.

Another key theme in this book is the importance of the arts in opening up spaces through which working-class children can develop the necessary courage, or audacity, to 'take flight'. Both Broadhead's (Chapter 10) and Hammond's (Chapter 2) chapters attest to the important role played by the arts in how we relate to the world around us and in how working-class people find ways of overcoming the barriers they face, or as Hammond recalls far more eloquently, 'through the abysmal schooling experiences, the tribulations and traumas of socio-economic precarity, and the realisation that as a consequence of my working-class positionality [...] I sought – and found – solace in an unconquerable and private world of music-hued reverie'. For Hammond, 'the important experience of imaginative flight and aerial escape' (which echoes in Shukie's having 'almost levitated upwards' in his university encounters with knowledge 'that resonated in my world') is key. It's something we should be mindful of in a climate where politicians like Tory Education Secretary Gavin Williamson can comment that 'the record number of people taking up science and engineering demonstrates that many are already starting to pivot away from dead-end courses that leave young people with nothing but debt' (Tidman, 2021). This theme is taken up by Broadhead, whose experiences of moving through the academy further indicate the power of snobbery and inequality that can dissuade working-class people from studying the arts. As Burnell Reilly attests in her chapter (Chapter 8), habitus is permeable, and can be 'altered and adapted, as a result of participating in higher education', a reality her work to support Further Education (FE) students in seeking HE opportunities confirmed. The arts can provide a route into that altered habitus, and in working-class art we frequently discover defiant pride where there had once been shame. As Shukie writes in Chapter 9, 'we were desperate for representation, for cultural depictions we could relate to [...] a sense of belonging denied us apart from fragments collected over decades'.

There is thus an important timeliness to this collection. Colin McCaig's piece (Chapter 3) notes how the intensification of demonisation of the working class in recent decades – the reminders of 'just how *thoroughly* undeserving we were' in popular culture – ought to be factored into our thinking on why class can be difficult to broach (even among working-class students) in the contemporary university. He furthermore observes, following Selina Todd's recent work (Todd, 2021), the dangers of a 'deficit model' of the working class and its undergirding ideology of meritocracy that actually hinders working-class students with hopes of entering HE – particularly its most prestigious institutions. As Maisuria (Chapter 1) reminds us, neoliberalism has encouraged us 'to think of ourselves as individual agents acting freely as consumers and rational beings', diminishing the ground for commonality and thus transformative collective action. HE can be 'used to further promote a narrative that celebrates education as an individualist escape route', as Shukie warns (Chapter 9). The marketisation of universities has encouraged students and staff to think in transactional terms, as 'consumers' and 'service providers' in a supposedly meritocratic and vigorously competitive model of HE (Tomlinson, 2018), but the goal of improving access and experiences for working-class students and scholars requires us to think in a radically different way. As Shukie writes above, 'the purpose/power, of knowledge, sharing, creating [...] is strangled by the weeds of aspirational, me-first, prestige riddled concepts of education as status'. Maisuria's conceptualisation of class in relational, rather than gradational, Weberian terms, also importantly foregrounds the necessary cognisance of 'the Capital-Labour Relation': while, as in Savage et al. (2015), describing classes as they are is both fascinating and instructive, the goal of transforming how we relate as classes and human beings makes praxis and con-scientisation key. As with Crew (Chapter 12), who notes how academics down-playing the importance of class produces 'indirect stigmatizations' of her research area, Maisuria writes of his own experiences of encountering resistance, within the academy, to his research on class – and many of those with analogous research interests will have encountered similarly dismissive remarks about research on class in general as 'old hat'. But such remarks, as Maisuria rightly discerns, reveal contemporary strategies of resistance and mystification in response to calls for social change. Maisuria's advice is wise: 'be strategic about when you pipe-up, do not believe that you can win all battles, and find pockets of solidarity with fellow intellectual travellers'. It chimes with Rowell and Walters' counsel to 'make visible your working-class identity when teaching and interacting with students'. The inclination of these chapters to find ways to advise and support working-class students and fellow academics echoes in recent initiatives by De Waal (2019) and McVeigh (2021) to publish and support working-class writers. As McVeigh puts it in his volume of 'working-class voices', 'successful working-class artists often travel between worlds and are likely to pull over and offer you a lift' (2021, p. 1). As Shukie (quoting Shadrick) advises in the present volume, in 'telling our stories we become "calling cards and quiet invitations" that encourage others to step from the silence'. This book, so ably edited by Burnell Reilly, will play a part in enabling working-class students and academics to find a voice, and it suggests that parallel, practical initiatives in mutual 'lifting' in HE could be a further step to emerge from the collaboration. As Wilson writes above, improving our self-care, allyship, mentoring and authenticity are key to 'leaving academia in a better state than when we found it'.

References

Austin, D. (2021). Leadership lapse: Laundering systemic bias through student eval-uations. *Villanova Law Review, 65*(5), 995–1009.

Baker, J., Lynch, K., Cantillon, S., & Walsh, J. (2009). *Equality: From theory to action.* Basingstoke: Palgrave.

Bourdieu, P. (1977). *Outline of a theory of practice* (Richard Nice, Trans.). Cambridge, MA: CUP.

Clegg, S. (2011). Cultural capital and agency: Connecting critique and curriculum in higher education. *British Journal of Sociology of Education, 32*(1), 93–108.

De Waal, K. (Ed.). (2019). *Common people: An anthology of working class writers.* London: Unbound.

Finnegan, F., & Merrill, B. (2017). "We're as good as anybody else": A comparative study of working-class university students' experiences in England and Ireland. *British Journal of Sociology of Education, 38*(3), 307–332.

Fourie, I. (2021). What is autoethnography? In I. Fourie (Ed.), *Autoethnography for librarians and information scientists.* London: Routledge.

Freire, P. (2005 [1968]). *Pedagogy of the oppressed.* London: Continuum.

Freire, P. (2021 [1997]). *Pedagogy of the heart.* London: Bloomsbury.

hooks, b. (1989). Choosing the margin as space of radical openness. *Framework*, *0*(36), 15–23.

hooks, b. (2003). Confronting class in the classroom. In A. Darder, M. Baltodano, & R. D. Torres (Eds.), *The critical pedagogy reader* (pp. 142–150). New York, NY: Routledge.

Keane, E. (2013). *Widening participation in higher education in the republic of Ireland*. Galway: NUIG.

Lynch, K. (2020). Opinion: Class and wealth, not merit, are rewarded in Ireland's education system. Online. Retrieved from https://www.thejournal.ie/readme/education-inequality-class-divide-5216581-Sep2020/

McVeigh, P. (2021). Introduction. In P. McVeigh (Ed.), *The 32: An anthology of Irish working-class voices* (pp. 1–7). London: Unbound.

Meehan, P. (2000). *Dharmakaya*. Manchester: Carcanet Press.

O'Brien, C. (2008). Adding up the real cost of free fees. *Irish Times*. 16 August. Online. Retrieved from https://www.irishtimes.com/news/adding-up-the-real-cost-of-free-fees-1.931247

Reay, D. (2005). Beyond consciousness?: The psychic landscape of social class. *Sociology*, *39*(5), 911–928.

Sanders, M. R., & Mahalingam, R. (2012). Under the radar: The role of invisible discourse in understanding class-based privilege. *Journal of Social Issues*, *68*(1), 112–127.

Savage, M., Cunningham, N., Devine, F., Friedman, S., Laurison, D., McKenzie, L., ... Wakeling, P. (2015). *Social class in the 21st century*. London: Pelican Books.

Scanlon, M., Leahy, P., Jenkinson, H., & Powell, F. (2020). 'My biggest fear was whether or not I would make friends': Working-class students' reflections on their transition to university in Ireland. *Journal of Further and Higher Education*, *44*(6), 753–765.

Sennett, R., & Cobb, J. (1972). *The hidden injuries of class*. Cambridge: Cambridge UP.

Skeggs, B., & Loveday, V. (2012). Struggles for value: Value practices, injustice, judgement, affect and the idea of class. *British Journal of Sociology*, *63*(3), 472–490.

Thompson, E. P. (1980). *The making of the English working class*. London: Penguin.

Tidman, Z. (2021). Gavin Williamson criticised for 'galling' comment on 'dead-end' university courses. *Independent*. 17 May. Online. Retrieved from https://www.independent.co.uk/news/education/education-news/gavin-williamson-deadend-courses-nus-b1848461.html

Todd, S. (2021). *Snakes and ladders: The great British social mobility myth*. London: Chatto & Windus.

Tokarczyk, M. M. (2014). Introduction. In *Critical approaches to American working-class literature*. New York, NY: Routledge.

Tomlinson, M. (2018). Conceptions of the value of higher education in a measured market. *Higher Education*, *75*, 711–727.

Afterword

above one's station

English

Prepositional phrase

> 1. Of higher <u>social status</u> than suitable for one's position, standing or rank.
>
> *The serf's ideas of equity were **above his station**.*

Wiktionary
(retrieved 26.4.22)

I am sitting in the university library reading journal articles when suddenly I think – 'Oh – is that all they want?' This is the first time I remember understanding what an academic argument was (not a row or a punch-up in the car park). I was in my 20s and had returned to university following a (then) non-degree teacher training. This light-bulb moment happened to me many times. Like many of the writers in this volume, I assumed that academic work was 'head-hurt' hard. I remember thinking at school that you had to have a big brain (as in *Brain of Britain*, a then popular radio programme – which led me to believe that all you needed to do was remember things). But every time, I thought this same 'oh! Is THAT all they want?', I realised that I had to put aside my idea that only very special people (mostly men) with big brains could possibly understand really hard things and therefore be let in. Because, I learnt that, when you understood the academic rules of the game, they were, in fact, easy. I can't say that the feeling of being found out as stupid disappeared quickly as in a puff of smoke. Occasionally it still comes to haunt me. But then, as now, it was the joy of ideas that kept me going. It was so exhilarating. Just like the beautiful scene of watching planes take off from Manchester Airport and wanting to fly, as described by one of the chapter authors.

As several people in this volume argue, this is not about having aspirations, of growing up without any dreams. But some dreams are often presented as ridiculous by teachers in school. I mean, I wanted to be Audrey Hepburn in *My Fair Lady* – already fanciful – and the idea that I should have aspired instead to be a professor was simply non-thinkable. For a start, I didn't know what one was, and, even if I had, nobody would have assumed it applied to the likes of me. This was the 1960s, a time when only 13% of 18-year-olds went on to *any* form of higher education.

This volume offers an enormously important set of accounts. What do we learn about becoming a working-class academic from them? The book covers a huge, diverse range of historical moments, and yet despite this, they routinely show similar experiences. In itself this alone is depressing and illustrates the continued significance of class, particularly when one understands that these accounts stem from the few people who actually achieved a PhD – something even more prescient when we understand that in the UK over 50% of 18-year-olds go on to higher education.

Given that, these accounts are also uplifting because they illustrate the courage and determination of those working-class students who do manage to gain entry to the academy.

For me then, these stories highlight the key significance of approaching class through embodied experience – that is, how class is lived and experienced through its affective resonances and discursive and material organisation.

But more than this, these stories also act as a key resource. The role of the ethnographer has traditionally been to understand how the 'ethnos' understand their world. But the world of working-class transition can only be auto-written because otherwise it tends to be ignored, misrepresented or pathologised. So many of us have felt alone in higher education and students need stories to connect with, stories that help them understand their own experience. In the light of the scant attention paid to class and classism within the academy, contained principally in patronising and usually broken attempts at 'widening participation' (Walkerdine, 2020), this collection functions as a crucial intervention.

I would go further and say that such work can form the basis of what is currently being called autotheory (Fournier, 2022). That is, the building of an account of class by theorising one's own life. We all know that class divisions are at the heart of much politics today, and building other accounts and other theories is such an important intervention into the politics of class.

The characteristics of these working-class academics is not therefore one of actual failure but rather a potent sense of fear of failure, of being an imposter, of not belonging, but crucially they are also a dream of possibility – of a desire for a different life – a dream and the difficult path of following that dream.

I was really struck by the longing contained in many of the stories. I recognise that longing – such a strong desire to be able to think and to dream. How I revelled in it and nothing and nobody could take this away from me. Just think what would happen if all the working-class children were actually supported in their dreaming (Morgan, 2021) – what a revolution that would be!

When my parents and grandparents were alive, getting above one's station was almost impossible. And when I was young, women's magazines were full of stories of finding a higher status husband. Although 50% of 18-year-olds now enter higher education, the situation is still replete with obstacles. The introduction of enormous fees, with their associated debts, the huge divisions in status between universities, academic staff under pressure just to give a few examples, all still mean that it is very difficult to give working-class students as much support as they deserve.

For all this, however, I am so happy that working-class academic work is now being widely developed, and I salute this and all attempts not only to bring class back onto the agenda but also to develop our own autotheorisations through which we might understand and engage with class in the present as it rears its head in all facets of social life.

Professor Valerie Walkerdine
School of Social Sciences
Cardiff University

References

Fournier, L. (2022). *Autotheory as feminist practice in art, writing, and criticism.* Cambridge, MA: MIT Press.

Morgan, R. (2021). *Young people's access to employment in disadvantaged communities in Wales.* PhD thesis, Cardiff University.

Walkerdine, V. (2020). What's class got to do with it? Discourse. *Does Class Still Matter? Conversations About Power, Privilege and Persistent Inequalities in Higher Education, 42*(1), 60–74.

Enriching Universities and Scholarship by Prohibiting Class Discrimination

Geraldine Van Bueren

There is a significant change occurring in academia, as this volume of autoethnography attests, because many of us who are from working-class heritages are questioning the reasoning behind university class ceilings.[1] Linking all these chapters is the conclusion that working-class heritage scholars enrich universities in their teaching, scholarship and impact, but that the obstacles, sometimes unconscious, and frequently unacknowledged, are hindering the progress both of scholarship and of individual scholars.

This prompts two questions: in order to improve universities, do we need a change in legislation such as, in the United Kingdom, amending the Equality Act 2010, to include a prohibition on class discrimination; and secondly, is there anything that can be done until such legislative amendment?

The first question is whether a change in the law will remove the class ceiling or at the very least breach it, so that class discrimination would be taken as seriously as other prohibited forms of prejudicial actions. By class, I mean the richly diverse and intersectional concept of class as the basis for discriminatory treatment. The advantage for universities in prohibiting class discrimination is that, by adding a prohibition on class discrimination, the law will be strengthened, not only in relation to class discrimination but also reinforcing all the other protected characteristics and their rich intersections.

The reasons behind the insufficient attention to class may have to do with the many myths surrounding class in universities and in the United Kingdom generally, which may also have contributed to the exclusion of class discrimination from legal prohibition. One of the challenges faced by those who confront class discrimination is that it is perceived as too difficult to define. In particular, there are issues such as fluidity, and attributed and self-attributed identity, and there are concerns with class being too loose to be capable of a satisfactory definition to constitute a category for protection in law. However, such arguments are open to challenge.[2] The right to change one's religion, recognised in international law, has not been regarded as an insurmountable obstacle to prohibiting religious discrimination.[3] Similarly, there is also fluidity in definitions of gender, and a change in gender is not regarded as a bar to gender equality, and in fact gender reassignment is a ground of protection.[4]

This is not to deny the complexities surrounding class and other forms of discrimination; however, law has always, since its inception, grappled with complex and challenging cases in both domestic and international contexts. The *travaux préparatoires* or working documents of the United Nations Convention on the Rights of Persons with Disabilities, 2006, for example, illustrate the challenges of defining 'disability' based on different conceptions or models of disability – medical, social and human rights.

In any event it ought to be questioned, why class discrimination should be placed on a higher definitional tier than other forms of discrimination. The prohibited grounds of race and sex discrimination have not been exhaustively defined in their specific international or domestic instruments; rather, they have been defined and explored on a case-by-case basis. In defining class, guidance can therefore be sought from the approach to the definitions of race and sex.

Interestingly, speaking about class discrimination in British universities, the question I am always asked is how I define working class. I have never, it should be noted, been asked to define middle class. This question is frequently followed with the question of whether a working class or classes still exist. The existence of the middle class or classes is never questioned.

Because of the nervousness surrounding class, universities have adopted other approaches including socio-economic status and social mobility. These approaches, however, have generally been adopted in relation only to students, and rarely to academics. However, neither social mobility nor socio-economic status captures the rich and valuable experiences of entering academia with a working-class heritage. The term 'socio-economic status', for example, does not provide positive definitions of identity, nor is it seen as autonomy-affirming. For example, I may choose to describe my origins as working class, which is an important facet of my identity, but I do not self-identify as being from a low socio-economic status. There is nothing positive about low socio-economic status, whereas many of us are proud either: (1) to be living working-class lives or (2) of coming from working-class heritages.

Social mobility is also a less accurate concept than class. A legal prohibition on class discrimination would mean that universities would have to prevent class discrimination across the entire university, whereas social mobility, despite the excellent work of universities, is generally optional, recommendatory, and, with some exceptions, it does not apply to everybody. Social mobility alone cannot rectify the salary gap that the Sutton Trust and others have evidenced in their reports, so that those from working-class backgrounds with identical qualifications are and will continue to be paid less, unless such a discrimination is prohibited by law.

There are also difficulties in universities gathering data about class discrimination because universities are not under a legal duty to collate such information, and priority is understandably given to data which universities are legally required to collect.

Yet class prejudice is also reflected in the curriculum. How many courses which focus on increasing and equalising human longevity include class in their analysis? Yet there is a significant and unacceptable difference in life expectancy in the United Kingdom between different classes in boroughs of the same city.[5]

Another change that this volume of autoethnography symbolises is that working-class heritage academics are gathering together to offer support to each other, and, equally importantly, to offer support to newer scholars and postgraduate students through regular seminars and mentoring. Much of this work is taking place under the auspices of the international Alliance of Working Class Academics.[6]

Similarly, rather than waiting for legislative change, the world's first University Code on Equal Opportunity for Working Class Students and Academics 2021 has been drafted by the international Alliance for Working Class Academics.[7] It is designed so that universities around the world can adapt it to their own cultures, with their own linguistic terminology, such as in America, blue collar heritages. The University Code calls upon universities to acknowledge that students and academics from a richly diverse range of working-class heritages add economic, social and cultural value to communities, to the state and the global community, and enhance the scholarship, work, productivity and research impact of university communities.

The University Code also requires university employment policies and practices to provide for equal treatment of working-class heritage staff in relation to their recruitment, retention, salaries and promotions policies. It also urges universities to guarantee equal treatment to working-class heritage students and to assist them in overcoming hurdles to full participation in university life and in seeking employment. Article 5 of the University Code requires universities to recognise that there may be additional economic and time-specific hurdles for students and staff with working-class heritages, not only in access to university but also in further university qualifications, research assistance and conference attendance. The Code requires universities to assist in overcoming these hurdles.

A part of the devaluation of working-class culture is that universities generally do not include the rich range of working-class histories and experiences in curricula content. In law, for example, emphasis has traditionally been placed on John Locke, a lawyer's son and slave profiteer, and on his concept of a social contract, and less on Tom Paine, a corset-maker's son and abolitionist. However, Paine's concept of humanity in his *Rights of Man* is one of the earliest scholarly arguments for a wide range of state-guaranteed human rights. The principle underlining the University Code is of a democracy of knowledge, so that such valuable scholarship is also included in curricula.

The University Code is drawn from international law, which increases its normative strength. This includes, as the Preamble states, that universities ought to be guided by United Nations Sustainable Development Goal four on education to ensure equal opportunity, improve equitable access, enhance mobility and accountability by the United Nations targeted date of 2030.

While an express prohibition of class discrimination is the desirable longer-term goal, in the interim, The University Code on Equal Opportunity for Working Class Students and Academics 2021 provides a practical and constructive beginning for dialogue, which is the reason that the Alliance is currently working with one British university, the Code is on the websites of universities regulators and also in the newsletter of Universities UK. Ultimately, however, universities ought to take class discrimination as seriously as all the other prohibited discriminations, and the only way this is possible is if it is prohibited by law.

© 2022 Professor Emerita Geraldine Van Bueren QC is a Visiting Fellow at Kellogg College Oxford, the Chair of the Alliance of Working Class Academics, and holds a Leverhulme Fellowship for her work on Class, Social Mobility and the Law (https://www.workingclassacademics.com).

Notes

1. I prefer the term heritage to background as it denotes something of value; see Jonathan Prangnell and Geraldine Mate, 'Kin, fictive kin and strategic movement: Working class heritage of the Upper Burnett' (2011) 17(4) *International Journal of Heritage Studies*, 318–330; *Carole Binns, Experiences of Academics From a Working-Class Heritage: Ghosts of Childhood Habitus* (Newcastle: Cambridge Scholars Publishing, 2011).
2. Geraldine Van Bueren QC 'Inclusivity and the law: Do we need to prohibit class discrimination?' 21 *European Human Rights Law Review*, 274–284.
3. Under the International Covenant on Civil and Political Rights and in regional treaties, including the European Convention on Human Rights.
4. Court of Justice of the European Union in *P v S and Cornwall County Council* (1996) Case C-13/94 recognised that discrimination on the basis of gender reassignment constituted discrimination under the EU Directive on equal treatment for men and women.
5. In relation to Glasgow, see 'Closing the Gap in a Generation: Health Equity Through Action on the Social Determinants of Health' (Commission on Social Determinants of Health Final Report, 2009), World Health Organization, https://www.who.int/social_determinants/thecommission/finalreport/en (Accessed 21 May 2021). See also S.D.S. Fraser and Steve George, 'Perspectives on differing health outcomes by city: Accounting for Glasgow's excess mortality' (2015) 8 *Risk Managed Healthcare Policy*, 99.

6. The Alliance's support sessions, initiated by Carole Binns and organised by Craig Johnston and Charlie Davis, found that there is only limited recognition of the scholastic importance of working-class culture. They also revealed many unacknowledged obstacles in the pursuit of doctoral studies (https://www.workingclassacademics.com).

7. https://www.workingclassacademics.com/universitycode.

Index

www.ingramcontent.com/pod-product-compliance
Lightning Source LLC
Chambersburg PA
CBHW050346270326
41926CB00016B/3627